Color Atlas & Textbook of

Oral Anatomy

Histology and Embryology

Color Atlas & Textbook of
Oral Anatomy
Histology and Embryology

Second Edition

B K B Berkovitz
Reader in Dental Anatomy
King's College
London

G R Holland
Professor of Restorative Dentistry
University of Alberta
Edmonton, Alberta, Canada

B J Moxham
Professor of Anatomy
University of Wales
Cardiff

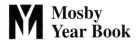 Mosby
Year Book

St. Louis   Baltimore   Boston   Chicago   London   Philadelphia   Sydney   Toronto

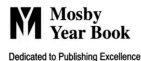
Mosby Year Book

Dedicated to Publishing Excellence

Copyright © B K B Berkovitz, G R Holland, B J Moxham, 1992
All rights reserved.
Published with rights in the USA, Canada and Puerto Rico by Mosby–Year Book, Inc.
A Year Book Medical Publishers imprint of Mosby–Year Book, Inc.
ISBN 0 8151 0697 1

First edition published in 1977, © Wolfe Publishing Ltd.

Library of Congress Cataloguing-in-Publication Data

Berkovitz, B.K.B.
    Color atlas & textbook of oral anatomy, histology, and embryology
    B.K.B. Berkovitz, G.R. Holland, B.J. Moxham. —2nd ed.
        p.   cm.
    Rev. ed, of: A colour atlas & textbook of oral anatomy. c1978.
    Includes index.
    ISBN 0-8151-0697-1
    1. Mouth—Anatomy.   2. Mouth—Histology.   3. Teeth—Anatomy.
4. Teeth—Histology.   5. Mouth—Atlases.   6. Teeth—Atlases.
I. Holland, G.R. (Graham Rex), 1946–   .   II. Moxham, B.J.
III. Berkovitz, B.K.B.   Color atlas & textbook of oral anatomy,
histology, and embryology.
    [DNLM: 1. Mouth—anatomy & histology—atlases.   2. Mouth—
embryology—atlases.   3. Neck—anatomy—atlases.   4. Tooth—
anatomy & histology—atlases.   WU 17 B513c]
RK280.B42   1992
611'.31'0222—dc20
DNLM/DLC
for Library of Congress   92-12712
                                                                    CIP

English edition first published by Wolfe Publishing Ltd., Brook House,
2–16 Torrington Place, London WC1E 7LT, UK.

Contents

Preface to the second edition

It is gratifying to be asked to produce a new edition of a text-book. Not only does the request signal the success of the original book but, more importantly, a new edition obviously allows the authors to update and to improve upon the original. One of the features from the first edition of this book which we have retained is the basic format, which combines colour atlas with textbook. Indeed, we believe firmly that anatomical and histological textbooks must present information primarily in 'visual' form. Others are of the same opinion; subsequent to the publication of the first edition of this book, many more books using this format have appeared in diverse medical and dental disciplines.

Although we have maintained the same approach, there are so many other changes that we are tempted to think of the second edition as a completely new book. It has been increased in size by approximately one-third, and the number of illustrations has risen from about six hundred to over seven hundred. Just over forty-five percent of the illustrations are new, and many of those retained have been enlarged. As for the first edition, we have kept the sudivision of our book into four sections — the macroscopic appearance of oro-dental tissues, the microscopic appearance of oro-dental tissues, the development of oro-dental structures, and comparative dental anatomy. However, all of these sections have undergone major revisions. Most change has occurred in the sections concerned with oral histology. Virtually all the chapters in these sections have been rewritten, with the inclusion of many new pictures. This befits an area of major research importance where, these days, progress relies upon advanced techniques such as autoradiography, histochemistry and immunohistochemistry, and transmission and scanning electronmicroscopy. The section dealing with the gross morphology of the oral cavity has also been re-organised and expanded. Chapters concerned with the functional anatomy of mastication, swallowing and speech are included, and the chapter concerned with sectional anatomy has been augmented with NMR scans. A major reorganisation has been undertaken for the section concerned with comparative dental anatomy. Although we deplore the recent trend to downgrade this topic in the dental under-graduate course, we have felt an obligation to rewrite this section in order to emphasise those aspects of comparative oral anatomy pertaining to the evolution of man and to the under-standing of the dentitions of the most commonly used laboratory animals in dental research. To provide some insight into the variety of dental tissues found in the vertebrates, brief descriptions of such tissues appear at various intervals in the section concerned with the microscopic appearance of oro-dental tissues. In all sections, we have highlighted some of the most controversial areas for which research has yet to provide definitive answers (for example, jaw movements during mastication, sensory mechanisms in dentine, the mechanisms of tooth support and tooth eruption, ectodermal/mesenchymal interactions during tooth development, mechanisms during palatogenesis). Finally, whilst we cannot claim that we are without bias in our selection of material for inclusion in this second edition, we trust that our sins will be seen as those of unwitting omission rather than of conscious commission.

BKB Berkovitz
GR Holland
BJ Moxham

London 1992

Preface to the first edition

The demands placed upon students of dentistry to assimilate information regarded as crucial to the satisfactory development of their careers increase as the tempo of scientific inquiry increases. It is unfortunate that this, together with the defects of compartmentalisation of the subject, has conspired against the dental student to make the learning of oral anatomy less easy than it should be. Our aim in writing this book has been to gather together the diverse elements of oral anatomy which, in the past, have been scattered throughout many different textbooks, and to arrive at an integrated perspective of the subject. We were further persuaded to our task by the feeling that the time was ripe for such an encyclopaedic approach to oral anatomy; it is not so much that the rapid advances in the subject seem to be abating but that the variety of experimental approaches used in dental research seem to be converging to produce fewer deficiencies in our interpretations.

We have subdivided our book into four sections — the macroscopic appearance of the oral cavity and related structures, the microscopic appearance of oro-dental tissues, the development of oro-dental tissues and comparative dental anatomy. Thus, the book covers all the basic material generally used to teach oral anatomy in most dental schools. Indeed, the material has formed the basis of our own course at Bristol University.

Since in our view oral anatomy occupies a central position in the dental curriculum, looking forward to much which is basic in the clinical world, we have included such topics as radiographic anatomy of the jaws and teeth, cephalometry and occlusion which, although anatomical, are not always taught to preclinical students (although it is our contention that they should be).

We have also striven to adopt the best features of the textbook and the atlas, without, we hope, their deficiencies. It may seem at times that we have adopted a dogmatic approach to the subject, preferring consensus views where there is uncertainty. However, we have not avoided controversy, merely avoided courting it. We have tried to suppress our own personal views where these are in the formative or hypothetical stages, although we appreciate that such views may come out if only through nuance of style. We hope that the suggestions for further reading at the back of the book will correct any bias.

Finally, in a book of this scope it is difficult to avoid errors. We crave the indulgence of the reader should he not agree with what is written, and trust that he will not hesitate to inform us of our mistakes.

B K B Berkovitz
G R Holland
B J Moxham

Bristol 1977

Acknowledgements

We wish to express our thanks to the following for allowing us to draw freely from their knowledge and experience: RF Brooks (King's College, London), C Dean (University College, London), CL Fox (University of Barcelona) JD Harrison (King's College, London), J Kirkhan, C Robinson, RC Shore (University of Leeds), AGS Lumsden (United Medical and Dental Schools, London), HN Newman (Institute of Dental Surgery, London), PR Shellis (University of Bristol), G Singh (University of Bristol), CD Stevens (University of Bristol), C Stringer (Natural History Museum), A Thexton (United Medical and Dental Schools, London).

We are indebted to the following colleagues who generously, and freely, provided us with the excellent photographic material which made possible the production of this book: D Adams, University of Wales, School of Medicine (**341, 481, 484, 489, 569, 623, 624, 631**); P Andrews, Natural History Museum (**694**); TR Arnett, University College, London (Table 16); EH Batten, University of Bristol (**513, 518, 529, 530**); DC Berry, University of Bristol (**99, 100**); AD Beynon, University of Newcastle (**382, 709**); Squadron Leader SCP Blease, Princess Alexandra Hospital, Wroughton (**180b, 181b, 182b, 183b, 184b**); A Boyde, University College, London (**213, 251, 601**); EW Bradford, University of Bristol (**273, 314**); BAW Brown, King's College, London (**230, 298, 556a, 620, 627**); MR Byers, University of Washington (**289, 332**); SJ Challacombe, United Medical and Dental Schools, London (**263**); NG El-Labban, Institute of Dental Surgery, London (**462**); S-Y Chen, Temple University (**463**); C Dean, University College, London (**695a, 696–699, 700a, 700b, 701a, 703–705, 708, 710–712**); BM Eley, King's College, London (**392**); MWJ Fergusson, University of Manchester (**545, 547, 549–554**); L Fonzi, University of Siena (**614**); SW Franey, King's College, London (**514, 521–523**); DL Franklin and NJ Severs, Queen Mary and Westfield College and Cardiothoracic Institute, London (**596**); LJ Gathercole and A Keller, University of Bristol (**378**); P Glick, University of Iowa (**608, 609, 611, 612**); DA Grant, University of Southern California (**633, 634**); AJ Gwinnett, State University of New York, Stoney Brook (**224**); RV Hawkins, University of Leeds (**301, 445–446**); JD Harrison, King's College, London (**392, 525, 526**); PF Heap, University of Bristol (**515–517, 519, 520, 524**); RJ Hillier and GT Craig, University of Sheffield (**220b, 226**); WJ Hume, University of Leeds (**496**); NW Johnson, Department of Dental Science, Royal College of Surgeons, London (**274, 309b**); SJ Jones, University College, London (**349, 350, 357, 379, 442–444, 447, 651**); S Kariyawasam, United Medical and Dental Schools, London (**200, 470–474, 578**); E Katchburian, University of São Paulo (**595–598**); J Kirkham, University of Leeds (**386**); Y Kishi and K Takahashi, Kanagawa Dental College (**323–325**); EJ Kollar, University of Connecticut (**589, 590**); D Lee, MR Sims, CW Dreyer and WJ Sampson, University of Adelaide (**411**); BGH Levers, University of Bristol (**235, 241, 300, 306, 641, 642, 652**); RWA Linden, King's College, London (**414**); A Loescher, University of Sheffield (**448**); DA Luke, United Medical and Dental Schools, London (**433, 436, 440, 502–504, 507–509, 534a**); AGS Lumsden, United Medical and Dental Schools, London (**278, 336a, 591–593, 647**); DA Lunt, University of Glasgow (**199, 361**); I Mackenzie, University of Texas, Houston (**459, 461**); B Matthews, University of Bristol (**193, 194**); JC Marks Jr. and DR Cahill, Universities of Massachusetts and Rochester (**655**); RMH McMinn (**19**); AH Meckel, WJ Griebstein and RN Neal, Proctor and Gamble, Cincinnati (**209**); BRRN Mendis, University of Peradeniya (**275–277**); HN Newman, Institute of Dental Surgery, London (**223a, 236, 242–245, 254–266**); HJ Orams, PP Phakey, and WA Rachinger, Universities of Melbourne and Monash (**206, 207a**); R O'Sullivan, University of Cork (**371**); PDA Owens, Queens University, Belfast (**353, 356, 397, 637, 640**); H Ozawa and H Nakamura, Nigata University (**580**); GW Parfitt, University of Alabama (**418**); CH Pearson, University of Alberta (**385**); RW Pigott, University of Bristol (**556b**); DGF Poole,

University of Bristol (**201, 208, 210, 211, 213, 218, 223a, 223b, 242–245, 248**); WDL Ride, Western Australia Museum (**580**); A Riske-Anderson and A Koling, University of Umeå (**287**); M Robins, King's College, London (**678**); C Robinson, University of Leeds (**386**, 'rose' diagrams, page 263); SM Royer and JC Kinnamon, University of Colorado (**500**); J Searles, University of Iowa (**299**); PR Shellis, University of Bristol (**219, 247, 310, 313, 421, 423, 424, 617**); CA Shuttleworth, University of Manchester (**391**); M Sigal, S Pitaru, J Aubin and AR Ten Cate, University of Toronto (**284, 285**); LM Silverstone, University of Colorado (**217**); G Singh, University of Bristol (**543, 544, 546, 548**); P Sloan, University of Manchester (**373, 375–377, 380, 431, 449**); JV Soames, University of Manchester (**483**); R Sprinz, University of Edinburgh (**232, 239, 272, 302, 402a**); CA Squier, University of Iowa (**454–458, 460, 464–467, 478, 480, 495**); C Stevens, University of Bristol (**3, 84**); PE Taylor and PE Redd, University of Washington (**332**); I Thesleff, University of Helsinki (**587, 588**); A Thexton, United Dental and Medical Schools, London (**187, 189**); S Wakisaka, University of Osaka (**331**); H Warshawsky, McGill University (**207b**); D Weber, University of Illinois (**316, 317**) and DK Whittaker, University of Wales, School of Medicine (**204, 227, 234, 240, 246, 354b**).

Acknowledgement is also owing to: American Dental Association (**661**), National Geographic Society (**702**), Natural History Museum (**695b, 701b, 706, 707**), Odontological Museum, Royal College of Surgeons of England (**27**), Wenner–Gren Foundation (**700c**).

We thank the Editors and Authors of the following publications for permission to reproduce illustrations: *Acta Anatomica* (**335**); *Acta Odontologica Scandinavika* (**287**); *Advances in Dental Research* (**207b**); *Anatomical Record* (a publication of the Wistar Press) (**284, 285**); *Archives of Oral Biology* (**264, 415–417, 420, 654, 655–657, 659, 660, 708, 711**); *Companion to Dental Studies*, Vol. 2, Blackwell's, Oxford (**349, 350, 570, 619**); *Development*, Company of Biologists Ltd. (**545, 547, 549–554, 591–593**); *Developmental Biology* (**587, 588**); *Dynamic Aspects of the Dental Pulp*, Chapman Hall, London (**325a, 332**); *European Journal of Orthodontics* (**414**, Table 16); *Histochemistry* (**331**); *Journal of Anatomy* (**395, 596**); *Journal of Comparative Neurology* (**500**); *Journal of Dental Research* (**323, 324, 325b, 392, 418**); *Journal of Dentistry* (by permission of the publishers, Butterworth–Heinmann Ltd.) (**262**); *Journal of Embryology and Experimental Morphology* (**588, 589**); *Journal of Human Evolution* (**710**); *Journal of Periodontology* (**633, 634**); *Journal of Zoology* (**425**); *Oral Histology: Development Structure and Function*, A R Ten Cate, Mosby, St Louis (**460, 464–467**); *Proceedings of the Finnish Dental Society* (**330**); *Structural and Chemical Organisation of Teeth*, Vol. 1, Academic Press, London (**224**); *Teeth* Vol. 6, *Handbook of Microscopic Anatomy*, Springer–Verlag, Berlin (**251, 601, 651**); *Tooth Enamel*, Vol. 1, Wrights, Bristol (**209**).

We have modified diagrams originally published by the following: J Ahlgren (**191**); RB Carter and EN Keen (**170**); BN Davies and KW Cross (**196**); JH Farrell (**185**, from the *British Dental Journal*, Volume 56); HRB Fenn, KP Liddlelow and EP Gimson (**469**); NJB Houston and WJ Tulley (**112**); BS Kraus, RE Jordan and L Abrams (**80**); JW Osborne (**229**); F Rushmer and GA Hendron (**195**); H Sicher and EL Dubrul (**192**); RC Wheeler (**29, 38, 43, 48**).

We are grateful to PF Hire and L Kelberman for photographic assistance, to B Hestbak for preparing diagrams, to E Pehowich for preparing electron micrographs, to Mrs SK Collins, Mrs C Cybil and Miss A Filice for secretarial assistance, and to Mrs S Berkovitz and Mrs RA Moxham for proof-reading.

Macroscopic anatomy of the oral cavity and related regions

The *in vivo* appearance of the oral cavity

1 The oral cavity extends from the lips and cheeks externally to the pillars of the fauces internally, where it continues into the oropharynx. It is subdivided into the vestibule external to the teeth and the oral cavity proper internal to the teeth. The palate forms the roof of the mouth and separates the oral and nasal cavities. The floor of the oral cavity is formed by the mylohyoid muscle and is occupied mainly by the tongue. The lateral walls of the oral cavity are defined by the cheeks and retromolar regions. The functions of the mouth include ingestion, mastication, speech and ventilation.

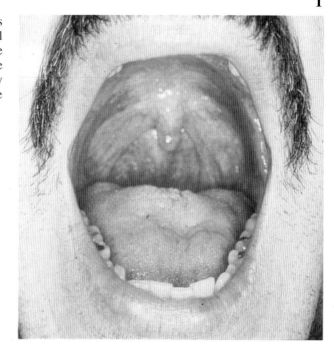

2 The lips are composed of a muscular skeleton (the orbicularis oris muscle) and connective tissue, and are covered externally by skin and internally by mucous membrane. The red zone of the lip (the vermilion zone) is a feature characteristic of man. The sharp junction of the red zone and the skin is termed the vermilion border. In the upper lip, the vermilion zone protrudes in the midline to form the tubercle (**A**). The lower lip shows a slight depression in the midline corresponding to the tubercle. From the midline to the corners of the mouth, the lips widen and then narrow. Laterally, the upper lip is separated from the cheeks by nasolabial grooves (**B**). Similar grooves appear with age at the corners of the mouth to delineate the lower lip from the cheeks (the labiomarginal sulci, **C**). The labiomental groove (**D**) separates the lower lip from the chin. In the midline of the upper lip runs the philtrum (**E**). The corners of the lips (the labial commissures, **F**) are usually located adjacent to the maxillary canine and mandibular first premolar teeth. The lips exhibit sexual dimorphism; as a general rule, the skin of the male is thicker, firmer, less mobile and hirsute. The lips illustrated are lightly closed at rest and are described as being 'competent'.

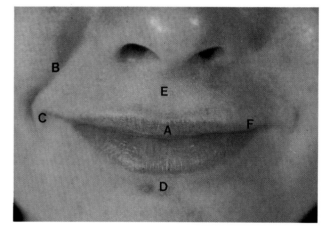

3 Incompetent lips describe a situation where at rest, with the facial muscles relaxed, a lip seal is not produced. It is of some importance that this is distinguished from conditions where the lips are merely held apart habitually (as often occurs with 'mouth breathers'). The lip posture illustrated here can be described as being 'potentially competent' because the lips would be capable of producing a seal at rest if there were no interference caused by the protruding incisors. Where the lips are incompetent, the pattern of swallowing is often modified to produce an anterior oral seal. Accordingly, an oral seal may be formed by contact between the lower lip (or the tongue) and the palatal mucosa, and there may even be a forcible tongue thrust. It has been estimated that in the UK and the USA about 50% of children at the age of 11 years have some degree of lip incompetence.

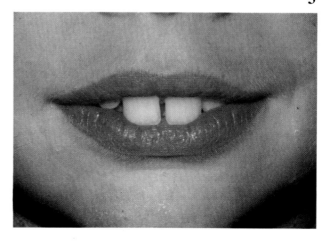

4 Lip posture and tooth position. The position and activity of the lips are important in controlling the degree of protrusion of the incisors. With competent lips (**A**), the tips of the maxillary incisors lie below the upper border of the lower lip, this arrangement helping to maintain the 'normal' inclination of the incisors. With incompetent lips (**B**), the maxillary incisors may not be so controlled and the lower lip may even lie behind them, thus producing an exaggerated proclination of these teeth. If there is tongue thrusting to provide an anterior oral seal, further forces that tend to protrude the incisors are generated. A tight, or overactive, lip musculature may be associated with retroclined incisors.

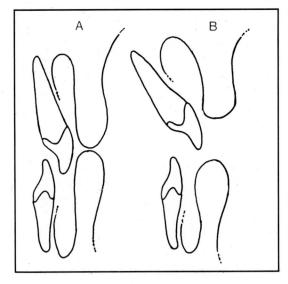

5 The oral vestibule is a slit-like space between the lips and cheeks and the teeth and alveolus. At rest, or with the mouth open, the vestibule and oral cavity proper directly communicate between the teeth. When the teeth bite together, the vestibule is a closed space which only communicates with the oral cavity proper behind the last molars (the retromolar regions). The mucosa covering the alveolus is reflected onto the lips and cheeks, forming a trough or sulcus called the fornix vestibuli (**A**). In some regions of the sulcus, the mucosa may show distinct sickle-shaped folds running from the cheeks and lips to the alveolus. The upper and lower labial frena or frenula (**B**) are such folds in the midline. Other folds of variable dimensions may traverse the sulcus in the regions of the canines or premolars (**C**). Such frena are said to be more pronounced in the lower sulcus. All folds contain loose connective tissue and are neither muscle attachments nor sites of large blood vessels. The upper labial frenum should be attached well below the alveolar crest. A large frenum with an attachment near the crest may be associated with a midline diastema between the maxillary first incisors. Prominent frena may also influence the stability of dentures.

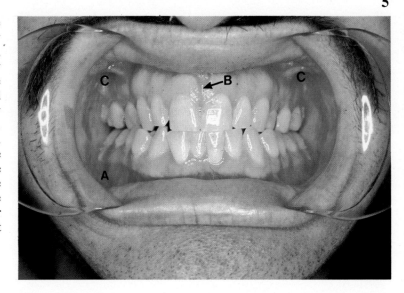

6 The gums or gingivae. The mucosa lining the lower part of the alveolus is loosely attached to the periosteum via a diffuse submucosa and is termed the alveolar mucosa (**A**). It is delineated from the gingiva (**B**) by the mucogingival junction (**C**). The alveolar mucosa appears dark red, the gingiva pale pink. These colour differences result from differences in the type of keratinisation and the proximity to the surface of underlying blood vessels. Indeed, small blood vessels may readily be seen coursing beneath the alveolar mucosa. The gingiva may be subdivided into the attached gingiva (**D**) and the free gingiva (**E**). The attached gingiva is firmly bound to the periosteum of the alveolus and to the teeth, and the free gingiva lies unattached around the neck (cervical margin) of the tooth. Between the free and attached gingiva a groove may be seen (the free gingival groove). The interdental papilla (**F**) is that part of the gingiva which fills the space

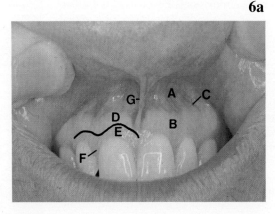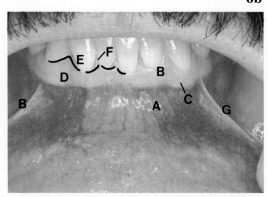

between teeth. A feature of the attached gingiva is its surface stippling. However, the degree of stippling varies from individual to individual and also according to age and sex and the health of the gingiva. The free gingiva is not stippled. On the lingual surface of the lower jaw, the attached

gingiva is sharply differentiated from the lining, non-keratinised mucosa of the floor of the mouth. On the palate, there is no obvious division between the attached gingiva and palatal mucosa. Note the frena (**G**) extending across the fornix vestibuli.

7 The cheek and mandibular retromolar region. The cheeks extend intra-orally from the labial commissures anteriorly to the ridge of mucosa overlying the ascending ramus of the mandible posteriorly. They are bounded superiorly and inferiorly by the upper and lower vestibular sulci. The mucosa is non-keratinised and, being tightly adherent to the buccinator muscle, is stretched when the mouth is opened and wrinkled when closed. Ectopic sebaceous glands may be evident as yellowish patches (Fordyce's spots). Few structural landmarks are visible. The parotid duct drains into the cheek opposite the maxillary second molar tooth and its opening may be covered by a small fold of mucosa termed the parotid papilla. A hyperkeratinised line called the linea alba may be seen at a position related to the occlusal plane. In the retromolar region, in front of the pillars of the fauces, a fold of mucosa containing the pterygomandibular raphe extends from the upper to the lower alveolus. The pterygomandibular space, in which the lingual and inferior alveolar nerves run, lies lateral to this fold and medial to the ridge produced by the mandibular ramus. **A**, cheek; **B**, ridge of mandibular ramus; **C**, pterygomandibular raphe; the arrow indicates a landmark for insertion of a needle for local anaesthesia of the lingual and inferior alveolar nerves.

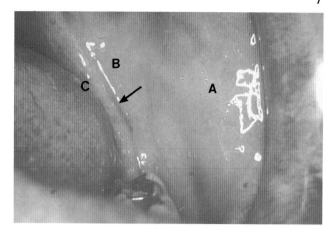

The palate is divided into the immovable hard palate anteriorly and the movable soft palate posteriorly. As their names suggest, the skeleton of the hard palate is bony while that of the soft palate is fibrous.

8 The hard palate is covered by a keratinised mucosa. It shows a distinct prominence immediately behind the maxillary central incisors, the incisive papilla (**A**), which covers the nasopalatine nerves as they emerge from the incisive foramen. Extending posteriorly in the midline from the papilla runs a ridge termed the palatine raphe (**B**). The palatine rugae (**C**) are irregular folds which radiate transversely from the incisive papilla and the anterior part of the palatine raphe. At the junction of the palate and the alveolus (**D**) lies a mass of soft tissue (submucosa) in which run the greater palatine nerves and vessels. The shape and size of the dome of the palate varies considerably, being relatively shallow in some cases and having considerable depth in others.

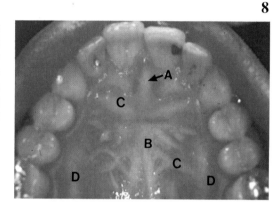

9 The soft palate and oropharyngeal isthmus. The boundary between the hard and soft palate is readily palpable and may be distinguished by a change in colour, the soft palate being a darker red with a yellowish tint. Extending laterally from the free border of the soft palate on each side are the palatoglossal (**A**) and palato-pharyngeal (**B**) folds, the palatoglossal fold being more anterior. These folds cover the palato-glossus and palatopharyngeus muscles and between them lies the tonsillar fossa housing the palatine tonsil (**C**). Extending backwards from the free edge of the soft palate in the midline is the palatal uvula (**D**). The oropharyngeal isthmus is where the oral cavity and the oropharynx meet. It is delineated by the palatoglossal and palatopharyngeal folds (i.e. the pillars of the fauces) and by the uvula and the pharyngeal surface of the tongue. The palatine tonsil is a collection of lymphatic material of variable size. It exhibits several slit-like invaginations (the tonsillar crypts), one of which is particularly deep and named the intratonsillar cleft.

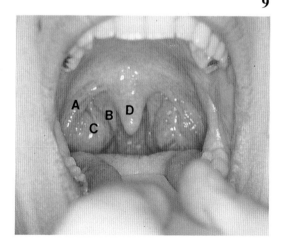

10 **The floor of the mouth** is a small horseshoe-shaped region above the mylohyoid muscle and beneath the movable part of the tongue. It is covered by a lining of non-keratinised mucosa. In the midline, near the base of the tongue, a fold of tissue called the lingual frenum (**A**) extends on to the inferior surface of the tongue. Rarely, the lingual frenum extends across the floor of the mouth to be attached to the mandibular alveolus. The sublingual papilla (**B**), onto which the submandibular salivary ducts open into the mouth, is a large centrally positioned protuberance at the base of the tongue. On either side of this papilla are the sublingual folds (**C**), beneath which lie the submandibular ducts and sublingual salivary glands.

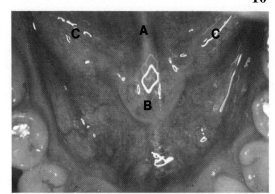

The tongue is a muscular organ with its base attached to the floor of the mouth.

11 **The inferior surface of the tongue**, related to the floor of the mouth, is covered by a thin lining of non-keratinised mucous membrane which is tightly bound to the underlying muscles. In the midline, extending onto the floor of the mouth, lies the lingual frenum (**A**). Lateral to the frenum lie irregular, fringed folds of mucous membrane, the fimbriated folds (**B**). Also visible through the mucosa are the deep lingual veins (**C**).

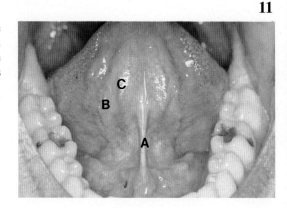

12a **12b**

12 **The dorsum of the tongue** may be sub-divided into the anterior two-thirds or palatal part and the posterior third or pharyngeal part. The junction of the palatal and pharyngeal parts is marked by a shallow V-shaped groove (the sulcus terminalis, **A**). The angle (or 'V') of the sulcus terminalis is directed posteriorly. In the midline, near the angle, may be seen a small pit called the foramen caecum (**B**). This is the primordial site of development of the thyroid gland. The mucosa of the palatal part of the tongue is partly keratinised and is characterised by the abundance of papillae. The most conspicuous papillae on the palatal surface of the tongue are the circumvallate papillae (**C**), which lie immediately in front of the sulcus terminalis. The pharyngeal surface of the tongue is covered with large rounded nodules termed the lingual follicles (**D**). These follicles are composed of lymphatic

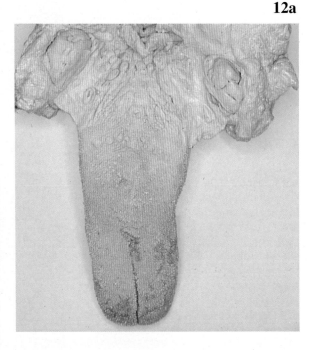

tissue, collectively forming the lingual tonsil. The posterior part of the tongue slopes towards the epiglottis, where three folds of mucous membrane are seen, the median and lateral glossoepiglottic folds. The anterior pillars of the fauces (the palatoglossal arches, **E**) extend from the soft palate to the sides of the tongue near the circumvallate papillae. **F**, palatal tonsil.

13 Dorsum of tongue showing filiform and fungiform papillae. The surface is covered with numerous whitish, conical elevations, the filiform papillae. Interspersed between the filiform papillae are isolated reddish prominences, the fungiform papillae (*arrowed*). The fungiform papillae are most numerous at the tip of the tongue.

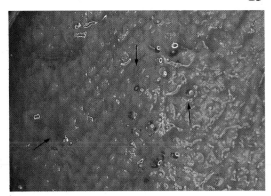

14 The circumvallate papillae (A) are considerably larger than either the filiform or fungiform papillae. They lie immediately in front of the sulcus terminalis. They do not project beyond the surface of the tongue. They are surrounded by a circular 'trench'. The surface of the posterior third of the tongue, lying behind the sulcus terminalis, is covered by a number of smooth elevations (**B**) produced by underlying lymphoid tissue.

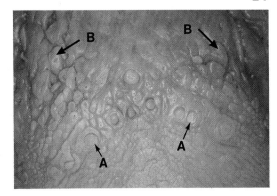

15 Foliate papillae. These appear as a series of parallel, slit-like folds of mucosa on each lateral border of the tongue, near the attachment of the palatoglossal fold (anterior pillar of the fauces). The foliate papillae are of variable length in man and are the vestige of large papillae found in many other mammals.

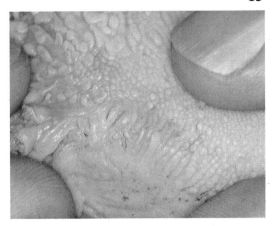

Dento-osseous structures
The jaws

The jaws are the tooth-bearing bones. They comprise three bones. The two maxillary bones form the upper jaw. The lower jaw is a single bone, the mandible.

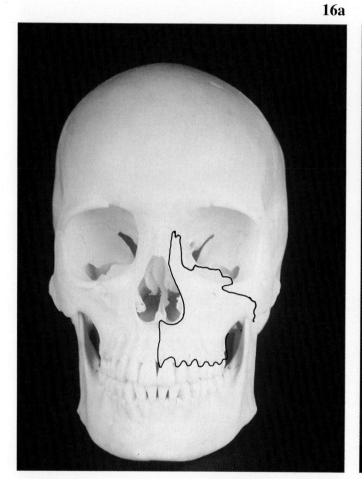
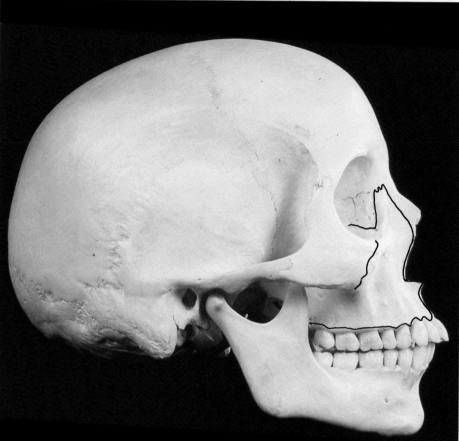

16 The relationship between the jaws and the remainder of the skull.
The black outline describes the boundaries of a maxillary bone.

The skull is the most complex osseous structure in the body. It protects the brain, the organs of special sense, and the cranial parts of the respiratory and digestive systems. The skull is divided into the neurocranium (which houses and protects the brain and the organs of special sense) and the viscerocranium (which surrounds the upper parts of the respiratory and digestive tracts). The jaws contribute the major part of the viscerocranium, comprising about 25% of the skull. The jaws have evolved from the gill arch elements of early *agnathan vertebrates*. It is probable that one or two anterior gill arches gradually disappeared with the expansion of the mouth cavity, so that the gill arch which developed phylogenetically into the jaws of ancestral gnathostomes was not the first of the series. Note that the upper jaw not only contains teeth, but also contributes to the skeleton of the nose, orbit, cheek and palate.

17 The maxilla (upper jaw) — lateral aspect. The maxilla consists of a body and four processes: the frontal (**A**), zygomatic (**B**), alveolar (**C**) and palatine processes. Only the palatine process cannot be seen from the lateral aspect of the maxilla. The anterolateral surface of the maxilla (the malar surface) forms the skeleton of the anterior part of the cheek. In the midline, the alveolar processes of the two maxillae meet at the intermaxillary suture whence they diverge laterally to form the opening into the nasal fossae (the piriform aperture). At the lower border of the piriform aperture, in the midline, lies the bony projection termed the anterior nasal spine (**D**). The malar surface of the body of the maxilla is concave, forming the canine fossa (**E**). Superiorly, the malar surface is continuous with the orbital plate of the maxilla (**F**) and forms the floor of the orbit. Anterior to the orbital plate, the frontal process extends above the piriform aperture to meet the nasal and frontal bones. Below the infraorbital rim lies the infraorbital foramen (*arrowed*) through which the infraorbital branch of the maxillary nerve and the infra-orbital artery from the maxillary artery emerge onto the face. The posterolateral surface of the maxilla (the infratemporal surface) forms the anterior wall of the infratemporal fossa. The malar and infratemporal surfaces meet at a bony ridge extending from the zygomatic process to the alveolus adjacent to the first molar tooth. This ridge is called the zygomaticoalveolar or jugal crest (**G**). The posterior convexity of the infratemporal surface is termed the maxillary tuberosity and presents several small foramina associated with the posterior superior dental nerves (which supply the posterior maxillary teeth). The zygomatic process extends both from the malar and infratemporal surfaces of the maxilla. From the entire lower surface of the body arises the alveolar process, which supports the maxillary teeth.

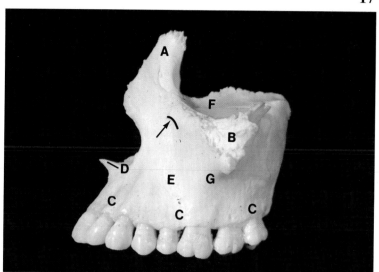
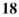

18 The maxilla (upper jaw) — medial aspect. This part of the maxilla forms the lateral wall of the nose. In the specimen illustrated, the central hollow of the body of the maxilla (the maxillary air sinus or antrum) is divided by a bony septum. In front of the antrum lies a deep vertical groove called the lacrimal sulcus (**A**). This sulcus meets the lower edge of the lacrimal bone to form the nasolacrimal canal. Behind the antrum lies the palatine groove (**B**). This groove is converted into a canal carrying the greater palatine nerve and artery by the perpendicular plate of the palatine bone. The maxillary palatine process (**C**) extends horizontally from the medial surface of the maxilla where the body meets the alveolar process.

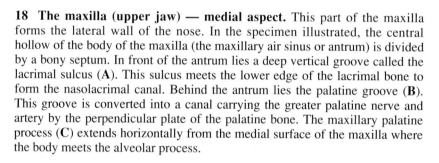
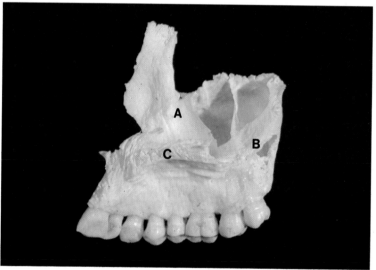

19 The osteology of the maxillary air sinus. The lateral wall of the nasal fossa consists mainly of the medial surface of the maxilla. This surface of the isolated bone is seen to be occupied mainly by the large maxillary hiatus (see **18**). To reduce the size of this space, the hiatus is overlapped by the lacrimal bone (**3**) and ethmoid bone above, the palatine bone (**4,5**) behind, and the inferior concha (**6**) below. **1**, lacrimal groove of maxilla; **2**, lacrimal groove.

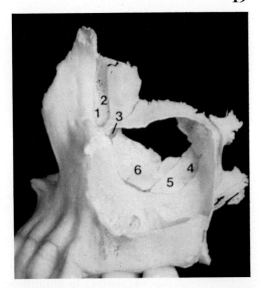

20 Inferior view of the maxillae and elements comprising the skeleton of the hard palate. The bones contributing to the hard palate are the palatine processes of the maxillae (**A**) and the horizontal plates of the palatine bones (**B**). The maxillary palatine processes arise as horizontal plates at the junction of the bodies and alveolar processes of the maxillae. The boundary between the palatine and alveolar processes is well defined in its posterior aspect only. Anteriorly, the angle between the two is less well defined. The junction between the palatine processes in the midline is termed the median palatine suture (**C**). Anteriorly, behind the central incisors, this junction is incomplete, thus forming the incisive fossa (**D**), through which pass the nasopalatine nerves. Unlike the nasal surface, the oral surface of the palatine process is rough and irregular.

The posterior edges of the palatine processes articulate with the horizontal plates of the two palatine bones to form the transverse palatine suture (**E**). Laterally, this junction is incomplete, forming the greater palatine foramina (**F**), through which pass the greater palatine nerves and vessels. Behind the greater palatine foramina lie the lesser palatine foramina (**G**), through which pass the lesser palatine nerves and vessels. The junction of the two palatine bones in the midline completes the median palatine suture. The posterior borders of the horizontal palatine plates are concave and in the midline form a sharp ridge of bone called the posterior nasal spine (**H**). To the posterior edge of the hard palate is attached the fibrous palatine aponeurosis of the soft palate, which is formed by the tendons of the tensor veli palatini muscles.

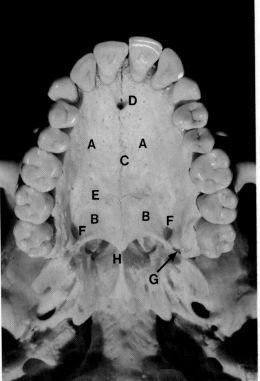

21 Lateral view of the maxillary teeth *in situ* within the alveolus, demonstrated by the removal of buccal bone around the roots of the teeth above the alveolar crests. Note the close relationship of the root apices of the premolars and molars to the floor of the maxillary antrum (red line), and those of the incisors and canine to the floor of the nasal fossa.

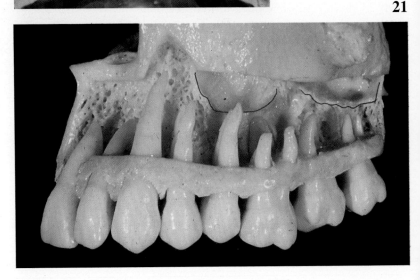

22 The maxillary alveolus and the arrangement of the tooth sockets. The maxillary alveolar processes extend inferiorly from the bodies of the maxillae and support the teeth within bony sockets. Each maxilla can contain a full quadrant of eight permanent teeth or five deciduous teeth. The form of the alveolus is related to the functional demands put upon the teeth. When the teeth are removed the alveolus resorbs. Essentially, the alveolar process consists of two parallel plates of cortical bone, the buccal (**A**) and palatal (**B**) alveolar plates, between which lie the sockets of individual teeth. Between each socket lie interalveolar or interdental septa (**C**). The floor of the socket has been termed the fundus, its rim the alveolar crest. The form and depth of each socket is defined by the form and length of the root it supports, and thus shows considerable variation. In multirooted teeth the sockets are divided by interradicular septa (**D**). The apical regions of the sockets of anterior teeth are closely related to the nasal fossae, while those of posterior teeth are closely related to the maxillary antra. The position of the sockets in relation to the buccal and palatal alveolar plates is shown in **27**.

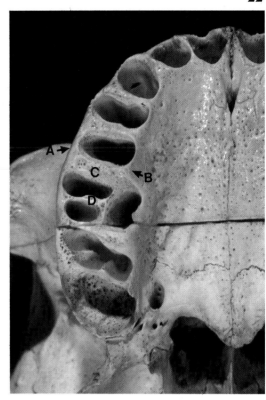

23 The mandible (lower jaw) — lateral aspect. The mandible consists of a horizontal horseshoe-shaped component, the body of the mandible (**A**), and two vertical components, the rami (**B**). The rami join the body posteriorly at obtuse angles. The body of the mandible carries the mandibular teeth and their associated alveolar processes. Before birth, the body consists of two lateral halves which meet in the midline at a symphysis. On either side of the midline, close to the inferior margin of the body, lies a distinct prominence called the mental tubercle. These tubercles constitute the mental protuberance or chin. Above the mental protuberance lies a shallow depression termed the incisive fossa (**C**). Behind this fossa, the canine eminence overlies the root of the mandibular canine. Midway in the height of the body of the mandible, related to the premolar teeth, is the mental foramen (**D**). The mental branches of the inferior alveolar nerve and artery pass onto the face through this foramen. The most common position for the mental foramen is on a vertical line passing through the mandibular second premolar. During the first and second years of life, as the prominence of the chin develops, the opening of the mental foramen alters in direction from facing forwards to facing upwards and backwards. Rarely, there may be multiple mental foramina. The inferior margin of the body meets the posterior margin of the ramus at the angle of the mandible (**E**). This area is irregular, being the site of insertion of the masseter muscle and stylomandibular ligament. The alveolus forms the superior margin of the mandibular body. The junction of the alveolus and

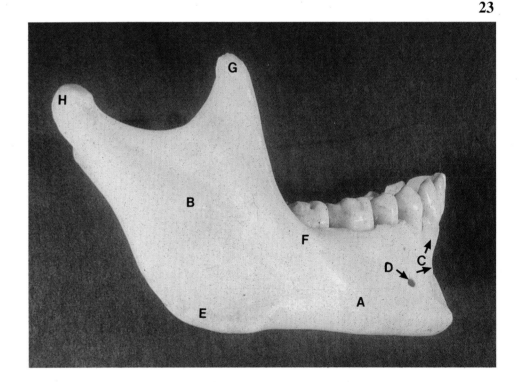

ramus is demarcated by a ridge of bone, the external oblique line (**F**), which continues downwards and forwards across the body of the mandible to terminate below the mental foramen. As this line progresses upwards, it becomes the anterior margin of the ramus and ends as the tip of the coronoid process. The coronoid (**G**) and the condylar (**H**) processes form the two processes of the superior border of the ramus. The coronoid process provides attachment for the temporalis muscle. The condylar process has a neck supporting an articular surface which fits into the mandibular fossa of the temporal bone to form a movable synovial joint (the temporomandibular joint). The concavity between the coronoid and condylar processes is called the mandibular notch.

24 Posterolateral aspect of the medial surface of the mandible. Close to the midline, on the inferior surface of the mandibular body, lie two shallow depressions called the digastric fossae. Into these fossae are inserted the anterior bellies of the digastric muscles. Above the fossae, in the midline, are the genial spines or tubercles (**A**). There are generally two inferior and two superior tubercles, which serve as attachments for the geniohyoid muscles and the genioglossus muscles respectively. Passing upwards and backwards across the medial surface of the body of the mandible is a prominent ridge. This is termed the mylohyoid or internal oblique ridge (**B**). From this ridge the mylohyoid muscle takes origin. The mylohyoid ridge arises between the genial tubercles and digastric fossa and increases in prominence as it passes backwards to end on the anterior surface of the ramus. Because the mylohyoid muscle forms the floor of the mouth, the bone above the mylohyoid ridge forms the anterior wall of the oral cavity proper, while that below the ridge forms the lateral wall of the submandibular space.

The following features may be seen on the medial surface of the ramus. Around the angle of the mandible, the bone is roughened (**C**) for the attachment of the medial pterygoid muscle. Commencing at the tip of the coronoid process, a

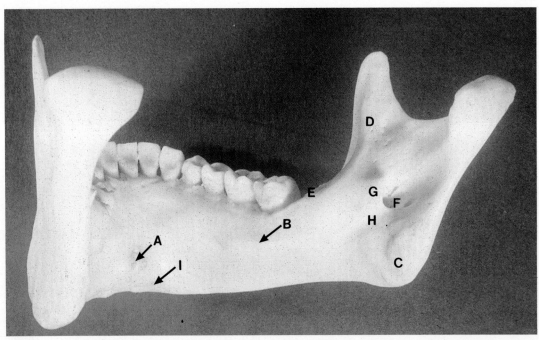

ridge of bone called the temporal crest (**D**) runs down the anterior surface of the ramus to end behind the mandibular molars at the retromolar triangle (**E**). In the centre of the medial surface of the ramus lies the mandibular foramen (**F**), through which the inferior alveolar nerve and

artery pass into the mandibular canal. A bony process, the lingula (**G**), extends from the anterosuperior surface of the foramen. The mylohyoid groove (**H**) may be seen running down from the posteroinferior surface of the foramen. **I**, digastric fossa.

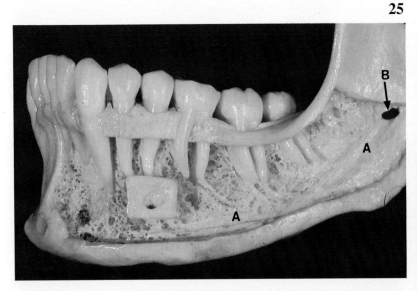

25 Lateral view of the mandibular teeth *in situ* within the alveolus and their relationship with the mandibular canal (**A**). The mandibular canal, which transmits the inferior alveolar nerve, artery and veins, begins at the mandibular foramen (**B**) and extends to the region of the premolar teeth, where it bifurcates into the mental and incisive canals. The course of the mandibular canal and its relationship with the teeth is variable and this variation is illustrated in connection with the course of the inferior alveolar nerve in **170**.

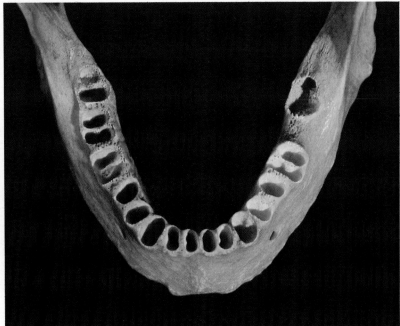

26 The mandibular alveolus and the arrangement of the tooth sockets. As for the maxilla, the mandibular alveolus consists of buccal and lingual alveolar plates joined by interdental and interradicular septa. In the region of the second and third molars the external oblique line is superimposed upon the buccal alveolar plate. The form and depth of the tooth sockets are related to the morphology of the roots of the mandibular teeth and the functional demands placed upon them.

27 Buccolingual sections through the teeth. These demonstrate the directional axes and bony relationships of the teeth and their alveoli and the relative thickness of the buccal and lingual alveolar plates.

a Maxillary incisor region.
b Maxillary canine region.
c Maxillary premolar region.
d Maxillary molar region.
e Mandibular incisor region.
f Mandibular canine region.
g Mandibular premolar region.
h Mandibular molar region.

Note the relationships of the mandibular teeth to the mandibular canal (**A**), and the maxillary teeth to the antrum (**B**).

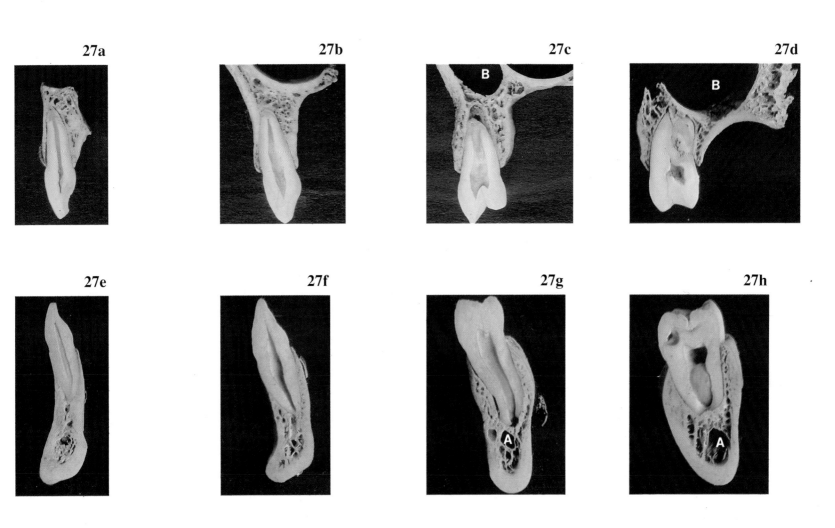

27a   27b   27c   27d

27e   27f   27g   27h

23

Tooth morphology

Man has two generations of teeth: the deciduous (or primary) dentition and the permanent (or secondary) dentition. There are no teeth in the mouth at birth, but by the age of 3 years the deciduous dentition is complete. By 6 years, the first permanent teeth appear and thence the deciduous teeth are exfoliated one by one to be replaced by their permanent successors. A complete permanent dentition is present at or around the age of 18 years. Thus, given the average life of 70 years, the functional lifespan of the deciduous dentition is only 6% of this total, while with care and luck it can be over 90% for the permanent dentition. In the complete deciduous dentition there are 20 teeth — 10 in each jaw. In the complete permanent dentition there are 32 teeth — 16 in each jaw. In both dentitions, there are three basic tooth forms: incisiform, caniniform and molariform. Incisiform teeth (incisors) are cutting teeth, having thin, blade-like crowns. Caniniform teeth (canines) are piercing or tearing teeth, having a single, stout, pointed, cone-shaped crown. Molariform teeth (molars and premolars) are grinding teeth possessing a number of cusps on an otherwise flattened biting surface. Premolars are bicuspid teeth; they are peculiar to the permanent dentition and replace the deciduous molars. Table 1 gives definitions of terms used for the descriptions of tooth form.

Table 1: Some terms used for the description of tooth form.

Crown	Clinical crown – that portion of a tooth visible in the oral cavity.	
	Anatomical crown – that portion of a tooth covered with enamel.	
Root	Clinical root – that portion of a tooth which lies within the alveolus.	
	Anatomical root – that portion of a tooth covered by cementum.	
Cervical margin	The junction of the anatomical crown and the anatomical root.	
Occlusal surface	The biting surface of a posterior tooth (molar or premolar).	
Incisal margin	The cutting edge of anterior teeth, analogous to the occlusal surface of the posterior teeth.	
Cusp	A pronounced elevation on the occlusal surface of a posterior tooth.	
Tubercle	A small elevation on the crown.	
Cingulum	A bulbous convexity near the cervical region of a tooth.	
Ridge	A linear elevation on the surface of a tooth.	
Marginal ridge	A ridge at the mesial or distal edge of the occlusal surface of posterior teeth. Some anterior teeth have equivalent ridges.	

Fissure	A long cleft between cusps or ridges.
Fossa	A rounded depression in a surface of a tooth.
Buccal	Towards or adjacent to the cheek. The term buccal surface is reserved for that surface of a premolar or molar which is positioned immediately adjacent to the cheek.
Labial	Towards or adjacent to the lips. The term labial surface is reserved for that surface of an incisor or canine which is positioned immediately adjacent to the lips.
Palatal	Towards or adjacent to the palate. The term palatal surface is reserved for that surface of a maxillary tooth which is positioned immediately adjacent to the palate.
Lingual	Towards or adjacent to the tongue. The term lingual surface is reserved for that surface of a mandibular tooth which lies immediately adjacent to the tongue.
Mesial	Towards the median. The mesial surface is that surface which faces towards the median line following the curve of the dental arch.
Distal	Away from the median. The distal surface is that surface which faces away from the median line following the curve of the dental arch.

The types and numbers of teeth in any mammalian dentition can be expressed using dental formulae. The type of tooth is represented by its initial letter, i.e. I for incisors, C for canines, P for premolars and M for molars. The deciduous dentition is indicated by the letter D. The formula for the deciduous dentition of man is $DI_2^2 DC_1^1 DM_2^2 = 10$, and for the permanent dentition $I_2^2 C_1^1 P_2^2 M_3^3 = 16$, where the numbers following each letter refer to the number of teeth of each type in the upper and lower jaws on one side only. Identification of teeth is made not only according to the dentition to which they belong and to basic tooth form, but also according to their anatomical location within the jaws. The tooth-bearing region of the jaws can be divided into four quadrants, the right and left maxillary and mandibular quadrants. A tooth may thus be identified according to the quadrant in which it is located, e.g. a right maxillary deciduous incisor or a left mandibular permanent molar. In both the permanent and deciduous dentitions, the incisors may be distinguished according to their relationship to the midline. Thus, the incisor nearest the midline is the central (or first) incisor, the incisor which is more laterally positioned being termed the lateral (or second) incisor. The permanent premolars and the permanent and deciduous molars can also be distinguished according to their mesiodistal relationships (see diagram below, 'Descriptive terms used in tooth morphology'). The molar most mesially positioned is designated the first molar, the one behind it being the second molar. In the permanent dentition, the tooth most distally positioned is the third molar. The mesial premolar is the first premolar, the premolar behind it being the second premolar.

A dental shorthand may be used in thé clinic to simplify tooth identification. The permanent teeth in each quadrant are numbered 1 to 8 and the deciduous teeth in each quadrant are lettered A to E. The symbols for the quadrants are derived from an imaginary cross, with the horizontal bar placed between the upper and lower jaws and the vertical bar running between the upper and lower central incisors. Thus, the

maxillary right first permanent molar is allocated the symbol 6⌋ and the mandibular left deciduous canine ⌈C. This system of dental shorthand is termed the Zsigmondy System. An alternative scheme has been devised by the *Fédération Dentaire Internationale,* in which the quadrant is represented by a number:

1 = maxillary right quadrant
2 = maxillary left quadrant
3 = mandibular left quadrant } Permanent
4 = mandibular right quadrant
5 = maxillary right quadrant
6 = maxillary left quadrant
7 = mandibular left quadrant } Deciduous
8 = mandibular right quadrant

In this system, the quadrant number prefixes a tooth number. Thus, the maxillary right first permanent molar is symbolised as 1,6 and the mandibular left deciduous canine as 7,3.

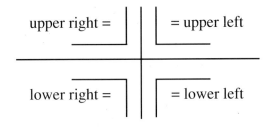

upper right = ⌋⌊ = upper left

lower right = ⌐¬ = lower left

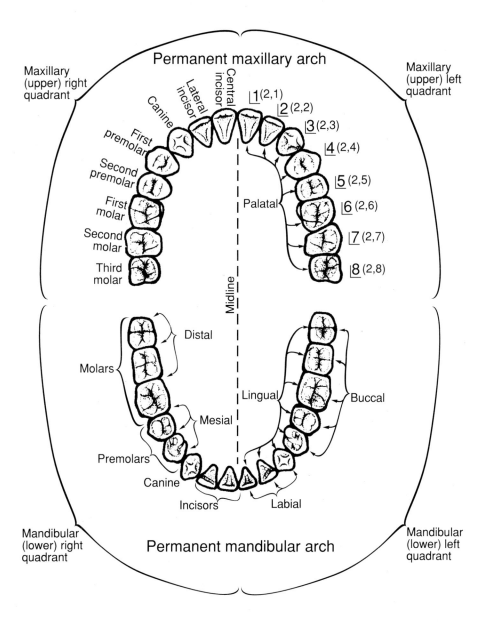

Descriptive terms used in tooth morphology, summarising the systems employed for the identification of teeth according to their location in the jaws.

Principal differences between the dentitions

28 Comparisons between models of deciduous (A) and permanent (B) dental arches and some examples of deciduous and permanent teeth. **C**, deciduous canine. **D**, permanent canine. **E**, deciduous second molar. **F**, permanent first molar.

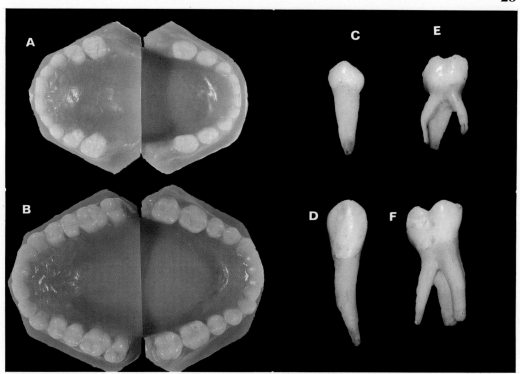

1. The dental formula for the deciduous dentition is:
$$DI\frac{2}{2}\,DC\frac{1}{1}\,DM\frac{2}{2} = 10$$
while that of the permanent dentition is:
$$I\frac{2}{2}\,C\frac{1}{1}\,P\frac{2}{2}\,M\frac{3}{3} = 16$$

2. The deciduous teeth are smaller than their corresponding permanent successors though the mesiodistal dimensions of the permanent premolars are generally less than those for the deciduous molars.

3. Deciduous teeth have a greater constancy of shape.

4. The crowns of deciduous teeth appear bulbous, often having pronounced labial or buccal cingula.

5. The cervical margins of deciduous teeth are more sharply demarcated and pronounced than those of the permanent teeth, the enamel bulging at the cervical margins rather than gently tapering.

6. Comparing newly-erupted teeth, the cusps of deciduous teeth are more pointed than those of the permanent teeth.

7. The crowns of deciduous teeth have a thinner covering of enamel (average width 0.5–1.0mm) than the crowns of permanent teeth (average width 2.5mm).

8. The enamel of deciduous teeth, being more opaque than that of permanent teeth, gives the crown a whiter appearance.

9. The enamel of deciduous teeth is softer than that of permanent teeth and is more easily worn.

10. Enamel of deciduous teeth is more permeable than that of permanent teeth.

11. The prismless layer of surface enamel (see **204**) is wider in deciduous teeth.

12. The enamel and dentine of *all* deciduous teeth exhibit neonatal lines (see **300**).

13. The roots of deciduous teeth are shorter and less robust than those of the permanent teeth.

14. The roots of the deciduous incisors and canines are longer in proportion to the crown than those of their permanent counterparts.

15. The roots of the deciduous molars are widely divergent, extending beyond the dimensions of the crown.

16. The pulp chambers of deciduous teeth are proportionally larger in relation to the crown than those of the permanent teeth. The pulp horns in deciduous teeth are more prominent.

17. The root canals of deciduous teeth are extremely fine.

18. The dental arches for the deciduous dentition are smaller.

The following descriptions of individual teeth will be considered according to tooth class (i.e. incisors, canines, premolars and molars) rather than by membership of either the permanent or deciduous dentitions. For each class, the permanent teeth will be described before the deciduous teeth. This arrangement allows emphasis of the basic features common to each class to be made.

To help visualise the tooth as a three-dimensional object, the illustrations of each tooth are arranged according to the 'third angle projection technique' which aligns each side of a tooth to its occlusal or incisal aspect.

The morphology of the pulp is treated independently of the morphology of the external surfaces of the teeth on pages 42 and 43. For the chronology of the developing dentitions see pages 288–291, for the average dimensions of the teeth see Tables 2 and 3 (page 40), and for ethnic variations in tooth morphology see page 41.

The incisors

The incisors of man have thin, blade-like crowns which are adapted for the cutting and shearing of food preparatory to grinding.

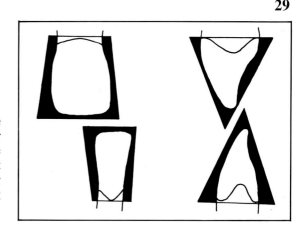

29

29 Schematic drawings of incisor crown form illustrating the relationship between anatomic and geometric form. Viewed mesially or distally, the crowns of the incisors are roughly triangular in shape, with the apex of the triangle at the incisal margin of the tooth. This shape is thought to facilitate the penetration and cutting of food. Viewed buccally or lingually, the incisors are trapezoidal, the shortest of the uneven sides being the base of the crown cervically.

30

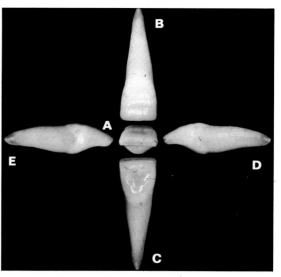

30 Maxillary first (central) permanent incisor. Of all the permanent incisors and canines, the maxillary first permanent incisor is the widest mesiodistally, the crown being almost as wide as it is long. Like all incisors, it is basically wedge- or chisel-shaped and has a single conical root. From the *incisal* view (**A**), the crown and incisal margin are centrally positioned over the root of the tooth. The incisal margin presents as a narrow, flattened ridge rather than as a fine, sharp edge. The incisal margin may be grooved by two troughs, the labial lobe grooves, which correspond to the divisions between three developmental lobes or mammelons seen on newly erupted incisors. The mammelons are lost by attrition soon after eruption. From the incisal aspect, the crown outline is bilaterally symmetrical, being triangular. However, the mesial profile may appear slightly larger than the distal profile. From the *labial* view (**B**), the crown length can be seen to be almost as great as the root length. The crown has a smooth, convex labial surface. It may be marked by two faint grooves which run vertically towards the cervical margin and which are extensions of the labial lobe grooves.

The convexity of the labial surface is especially marked cervically, the labial surface sometimes being flat at its middle and incisal regions. The mesial surface is straight and approximately at right angles to the incisal margin. The distoincisal angle, however, is more rounded and the distal outline more convex. A line drawn through the axial centre of the tooth lies roughly parallel to the mesial outline of the crown and root. Viewed *palatally* (**C**), the crown is more irregular, its middle and incisal regions being concave, giving a slightly shovel-shaped appearance to the incisor. The palatal surface of the crown is bordered by mesial and distal marginal ridges. Near the cervical margin lies a prominent cingulum. The cingulum may be single, divided or replaced by prominent portions of the marginal ridges. Occasionally, a slight ridge of enamel may run towards the incisal margin, dividing the palatal surface into two shallow depressions. The *mesial* (**D**) and *distal* (**E**) views of the crown illustrate the fundamental wedge-shaped or triangular crown form of the incisor.

The sinuous cervical margin is concave towards the crown on the palatal and labial surfaces and convex towards the crown on the mesial and distal surfaces, the curvature on the mesial surface being the most pronounced of any tooth in the dentition. The single root of the central incisor tapers towards the apex. The root is conical in cross-section and appears narrower from the palatal than from the labial aspect.

31 Maxillary second (lateral) permanent incisor. The lateral incisor is one of the most variable teeth in the dentition, though generally it is morphologically a diminutive form of the maxillary central incisor with slight modifications. The lateral incisor crown is much narrower and shorter than the central incisor, though the crown:root length ratio is considerably decreased. From the *incisal* aspect (**A**), the crown has a more rounded outline than the adjacent central incisor. Viewed *labially* (**B**), the mesioincisal and distoincisal angles and the mesial and distal crown margins are more rounded than those of the central incisor. The *palatal* aspect (**C**) of the crown is similar to that of the central incisor, though the marginal ridges and cingulum are often more pronounced. Consequently, the palatal concavity appears deeper. Lying in front of the cingulum is a pit, the foramen cacumen, which may extend some way into the root. The *mesial* (**D**) and *distal* (**E**) aspects of the lateral incisor differ little from those of the central incisor. A common morphological variation is the so-called peg-shaped lateral incisor, which has a thin root surmounted by a small conical crown.

The course of the cervical margin and the shape of the root are similar to those of the central incisor. However, the root is often slightly compressed and grooved on the mesial and distal surfaces.

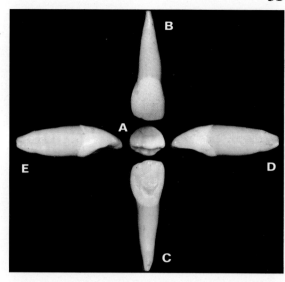

The mandibular incisors have the smallest mesiodistal dimensions of any teeth in the permanent dentition. They can be distinguished from the maxillary incisors not only by their size, but also by the marked lingual inclination of the crowns over the roots, the mesiodistal compression of their roots and the poor development of the marginal ridges and cingula.

32 Mandibular first (central) permanent incisor. Viewed *incisally* (**A**), the tooth has a bilaterally symmetrical triangular shape. The incisal margin in this specimen has been worn and appears flat, though in the newly-erupted tooth three mammelons are usually present. The incisal margin is at right angles to a line bisecting the tooth labiolingually. Viewed *labially* (**B**), the crown of the incisor is almost twice as long as it is broad. The unworn incisal margin is straight and approximately at right angles to the long axis of the tooth. The mesioincisal and distoincisal angles are sharp and the mesial and distal surfaces are approximately at right angles to the incisal margin. The profiles of the mesial and distal surfaces appear very similar, being convex in their incisal thirds and relatively flattened in the middle and cervical thirds. The *lingual* surface (**C**) is smooth and slightly concave, the lingual cingulum and mesial and distal marginal ridges appearing less distinct than those of the maxillary incisors. The *mesial* (**D**) and *distal* (**E**) views show the characteristic wedge shape of the incisor and the inclination of the crown lingually over the root.

The cervical margins on the labial and lingual surfaces show their maximum convexities midway between the mesial and distal borders of the root. The cervical margin on the distal surface is said to be less curved than that on the mesial surface. The root is narrow and conical, though flattened mesiodistally. It is frequently grooved on the mesial and distal surfaces, the distal groove generally being more marked and deeper.

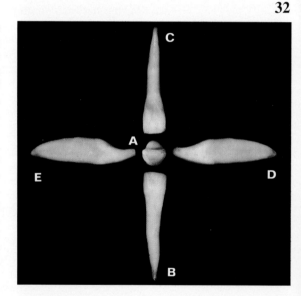

33 The mandibular second (lateral) permanent incisor closely resembles the mandibular central incisor. However, it is slightly wider mesiodistally and is more asymmetrical in shape. The distal surface diverges at a greater angle from the long axis of the tooth, giving it a fan-shaped appearance, and the distoincisal angle is more acute and rounded. Another distinguishing characteristic is the angulation of the incisal margin relative to the labiolingual axis of the root. In the central incisor, the incisal margin forms a right angle with the labiolingual axis, whereas that of the lateral incisor is 'twisted' distally in a lingual direction.

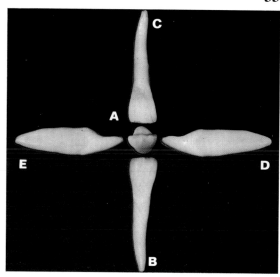

34 Maxillary first (central) deciduous incisor. This tooth is similar morphologically to the corresponding permanent tooth. However, since the transverse diameter of the crown of the deciduous incisor nearly equals the vertical diameter, it appears plumper than its permanent successor. From the *incisal* view (**A**), the straight incisal margin appears to be centred over the bulk of the crown. Unlike the permanent teeth, no mammelons are seen on the incisal margin of the newly-erupted deciduous incisor. The *labial* surface (**B**) is slightly convex in all planes and unmarked by grooves, lobes or depressions. The mesioincisal angle is sharp and acute, while the distoincisal angle is more rounded and obtuse. On the *palatal* surface (**C**), the cingulum is a very prominent bulge which extends some way up the crown (sometimes to the incisal margin to form a ridge). Unlike its permanent successor, the marginal ridges are ill-defined and the concavity of the palatal surface is shallow. *Mesial* (**D**) and *distal* (**E**) views show the typical incisal form of the crown. Note the low, rounded cingulum at the margin of the labial surface.

As with all deciduous teeth, the cervical margins are more pronounced but less sinuous than those of their permanent successors. The fully-formed root is conical in shape, tapering apically to a rather blunt apex. Compared with the corresponding permanent tooth, the root is longer in proportion to the crown. Note that for the four deciduous incisors illustrated in this book, the roots have not fully formed.

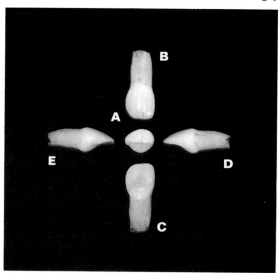

35 The maxillary second (lateral) deciduous incisor is similar in shape to the maxillary first deciduous incisor, though smaller. One obvious difference is the more acute mesioincisal angle and the more rounded distoincisal angle. The palatal surface is more concave and the marginal ridges are more pronounced. Viewed *incisally* (**A**), the crown appears almost circular in contrast to the central incisor, which appears diamond-shaped. As with the first deciduous incisor, there is a rounded, labial cingulum cervically. The palatal cingulum is generally lower than that of the central incisor.

The course of the cervical margin and the shape of the root is similar to the first deciduous incisor.

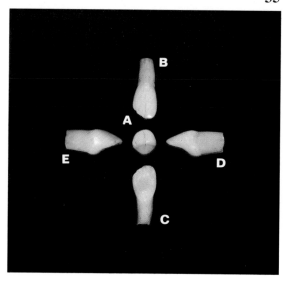

36 The mandibular first (central) deciduous incisor is morphologically similar to its permanent successor. However, it is much shorter and has a low labial cingulum. The mesioincisal and distoincisal angles are sharp right angles and the incisal margin is straight in the horizontal plane. While there are generally no mammelons or grooves on the incisal margin, in this specimen three mammelons may be discerned. The lingual cingulum and the marginal ridges are poorly defined.

The single root is more rounded than that of the corresponding permanent tooth and, when complete, tapers and tends to incline distally.

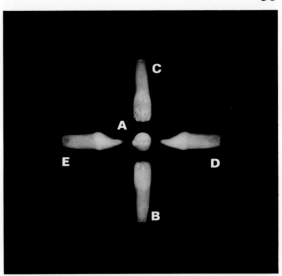

37 The mandibular second (lateral) deciduous incisor is a bulbous tooth which resembles its permanent successor. It is wider than the mandibular first deciduous incisor and is asymmetrical. The mesioincisal angle is more obtuse and rounded than that of the mandibular first deciduous incisor and the incisal margin slopes downward distally. Should the distoincisal angle be markedly rounded then the tooth may be difficult to distinguish from a maxillary second deciduous incisor.

Unlike the permanent successor, the root is rounded. When complete, it is longer than the root of the mandibular first deciduous incisor.

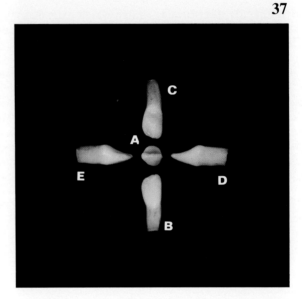

The canines

Canines are the only teeth in the dentition with a single cusp. Morphologically, they can be considered transitional between incisors and premolars.

38 Schematic drawings of canine crown form illustrating the relationship between anatomic and geometric form. Like the incisors, the crowns of canines are roughly triangular in shape when viewed mesially or distally, and trapezoidal buccally and lingually.

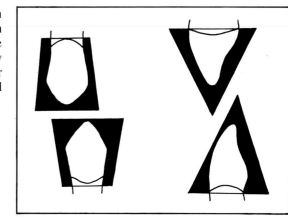

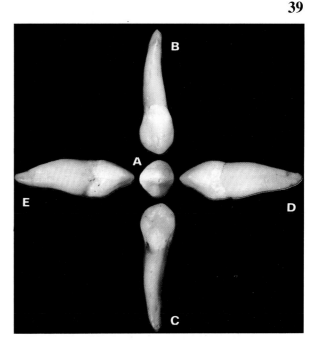

39 Maxillary permanent canine. This is a stout tooth with a well-developed cingulum and the longest root of any tooth. Viewed from its *incisal* aspect (**A**), it appears asymmetrical. If a plane is envisaged passing through the apex of the cusp to the cingulum on the palatal surface, then the distal portion of the crown is much wider than the mesial portion. It is thought that the pointed shape of the canine tooth is related to an increase in size of a central mammelon at the expense of mesial and distal mammelons. Prominent longitudinal ridges pass from the cusp tip down both the labial and palatal surfaces. A relatively frequent variation in the morphology of the incisal ridge is the development of an accessory cusp on its distal arm. The *labial* surface (**B**) of the canine is marked by the longitudinal ridge, which extends from the cusp towards the cervical margin. The incisal part of the crown occupies at least one-third of the crown height. Note that, from this view, the mesial arm of the incisal margin is shorter than the distal arm, and the distoincisal angle is more rounded than the mesioincisal angle. The profiles of the mesial and distal surfaces converge markedly towards the cervix of the tooth. The mesial profile is slightly convex, the distal profile markedly convex. The mesial surface of the crown forms a straight line with the root. The distal surface meets the root at an obtuse angle. The *palatal* surface (**C**) shows distinct mesial and distal marginal ridges and a well-defined cingulum. The longitudinal ridge from the tip of the cusp meets the cingulum and is separated from the marginal ridges on either side by distinct grooves or fossae. Viewed *mesially* (**D**) or *distally* (**E**), the distinctive feature is the stout character of the crown and the great width of the cervical third of both the crown and root.

The cervical margin of this tooth follows a similar course to the incisors, though the curves are less pronounced. The curvature of the cervical margin on the distal surface is less marked than that on the mesial surface. The root is the largest and stoutest in the dentition and is triangular in cross-section (its labial surface being wider than its palatal surface). The mesial and distal surfaces of the root are often grooved longitudinally.

40 The mandibular permanent canine is similar to the maxillary canine, but is smaller, more slender, and more symmetrical. The cusp is generally less well developed. Indeed, with attrition, the low cusp may be lost and the tooth may resemble a maxillary second permanent incisor. From the *incisal* aspect (**A**), no distinct longitudinal ridges can be seen running from the tip of the cusp onto the labial and lingual surfaces. Viewed *labially* (**B**), the incisal margin occupies only one-fifth of the crown height and the cusp is less pointed. The crown is narrower mesiodistally than the maxillary canine so that it appears longer, narrower and more slender. The mesial and distal profiles tend to be parallel or only slightly convergent towards the cervix. The labial and mesial surfaces are clearly defined, being inclined acutely to each other, whereas the labial surface merges gradually into the distal surface. On the *lingual* surface

(**C**), the cingulum, marginal ridges and fossae are indistinct. The lingual surface is flatter than the corresponding palatal surface of the maxillary permanent canine and simulates the lingual surface of the mandibular incisors. Viewed *mesially* (**D**) and *distally* (**E**), the wedge-shaped appearance of the canine can be clearly seen. These proximal surfaces are longer than those of the maxillary canine. The labiolingual diameter of the crown near the cervix is less than the corresponding labiopalatal diameter of the maxillary canine.

The cervical margin of this tooth follows a similar course to the incisors. The crownward convexity on the mesial surface is generally more marked than that on the distal surface. The root is normally single, though occasionally it may bifurcate. In cross-section the root is oval, being flattened mesially and distally. The root is grooved longitudinally on both its mesial and distal surfaces.

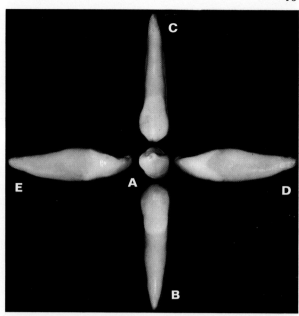

41 The maxillary deciduous canine has a fang-like appearance, being similar morphologically to its permanent successor (though more bulbous). It is generally symmetrical, but where there is asymmetry it is usual for the mesial slope of the cusp to be longer than the distal slope. Bulging of the tooth gives the crown a diamond-shaped appearance when viewed *labially* (**B**) or *palatally* (**C**), with the crown margins overhanging the root profiles. The mesiodistal dimension of the crown is

greater than its height. On the labial surface there is a low cingulum cervically, from which runs a longitudinal ridge up to the tip of the cusp. A similar longitudinal ridge also runs on the palatal surface. This ridge extends from the cusp apex to the palatal cingulum and divides the palatal surface into two shallow pits. The marginal ridges on the palatal surface are low and indistinct.

The root is long compared with the crown height and is triangular in cross-section.

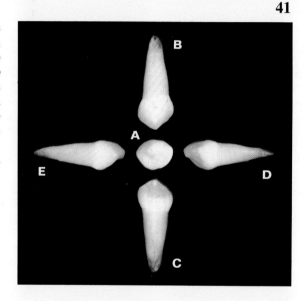

42 The mandibular deciduous canine is more slender than the maxillary deciduous canine. The crown is asymmetrical with the cusp tip displaced mesially. Consequently, the mesial arm is shorter and more vertical than the distal arm. On the *labial* surface (**B**), there is a low, labial cingulum. On the *lingual* surface (**C**), the cingulum and marginal ridges are less pronounced than the corresponding

structures on the palatal surface of the maxillary deciduous canine. The longitudinal ridges on both the labial and lingual surfaces are poorly developed. The mesiodistal dimension is less than the height.

The root is single and tends to be triangular in cross-section. Note the root resorption, which would be associated with the shedding of the tooth.

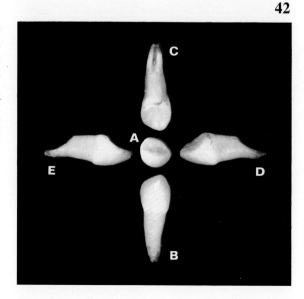

The premolars

Premolars are unique to the permanent dentition. They are sometimes referred to as 'bicuspids', having two main cusps — a buccal and a palatal (or lingual) cusp — which are separated by a mesiodistal occlusal fissure. The buccal surface of the buccal cusp is similar in shape to the cusp of a canine, to which it may be considered analogous, while the palatal or lingual cusp corresponds developmentally to the cingulum of the anterior teeth. Thus, premolars are considered to be transitional between canines and molars.

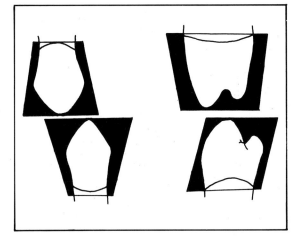

43 Schematic drawings of premolar crown form illustrating the relationship between anatomic and geometric form. Viewed mesially or distally, the maxillary premolars are trapezoidal in shape, the longest side of the trapezoid being the base of the crown at the cervical margin. Functionally, it is thought that, because the occlusal surface is not as wide as the base of the crown, the tooth can penetrate the food more easily, while minimising the occlusal forces. The mandibular premolars, however, are roughly rhomboidal in shape. The rhomboidal outline is inclined lingually, thus allowing correct intercuspal contact with their maxillary antagonists. Viewed buccally or lingually, all the premolars are trapezoidal, the shortest of the uneven sides being the bases of the crowns cervically.

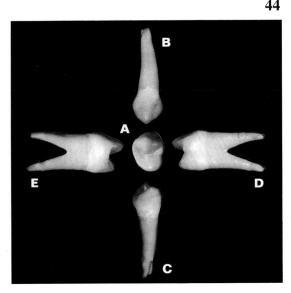

44 Maxillary first premolar. From the *occlusal* aspect (**A**), the crown appears ovoid, being broader buccally than palatally. Thus, the profiles of the mesial and distal surfaces converge palatally. The mesiobuccal and distobuccal corners are less rounded than the mesiopalatal and distopalatal corners. The mesial and distal borders of the occlusal surface are marked by distinct ridges, the mesial and distal marginal ridges. The buccal and palatal cusps are separated by a central occlusal fissure which runs in a mesiodistal direction. The occlusal fissure crosses the mesial marginal ridge onto the mesial surface. On the distal side, the fissure terminates in a fossa before the distal marginal ridge. Supplementary grooves from the central fissure are rare. Viewed *buccally* (**B**), the first premolar bears a distinct resemblance to the adjoining canine. A longitudinal ridge may be seen passing down the buccal cusp. The mesial and distal ridges of the buccal cusp each form a 30° slope and the mesio- and disto-occlusal angles are prominent, giving the crown a 'bulging-shouldered' ovoid appearance. The mesial slope is generally longer than the distal slope. Viewed *palatally* (**C**), the buccal part of the crown appears larger in all dimensions than the palatal part so that the entire buccal profile of the crown is visible from the palatal aspect. The palatal cusp is lower, and its tip lies more mesially than the tip of the buccal cusp. From the *mesial* aspect (**D**), the unequal height of the cusps is clearly seen. Note the canine groove extending across the marginal ridge from the occlusal surface. The cervical third of the mesial surface is marked by a distinct concavity, the canine fossa. The *distal* aspect (**E**) of the crown differs from the mesial aspect in that it lacks a canine groove and canine fossa.

The cervical margin follows a fairly level course around the crown, deviating slightly towards the root on the buccal and palatal surfaces and away from the root on the mesial and distal surfaces. There are usually two roots, a buccal and palatal root, though sometimes there may be a single root. However, even when it is single it is deeply grooved on its mesial and distal surfaces.

45 The maxillary second premolar is similar in shape to the maxillary first premolar except for the following features. Viewed *occlusally* (**A**), the mesiobuccal and distobuccal corners are more rounded and the mesial and distal profiles do not converge lingually, being nearly parallel. The occlusal surface appears more compressed, the mesiodistal dimension of the crown being smaller. The central fissure appears shorter and does not cross the mesial marginal ridge. From the *buccal* aspect (**B**), the mesio- and disto-occlusal angles are less prominent. These features give the crown a 'narrow-shouldered' appearance. The two cusps are smaller and more equal in size than those of the first premolar. The height of the buccal cusp is one-quarter of the height of the crown measured from the base of the occlusal fissure, while the height of the buccal cusp of the first premolar is up to one-half the height of the crown. Viewed *palatally* (**C**), less of the buccal profile is visible. *Mesially* (**D**) and *distally* (**E**), the tooth appears similar to the first premolar but there is no canine fossa or canine groove on the mesial surface. Note also the more equal size of the cusps.

The cervical margin appears similar to that of the maxillary first premolar but is slightly less undulating. The root is single.

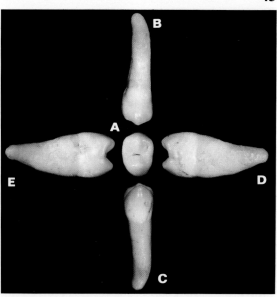

The mandibular premolars differ from the maxillary premolars in that, occlusally, the crowns appear rounder and the cusps are of unequal size, the buccal cusp being the most prominent. Furthermore, unlike the maxillary premolars, the first and second premolars differ more markedly.

46 The mandibular first premolar is the smallest premolar. Since it is comprised of a dominant buccal cusp and a very small lingual cusp which appears not unlike a cingulum, some consider it to be a modified canine. From the *occlusal* aspect (**A**), more than two-thirds of the buccal surface is visible, though only a small portion of the lingual surface can be seen. The occlusal outline is diamond-shaped and the occlusal table, outlined by the cusps and marginal ridges, is triangular. The buccal cusp is a broad cusp with its apex approximately overlying the midpoint of the crown. The lingual cusp is less than half the size of the buccal cusp. The buccal and lingual cusps are connected by a blunt, transverse ridge which divides the poorly developed mesiodistal occlusal fissure into mesial and distal fossae. The mesial fossa is generally smaller than the distal fossa. A canine groove often extends from the mesial fossa over the mesial marginal ridge onto the mesiolingual surface of the crown. Viewed *buccally* (**B**), the crown is seen to be nearly symmetrical, though the mesial profile is more curved than the distal. The buccal surface is markedly convex in all planes. From the *lingual* aspect (**C**), the entire buccal profile and the occlusal surface are visible. Thus, the mandibular first premolar differs from other premolars in that the occlusal plane does not lie perpendicular to the long axis of the tooth but is included lingually. The tilt of the occlusal plane can also be appreciated from the *mesial* (**D**) and *distal* (**E**) aspects. Note also the pronounced convexity of the buccal surface and the position of the apex of the buccal cusp over the crown.

The cervical line follows an almost level course around the tooth. The root is single, conical, and oval to nearly round in cross-section. The root is grooved longitudinally both mesially and distally, the mesial groove being the more prominent.

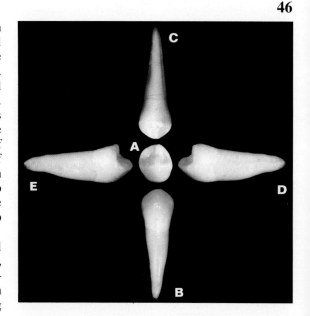

47 The mandibular second premolar differs from the mandibular first premolar in the following respects. Its crown is generally larger. The lingual cusp is better developed, although it is not quite as large as its buccal cusp. From the *occlusal* aspect (**A**), its outline appears round or square, the mesial and distal profiles being straight and parallel. The mesiodistal occlusal fissure between the cusps is well defined. However, like the first premolar, the fissure ends in mesial and distal fossae, the distal fossa being generally larger than the mesial fossa. Unlike the first premolar, the apices of the cusps are not usually joined by a transverse ridge. Accessory cusplets are frequent on both buccal and lingual cusps. Usually, the lingual cusp is subdivided into mesiolingual and distolingual cusps, the mesiolingual cusp being wider and higher than the distolingual cusp. The groove separating the mesiolingual and distolingual cusps lies opposite the tip of the buccal cusp. From the *buccal* aspect (**B**), the crown of the second premolar is symmetrical. From this view, the buccal cusp generally appears shorter and more rounded than that of the mandibular first premolar. *Lingually* (**C**), little if any of the occlusal surface and the buccal profile is visible. From the *mesial* (**D**) and *distal* (**E**) aspects, note that the occlusal surface is horizontal to the long axis of the tooth, unlike the mandibular first premolar. The crown appears wider buccolingually than that of the first premolar and the buccal cusp does not incline so far over the root. Note the relative size of the lingual cusp(s) from this view, and that the mesial marginal ridge is higher than the distal ridge.

The cervical margin follows an almost level course around the tooth. The root is single, conical, and nearly round in cross-section.

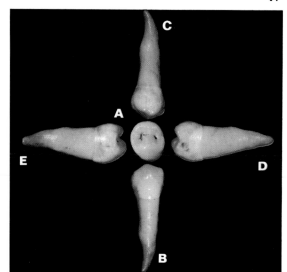

The molars

Molars present the largest occlusal surfaces of all teeth. They have three to five major cusps (though the maxillary first deciduous molar has only two). Molars are the only teeth that have more than one buccal cusp. Generally, the lower molars have two roots while the upper have three. The permanent molars do not have deciduous predecessors.

48 Schematic drawings of molar crown form illustrating the relationship between anatomic and geometric form. Like the premolars, the maxillary molars are roughly trapezoidal when viewed mesially and distally, while the mandibular molars are rhomboidal. Viewed buccally or lingually, the molars are trapezoidal.

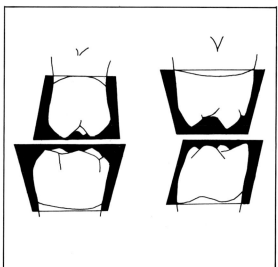

49 Maxillary first permanent molar. The first permanent molar is usually the largest molar in each quadrant. Viewed *occlusally* (**A**), the crown is rhombic in outline. The mesiopalatal and distobuccal angles are obtuse. The longest diameter of the crown runs from the mesiobuccal to the distopalatal corners. It has four major cusps separated by an irregular H-shaped occlusal fissure. The occlusal table may be divided into two distinct components (the trigon and talon) by an oblique ridge, which passes diagonally across the occlusal table from the mesiopalatal cusp to the distobuccal cusp. The trigon bears the mesiobuccal, mesiopalatal and distobuccal cusps, and the talon bears the distopalatal cusp. The trigon is characteristically triangular in shape, the apex of the triangle being directed palatally. The mesiopalatal cusp is the largest, the buccal cusps being smaller and of approximately equal size. The buccal cusps form the base of the trigon. The mesial marginal ridge forms the mesial side of the trigon and its distal side is formed by the oblique ridge. An accessory cusplet of variable size may be seen on the palatal surface of the mesiopalatal cusp. This cusplet is termed the tubercle of Carabelli and is found on about 60% of maxillary first permanent molars. The trigon has a central fossa from which a fissure extends mesially to terminate in a mesial pit before the mesial marginal ridge. Another fissure extends buccally from the central fossa to pass onto the buccal surface of the crown between the two buccal cusps. The distopalatal cusp of the talon is generally the smallest cusp of the tooth and is separated from the mesiopalatal cusp by a distopalatal fissure, which curves distally to end in a distal pit before the distal marginal ridge. The oblique ridge may be crossed by a shallow fissure, which thus connects the central fossa of the trigon with the distopalatal fissure and distal pit of the talon, completing the H-shaped fissure pattern. That the tips of the palatal cusps are situated nearer the mid-mesiodistal diameter of the crown than those of the buccal cusps is characteristic of maxillary molars. From the *buccal* aspect (**B**), the buccal cusps are seen to be approximately equal in height, though the mesiobuccal cusp is wider than the distobuccal cusp. The buccal surface is convex in its cervical third but relatively flat in its middle and occlusal thirds. Note the buccal groove extending from the occlusal table, passing between the cusps to end about halfway up the buccal surface. The mesial profile is convex in its occlusal and middle thirds but flat, or even concave, in the cervical third. The distal profile, on the other hand, is convex in all regions. Viewed *palatally* (**C**), the disproportion in size between the mesiopalatal and distopalatal cusps is most evident. The mesiopalatal cusp is blunt and occupies approximately three-fifths of the mesiodistal width of the palatal surface. The palatal surface is more or less uniformly convex in all regions. A palatal groove extends from the distal pit on the occlusal surface between the palatal cusps to terminate approximately halfway up the palatal surface. From the *mesial* (**D**) and *distal* (**E**) aspects, the maximum buccopalatal dimension is at the cervical margin, from which the buccal and palatal

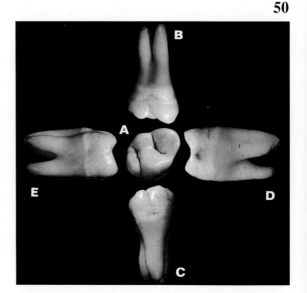

profiles converge occlusally. The mesial marginal ridge is more prominent than the distal ridge. The mesial marginal ridge may have a number of distinct tubercles. Such tubercles are rare on the distal marginal ridge.

The cervical margin follows a fairly even contour around the tooth. There are three roots, two buccal and one palatal, which arise from a common root stalk. The palatal root is the longest and strongest and is circular in cross-section. The buccal roots are more slender and are flattened mesiodistally; the mesiobuccal root is usually the larger and wider of the two. At the root stalk, the palatal root is more commonly related to the distobuccal root than to the mesiobuccal root.

50 The maxillary second permanent molar closely resembles the maxillary first permanent molar but shows some reduction in size and slightly different cusp relationships. Viewed *occlusally* (**A**), the rhomboid form is more pronounced than the first molar and the oblique ridge is smaller. The talon (distopalatal fissure cusp) is considerably reduced. The occlusal fissure pattern is similar to the first molar but is more variable, and supplemental grooves are more numerous. Two features of the *buccal* surface (**B**) differentiate the second molar, namely the smaller size of both the crown and the distobuccal cusp. From the *palatal* view (**C**), note the reduction in size of the distopalatal cusp. A tubercle of Carabelli is not usually found on the mesiopalatal cusp. The *mesial* (**D**) and *distal* (**E**) surfaces differ little from those of the first molar, except that the tubercles on the mesial marginal ridge are less numerous and less pronounced.

Like the first molar, the second molar has three roots, two buccal and one palatal. However, they are shorter and less divergent than those of the first molar and may be partly fused. The apex of the mesiobuccal root is generally in line with the centre of the crown, unlike that of the first molar, which generally lies in line with the tip of the mesiobuccal cusp.

Variations in morphology of the maxillary second permanent molar are quite common. Total reduction of the distopalatal cusp is frequent such that only the trigon remains. Less frequently, the crown may appear compressed because of fusion of the mesiopalatal and distobuccal cusps, resulting in an oval crown possessing three cusps in a straight line.

Maxillary third permanent molar. This tooth, being the most variable in the dentition, is not illustrated. Its morphology may range from that characteristic of the adjacent maxillary permanent molars to a rounded, triangular crown with a deep central fossa from which numerous irregular fissures radiate outwards. Most commonly, the crown is triangular in shape, having the three cusps of the trigon but no talon. The roots are often fused and irregular in form.

The mandibular molars differ from the maxillary molars in the following respects:

1. The mandibular molars have two roots, one mesial and one distal.
2. They are considered to be derived from a five-cusped form.
3. The crowns of the lower molars are oblong, being broader mesiodistally than buccolingually.
4. The fissure pattern is cross-shaped.
5. The lingual cusps are of more equal size.
6. The tips of the buccal cusps are shifted lingually so that, from the occlusal view, the whole of the buccal surface is visible.

51

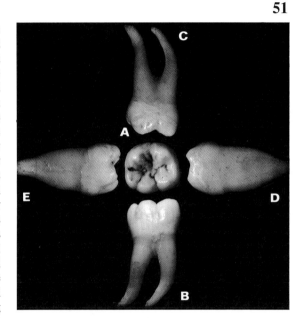

51 Mandibular first permanent molar. Viewed *occlusally* (**A**), the crown of this tooth is somewhat pentagonal in outline. It is broader mesiodistally than buccolingually. The occlusal surface is divided into buccal and lingual parts by a mesiodistal occlusal fissure, which arises from a deep central fossa. The buccal side of the occlusal table has three distinct cusps: mesiobuccal, distobuccal and distal. Each cusp is separated by a groove, which joins the mesiodistal fissure. On the lingual side are two cusps: mesiolingual and distolingual. The fissure separating the lingual cusps joins the mesiodistal fissure in the region of the central fossa. The lingual cusps tend to be the larger and more pointed, though they are not disproportionately larger than the mesiobuccal and distobuccal cusps. The tips of the buccal cusps are displaced lingually, are rounded and are lower than the lingual cusps. The smallest cusp is the distal cusp, which is displaced slightly towards the buccal surface. In 90% of cases, the mesiolingual cusp is joined to the distobuccal cusp across the floor of the central fossa. This feature and the five-cusped pattern is termed the *Dryopithecus* pattern. This 'primitive' pattern is characteristic of all the lower molars of the anthropoid apes and their early ancestors, the dryopithecines. Because of the resulting Y-shaped tissue pattern and the five cusps, the *Dryopithecus* pattern is sometimes referred to as a 'Y 5' pattern. In the 10% of cases where the mesiobuccal and distolingual cusps meet, a more cruciate system of fissures is produced. This is sometimes referred to as a '+5' pattern. From the *buccal* aspect (**B**), note the three cusps, the distal cusp being the smallest. The fissure separating the mesiobuccal and distobuccal cusps arises from the central fossa on the occlusal surface and terminates halfway up the buccal surface in a buccal pit. The buccal surface appears markedly convex especially at the cervical third of the crown. This convexity is associated with the characteristic lingual inclination of the buccal cusps. From the *lingual* aspect (**C**), note that although the two lingual cusps are nearly equal in size, the mesiolingual cusp is slightly larger. The fissure between the lingual cusps arises from the central fossa on the occlusal surface but does not extend a significant way down the lingual surface. The lingual surface is convex in its occlusal and middle thirds but is flat or concave cervically. From the lingual aspect, part of the buccal profiles and proximal surfaces may be seen. Viewed *mesially* (**D**), the mesial marginal ridge joining the mesiobuccal and mesiolingual cusps is V-shaped, being notched at its midpoint. The mesial surface is flat or concave cervically and convex in its middle and occlusal thirds. From the *distal* aspect (**E**), the distal marginal ridge joining the distal and distolingual cusps also appears V-shaped. The cervical third of the distal surface is relatively flat, the middle and occlusal thirds being highly convex. Thus, the distal surface is more convex than the mesial surface due to the distal cusp. From the proximal views, note the highly convex slope of the buccal surface compared to the lingual surface.

The cervical margin follows a uniform contour around the tooth. The two roots, one mesial and one distal, arise from a common root stalk. They are both markedly flattened mesiodistally and the mesial root is usually deeply grooved. Both roots curve distally.

52 Mandibular second permanent molar.
Viewed *occlusally* (**A**), the crown has a regular, rectangular shape. Thus, unlike the mandibular first permanent molar, the buccal profile is nearly equal in length to the lingual profile. There are four cusps, the mesiobuccal and mesiolingual cusps being slightly larger than the distobuccal and distolingual cusps. The cusps are separated by a cross-shaped occlusal fissure pattern, though it may be complicated by numerous supplemental grooves. From the *buccal* aspect (**B**), the crown appears smaller than that of the first molar. A fissure extends between the buccal cusps from the occlusal surface and terminates approximately halfway up the buccal surface. Like the mandibular first molar, the buccal surface is highly convex.

From the *lingual aspect* (**C**), the buccal profiles and proximal surfaces are not visible and the crown is noticeably shorter than the first molar. The *mesial* (**D**) and *distal* (**E**) aspects of the second molar resemble those of the first molar, although because there is no distal cusp the proximal surfaces are more equal in terms of their convexity. Note that the mesial and distal marginal ridges do not converge and are not so markedly notched at their midpoint.

The mesial and distal roots are flattened mesiodistally, and are smaller and less divergent than those of the first molar. Indeed they may be partly fused. The mesial root is not as broad as that of the first molar, and the distal inclination of the roots is usually more marked.

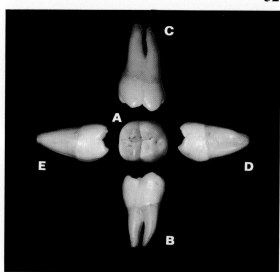

Mandibular third permanent molar. The morphology of this tooth is variable, though not as variable as that of the maxillary third permanent molar. The crown is usually the smallest of the mandibular molars but occasionally it may be as large as the mandibular first molar. The crown usually has four or five cusps. In shape, it is normally a rounded rectangle or is circular. Its occlusal fissure pattern is generally very irregular. As a rule, the roots are greatly reduced in size and are fused. They show a marked distal inclination.

53 Maxillary first deciduous molar. This tooth is the most atypical of all molars, deciduous or permanent. In form, it appears to be intermediate between a premolar and a molar. It is the smallest molar. Viewed *occlusally* (**A**), the crown is an irregular quadrilateral with the buccal and palatal surfaces lying parallel to one another. However, the mesiobuccal corner is extended to produce a prominent bulge, the molar tubercle, and the mesiopalatal angle is markedly obtuse. The tooth is generally bicuspid; the buccal (more pronounced) and palatal cusps are separated by an occlusal fissure which runs mesiodistally. A shallow buccal fissure may extend from the central mesiodistal fissure to divide the buccal cusp into two, the mesial part being the larger. The lingual cusp also may be sub-divided into two. The tips of the cusps converge towards the midline, so reducing the occlusal surface of the tooth. From the *buccal* aspect (**B**), the crown appears squat, its height being less than its width. On the mesial side lies the buccal cingulum which extends to the molar tubercle. From the *palatal* aspect (**C**), note that the palatal surface is shorter mesiodistally than the buccal surface, whose profile can be seen from this view. The views from the *mesial* (**D**) and *distal* (**E**) aspects show the cervical bulbosity of the buccal and palatal surfaces. Note the prominent molar tubercle mesially. Marginal ridges link the buccal and palatal cusps. No fissure crosses the marginal ridges.

The tooth has three roots (two buccal and one palatal) which arise from a common root stalk. The mesiobuccal root is flattened mesiodistally. The distobuccal root is smaller and more circular. The palatal root is the largest and is round in cross-section. The distobuccal and palatal roots may be partly fused.

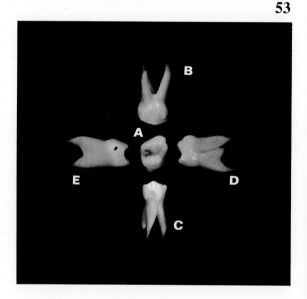

54 Maxillary second deciduous molar. This tooth closely resembles the maxillary first permanent molar (see **49**), though its size, whiteness, widely diverging roots and low buccal cingulum ought to distinguish it. A tubercle of Carabelli on the mesiopalatal cusp is often well developed.

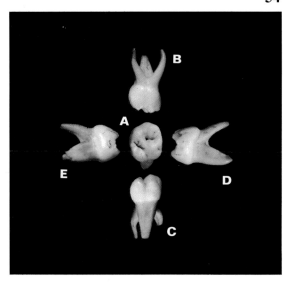

55 Mandibular first deciduous molar. Unlike the maxillary first deciduous molar, this tooth is molariform but has a number of unique features. From the *occlusal* aspect (**A**), the crown appears elongated mesiodistally and is an irregular quadrilateral, the buccal and lingual surfaces being parallel. Note that the mesiobuccal corner is extended, forming a molar tubercle, and that the mesiolingual angle is markedly obtuse. The occlusal table can be divided into buccal and lingual parts by a mesiodistal fissure. The buccal part consists of two cusps, the mesiobuccal cusp being larger than the distobuccal cusp. The lingual part of the tooth is narrower than the buccal part and has two cusps separated by a lingual fissure, the mesiolingual cusp being larger than the distolingual cusp. The buccal cusps are larger than the lingual cusps. A transverse ridge may connect the mesial cusps, dividing the mesiodistal fissure into a distal fissure and a mesial pit. Often a distal pit may be found just mesial to the distal marginal ridge. A supplemental groove from the mesial pit may extend over the mesial marginal ridge. From the *buccal* aspect (**B**), the mesiobuccal cusp occupies at least two-thirds of the crown area and projects higher occlusally than the distobuccal cusp. The distal slopes of the buccal cusps are longer than the mesial. The profile of the mesial surface appears flat, that of the distal surface convex. Note the molar tubercle on the mesial corner of the buccal surface. From the *lingual* aspect (**C**), note the conical shape of the cusps. The distolingual cusp appears only as a bulging protuberance on the distal margin. *Mesially* (**D**) and *distally* (**E**), the buccal and lingual aspects are seen to converge towards the midline of the crown. The mesial marginal ridge is more prominent than the distal marginal ridge. Note the bulge associated with the buccal cingulum near the cervical margin of the mesiobuccal cusp.

The mandibular first deciduous molar has two divergent roots, mesial and distal, which are flattened mesiodistally. The mesial root is often grooved.

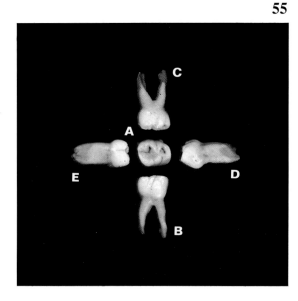

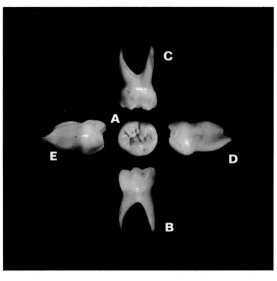

56 Mandibular second deciduous molar. This tooth is a smaller version of the mandibular first permanent molar (see **51**), though it is narrower, whiter and has widely diverging roots. Other distinguishing features are the cingulum on the mesiobuccal corner of the crown, the greater convexity of the mesial and distal surfaces, and the more extensive central fossa on the occlusal surface. The mesiolingual and distobuccal cusps are not usually joined to give the *Dryopithecus* pattern.

Table 2: Average dimensions of permanent teeth.

Tooth	Crown height (mm)	Length of root (mm)	Mesiodistal crown diameter (mm)	Labiolingual crown diameter (mm)
Maxillary				
1	10.5	13.0	8.5	7.0
2	9.0	13.0	6.5	6.0
3	10.0	17.0	7.5	8.0
4	8.5	14.5	7.0	9.0
5	8.5	14.0	7.0	9.0
6	7.5	12.5	10.5	11.0
7	7.0	11.5	9.5	11.0
8	6.5	11.0	8.5	10.0
Mandibular				
1	9.0	12.5	5.0	6.0
2	9.5	14.0	5.5	6.5
3	11.0	15.5	7.0	7.5
4	8.5	14.0	7.0	7.5
5	8.0	14.5	7.0	8.0
6	7.5	14.0	11.0	10.0
7	7.0	12.0	10.5	10.0
8	7.0	11.0	10.0	9.5

Table 3: Average dimensions of deciduous teeth.

Tooth	Crown height (mm)	Length of root (mm)	Mesiodistal crown diameter (mm)	Labiolingual crown diameter (mm)
Maxillary				
A	6.0	10.0	6.5	5.0
B	5.6	10.2	5.2	4.0
C	6.5	13.0	6.8	7.0
D	5.1	10.0	7.1	8.5
E	5.7	11.7	8.4	10.0
Mandibular				
A	5.0	9.0	4.0	4.0
B	5.2	9.8	4.5	4.0
C	6.0	11.2	5.5	4.9
D	6.0	9.8	7.7	7.0
E	5.5	12.5	9.7	8.7

Ethnic and racial differences in tooth morphology

The preceding description of the morphology of teeth is, of necessity, only generalised and is related to caucasians. Superimposed on the basic shapes of teeth are minor morphological variations affecting both deciduous and permanent teeth. Such variations are inherited, depend on many genes, and vary minimally in response to environmental factors. Their presence and degree of penetrance form the foundation of dental anthropology and have been utilised in distinguishing human races on a dental basis. The results of such studies enable us to trace the relationships between races and the racial affinity between human populations. A race may be defined as a subdivision of a species containing members sharing common biological and cultural characteristics. Thus, if the same highly heritable dental variants occur with a similar frequency in two populations, then the populations are likely to have a high degree of affinity. These anthropological studies generally utilise complex statistical analysis on groups of traits, rather than a single feature. Where frequencies of the features are low, a large sample size is necessary.

The following is a list of the more common secondary dental traits encountered in dental anthropology, although many more are encountered in the literature:

1. Winging of maxillary central incisors. Instead of the central incisors being straight and arranged along the dental arch, they are inclined mesially, and their incisal edges form a V-shape.
2. Shovel-shaped maxillary central incisors. Exaggerated and extensive marginal ridges give the tooth a shovel appearance. The palatal concavity is thus exaggerated. Indeed, the depth of the palatal fossa is the best indicator of the degree of shovelling. This may vary and, at its most pronounced, also involves the labial surface, giving rise to a 'double-shovelled' appearance. While predominantly found in the maxillary incisors, it can affect the mandibular incisors. This trait is particularly common in Chinese, Japanese and Eskimos, and low in Negroes and Europeans.
3. The frequency of peg-shaped maxillary second (lateral) permanent incisors.
4. The presence of only a single root on the maxillary first permanent premolar.
5. The presence of accessory cusps on the maxillary first permanent molar. Accessory cusps regularly occur on the buccal and palatal surfaces. As mentioned on page 36, there is often a cusplet on the palatal surface of the mesiopalatal cusp known as the tubercle of Carabelli. It may vary from a large elevation to a mere groove. It has a low incidence in Negroes. When present on the buccal surface, accessory cusps are known as paramolar cusps.
6. The reduced size or absence of a distopalatal cusp on the maxillary second permanent molar.
7. The presence of a reduced, peg-shaped maxillary third permanent molar.
8. The presence of an additional cusp on the mandibular second premolar. Although the lingual cusp on this tooth is generally sub-divided into two, an additional cusp may be present, giving a total of four for the tooth.
9. The pattern of fissures on the mandibular first permanent molar. The fissure pattern may either have the configuration of a 'Y' or a '+' (see page 37). Further subdivisions are 'X' or 'C' (crenulated — where the occlusal surface does not exhibit a clear groove pattern but is covered with fine dendritic crenulations as in third molars).
10. The number of cusps on the mandibular molars. There may be six, five, or four cusps present. The additional sixth cusp is known as the protostylid and is associated with the mesiobuccal cusp. Where four cusps are present, there has been a loss of the distal cusp.
11. The presence of three roots on the mandibular first permanent molar.
12. The number of cusps present on the mandibular permanent second molar. This tooth may exhibit four or five cusps.

Two additional features are often incorporated into anthropological investigations of dental variation, even though they are not strictly morphological features. These are hypodontia (the frequency of missing teeth) and hyperdontia (the frequency of supernumerary teeth).

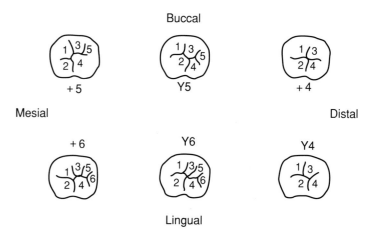

41

Pulp morphology

The pulp cavity consists of a pulp chamber in the crown from which canal(s) pass down into the root(s). As a general rule, the pulp cavities follow the contours of the teeth. Each root canal opens by a foramen or foramina at the apex of the root.

57–70 Pulp morphology in teeth of the permanent dentition. The red outline shows the pulp cavity in the young tooth, the blue outline shows the pulp in the old tooth. Labial/buccal and distal views of the teeth are shown. The descriptions of the pulp cavities are not always borne out in detail in individual teeth, there being much variation. As a general rule, in anterior teeth the pulp chambers merge imperceptibly into the root canals. In the cheek teeth, the pulp chambers and root canals are morphologically distinct. Pulp horns or cornua extend from the pulp chambers to the mesial and distal angles of the incisor teeth and towards the cusps of cheek teeth. Each root generally contains one root canal. However, the mandibular molars have two root canals in their mesial roots. Where roots are fused, the tooth still maintains the usual number of root canals. The size of the pulp cavity decreases significantly with age. When the tooth first erupts into the oral cavity the apical foramen is wide. The apical foramen narrows with subsequent development of the root.

The morphology of the pulp cavities of deciduous teeth is extremely variable, especially once root resorption has begun. The pulp cavities of deciduous teeth are proportionally larger than those of permanent teeth, and pulp horns may extend some way into the cusps.

57 Maxillary first incisor. Viewed from the labial aspect, the pulp chamber follows the general outline of the crown and is usually widest towards the incisal ridge. In a young tooth the pulp chamber has three pulp horns, which correspond to the mammelons; viewed distally, the pulp tapers towards the incisal ridge edge and widens cervically. Following a constriction, the (usually) single and centrally placed root canal tapers towards the apical foramen where it occasionally bends distally or labially. In cross-section the root canal tends to be roughly circular but tapers palatally. With age, the dimensions of the pulp cavity diminish as secondary dentine is laid down. The tip of the pulp chamber recedes until it may come to lie almost at the cervical level, and the root canal narrows especially in the mesiodistal plane.

57

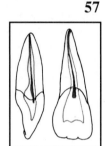

58 Mandibular first incisor. The pulp chamber is similar to that described for the upper central incisor, being broadest incisally with three pulp horns, although the pulp horns are less well developed. The pulp chamber is oval in cross-section, being wider labiolingually than mesiodistally, and is constricted at the cervical margin. Viewed distally, the root canal in the young only narrows in the middle third of the root. The root canal is oval in cross-section, being compressed mesiodistally. With age, the pulp cavity becomes considerably constricted and ultimately its roof lies at the level of the cervical margin. However, the root canal remains rather wide in its labiolingual dimension except near the apex of the tooth.

58

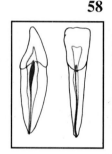

59 Maxillary second incisor. The pulp cavity of this tooth is similar to, but smaller than, that of the maxillary central incisor.

59

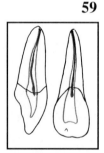

60 Mandibular second incisor. This differs little from the mandibular central incisor although being slightly longer. However, the root canal often divides in the middle third of the root to give a labial and lingual branch.

60

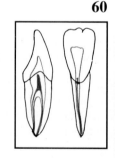

61 Maxillary canine. The pulp cavity of this tooth resembles that of the maxillary permanent canine, though it tends to be slightly smaller in all dimensions. The root canal is oval in cross-section, being wider buccopalatally. As with the mandibular incisors, it may divide into two branches towards the apex of the tooth.

61

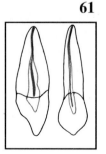

62 Mandibular canine. The pulp chamber is narrow with one pulp horn which points cuspally. Both the pulp chamber and the single root canal are wider labiopalatally than they are in the mesiodistal plane. The root canal does not constrict markedly until the apical third of the root is reached. The root canal is oval or triangular in cross-section except in its apical third, where it is circular. About 20% of single-rooted mandibular canines have two root canals.

62

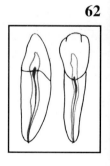

63 Maxillary first premolar. Whether the tooth has one or two roots, it has two root canals leaving a single pulp chamber. If the tooth is single-rooted the two root canals may merge to form a common apical foramen. The pulp chamber is wide buccopalatally with two distinct pulp horns pointing towards the cusps. From the buccal view, the pulp chamber is much narrower. The floor of the pulp chamber is rounded with the highest point in the centre. It usually lies within the root just apical to the cervix. Where the root canals arise from the pulp chamber the orifices are funnel-shaped. The root canals are usually straight and taper evenly from their origin to the apical foramina. In cross-section the root canals are generally round. With age the general shape of the pulp cavity remains the same but its dimensions, particularly the height of the pulp chamber, are reduced.

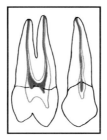

64 Mandibular first premolar. The pulp chamber in this tooth, like the maxillary premolars, is wider buccolingually than it is mesiodistally. Unlike the pulp chamber of the maxillary premolars, there is usually only one pulp horn which extends into the buccal cusp. Occasionally a small pulp horn may pass to the lingual cusp. There is a single root canal which becomes constricted towards the middle third of the root. The canal may temporarily branch in the middle third to form two separate root canals, which rejoin near the apical foramen. In cross-section the root canal is round.

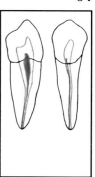

65 Maxillary second premolar. The second premolar has a single root with a single root canal and its pulp chamber extends apically well below the cervical margin. Variations are frequent. Sometimes the root canal branches in its apical third to form two apical foramina. Frequently (40%) the tooth has two root canals which join to form a common apical foramen. The appearance of the pulp cavity viewed from the buccal aspect is similar to that in the adjacent first premolar. In cross-section the root canal is oval.

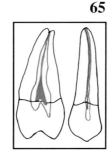

66 Mandibular second premolar. This differs little from that described for the mandibular first premolar. However, the pulp chamber of this tooth usually has two well-developed pulp horns projecting towards its cusps.

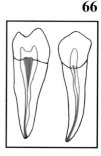

67 Maxillary first molar. The pulp chamber is quadrilateral in shape, being wider buccopalatally than mesiodistally. From the roof arise four pulp horns, one to each of the major cusps. The pulp horn to the mesiobuccal cusp is the longest. The floor of the pulp chamber generally lies below the cervical margin. From the floor arise three root canals, their orifices being funnel-shaped. The root canal of the mesiobuccal root leaves the pulp chamber in a mesial direction. In cross-section it appears as a narrow slit, being wider buccopalatally. Its anatomy may be complicated by irregular branching or bifurcation near the apical foramen. The palatal root canal is the widest and longest of the three root canals.

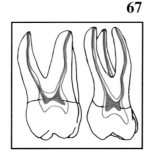

68 Mandibular first molar. The pulp chamber is wider mesiodistally than it is buccolingually. It is also wider mesially than distally. There are five pulp horns projecting to the cusps, the lingual pulp horns being longer and more pointed. The floor of the pulp chamber lies at, or just below, the level of the cervical margin. The root canals leave the pulp chamber through funnel-shaped orifices, of which the mesial are finer than the distal. The mesial root has two root canals, mesiobuccal and mesiolingual. Generally, the mesiobuccal root canal follows a tortuous path. The mesiolingual canal is straighter. Both are circular in cross-section. The distal root generally has a single root canal. This is considerably larger and more oval in cross-section than the mesial root canals. It generally follows a straight course.

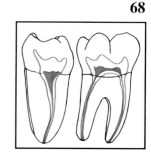

69 Maxillary second molar. The pulp cavity of the upper second molar may be regarded essentially as a smaller replica of that of the neighbouring first molar. The differences are due to the more convergent roots of the second molar.

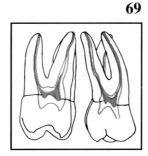

70 Mandibular second molar. This closely resembles that of the adjacent first molar, though there are only four pulp horns.

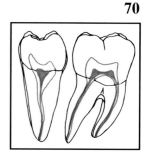

The alignment and occlusion of the permanent teeth

Tooth alignment may be defined as the arrangement of the teeth within the dental arches. Occlusion may be defined as the relationship of the dental arches when tooth contact is made.

Traditionally, textbooks describe a standard set of tooth relationships which is called 'normal'. Normal is a term that is generally used to describe situations which are the ordinary or most frequent. Alternatively, normal may define an authoritative standard or ideal which, in medical terms, is the healthy state. In these terms, malocclusions could be regarded as normal for they are more commonly found in the population than 'normal occlusion'; they rarely predispose to dental disease and in most cases are not associated with masticatory dysfunction. Our knowledge of the relationship between the structure and function of the dental arches during mastication is not yet sufficient to provide an authoritative standard for tooth relationships; in structural terms, the ideal occlusion is a rather subjective concept. If there is an ideal occlusion, it can only be defined at present in broad functional terms. We believe that the characteristics of an ideal occlusion are the following:

1. The teeth are aligned such that the masticatory loads are within physiological range and act through the long axes of as many teeth in the arch as possible.
2. Lateral jaw movements occur without undue mechanical interference.
3. In the rest position of the jaw, the gap between teeth (the freeway space) is correct for the individual concerned.
4. The tooth alignment is aesthetically pleasing to its possessor.

Despite these criticisms, the traditional descriptions of 'normal' tooth relationships provide a convenient *type* for the classification of malocclusions in clinical situations. In order to avoid the difficulties of defining normality with respect to tooth relationships, we have chosen to use the terms anatomical alignment and anatomical occlusion instead of normal alignment and normal occlusion. The occlusion of the deciduous dentition and the development of occlusion is considered on pages 292–294.

The anatomical alignment of teeth

71 **The dental arches** generally take the form of catenary curves. The well-aligned arch may be divided into three segments. A curved line in the coronal plane describes the anterior segment (**A**), which extends across the midline from canine to canine. A straight line describes the middle segments (**B**), which extend from the distal edge of the canines to the mesiobuccal cusps of the first molars. The posterior segments (**C**) extend from the mesiobuccal cusps of the first molars backwards. Both the middle and posterior segments lie in the sagittal plane, the posterior segments being more nearly parallel to this plane than the middle segments.

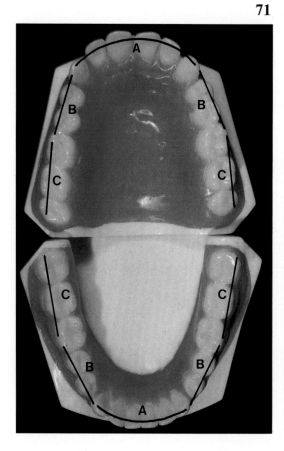

The size of the dental arches varies considerably between individuals. Table 4 below lists the average widths of the dental arches for the completed deciduous dentition (6 years) and the completed permanent dentition (18 years) for males. Averages for females are usually 1mm less.

Table 4: Average widths of the dental arches.

Age (years)	Between maxillary canines (mm)	Between mandibular canines (mm)	Between maxillary first molars (mm)	Between mandibular first molars (mm)
6	28	23	42	40
18	32	25	47	43

The angulation or axial positioning of individual teeth within the alveolus relative to perpendiculars dropped from a hypothetically flat occlusal plane

In the following series of diagrams, the angles quoted are average figures, though variation is considerable. The teeth are not drawn to scale and the numerical dental shorthand is used to identify the tooth (**M** = mesial).

72

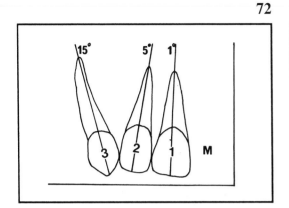

72 Alignment of the maxillary incisors and canine viewed labially.

73

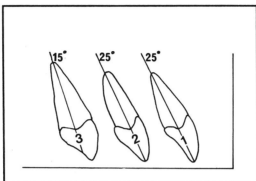

73 Alignment of the maxillary incisors and canine viewed distally.

74

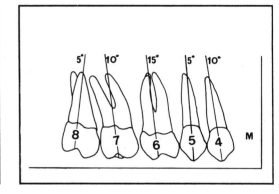

74 Alignment of the maxillary premolars and molars viewed buccally.

75

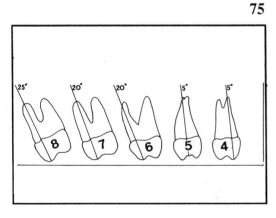

75 Alignment of the maxillary premolars and molars viewed distally.

76

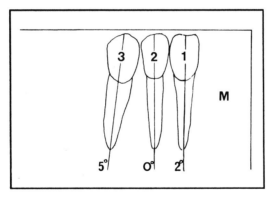

76 Alignment of the mandibular incisors and canine viewed labially.

77

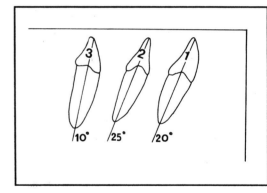

77 Alignment of the mandibular incisors and canine viewed distally.

78

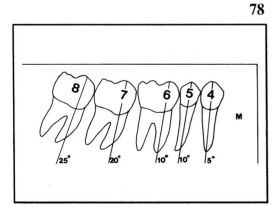

78 Alignment of the mandibular premolars and molars viewed buccally.

79

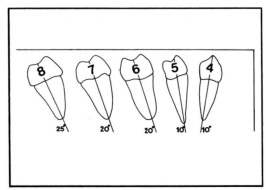

79 Alignment of the mandibular premolars and molars viewed distally.

80 The neutral zone. The spatial configuration of the arches is dependent upon an interaction between the eruptive movements carrying the teeth into their functional positions and, once erupted, the forces brought to bear upon each tooth. The term neutral zone is used to describe that space in which there is an equilibrium of forces such that the teeth attain a position of relative stability. A change in balance in this system, such as that produced by abnormal tongue thrusting behaviour during swallowing and abnormal lip posture (page 14, figure **4**), can result in malalignment of the teeth. The diagram shows the configuration of the neutral zone (the stippled area) in the incisor region (**A**) and the molar region (**B**). The tongue is labelled **1**, the lips **2**, and the cheek **3**.

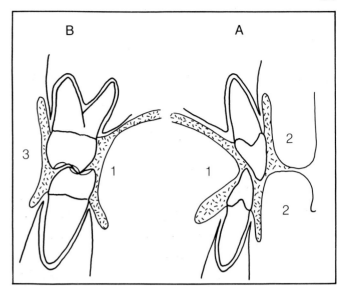

The curvatures of the teeth and arches

81a **81b**

81 The curvatures of the teeth and their functional significance. **72** to **79** may give the impression that the axes of the teeth are straight and run perpendicular to a horizontal, flat, occlusal plane. However, as shown in these dissected specimens of the jaws, neither the axes of the teeth nor the occlusal planes are straight but are curved in all directions. The curved axes of the teeth have a tendency to parallelism and are inclined mesially. It is often thought, mistakenly so, that the forces of mastication are at right angles to the occlusal surfaces of the teeth. If this were so and if the occlusal plane and axes of the teeth were not curved, the arches might not be stable and the masticatory loads might be at an unfavourable angle to the teeth. Indeed it has been suggested that during mastication the loads strike the teeth such that there is a mesial component of force.

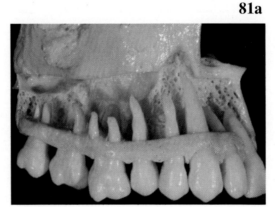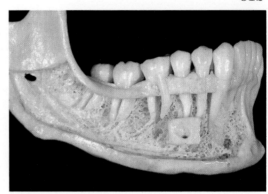

82

82 Curvatures of the occlusal plane – the curve of Spee. The teeth align themselves such that the occlusal plane is not flat but describes a relatively linear curve in the anteroposterior direction, the curve of Spee. The mandibular curve of Spee is concave whereas the maxillary curve is convex. An appreciation of the contribution of each tooth to the curve of Spee may be gained from analysis of the alignment of the long axes of the posterior teeth viewed buccally (**74** and **78**). The curves of Spee may help the achievement of occlusal balance during mastication by encouraging simultaneous contact in more than one area of the dental arches.

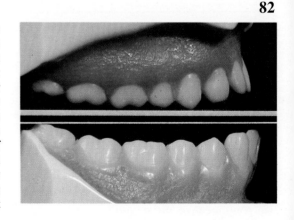

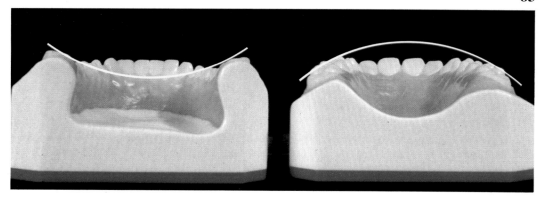

83 Curvatures of the occlusal plane — the curves of Wilson. The occlusal curves of Wilson are aligned in the transverse plane. Analysis of the alignment of the long axes of the posterior teeth (**75** and **79**) shows that the curves of Wilson are such that the occlusal surfaces of the mandibular molars are directed lingually, while those of the maxillary molars are directed buccally. The curves of Spee and Wilson were once thought to be related three-dimensionally, the occlusal surfaces of the teeth being aligned on the curved surface of a segment of a sphere having a radius of about 10cm. However, attempts to demonstrate and then measure the spherical curves (of Monson) have been unsuccessful.

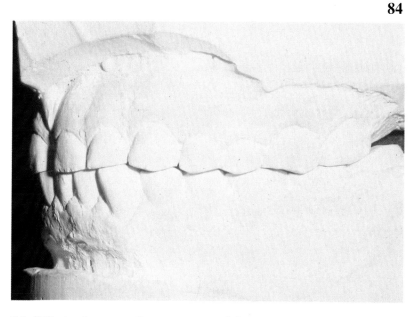

84 Effects of wear on the curvatures of the occlusal plane.

The anatomical occlusion of teeth

The relationships of the jaws in function are so variable that our understanding of the functional articulation of teeth remains poor. To simplify analysis, several occlusal positions have been strictly defined. These positions may be classified into those which are symmetric and those which are asymmetric. This corresponds with the classification of mandibular movements into symmetric and asymmetric movements (see page 100). The symmetric occlusal positions include centric occlusion and bilaterally protrusive position. The asymmetric occlusal positions are those associated with lateral (side-to-side) movements.

Centric occlusal position

85 Lateral view of the arrangement of teeth in anatomical centric occlusion. The centric occlusal position has been defined as the terminal position of physiological jaw movements. It is the relationship between the two arches when the teeth are brought into contact with the mandibular condyles centrally positioned at rest in the mandibular fossae. According to Angle, the key to the intercuspal relationships between the teeth in the centric occlusal position is to be found in the relative positions of the maxillary and mandibular first permanent molars. In the 'normal' or anatomical condition, each arch is bilaterally symmetrical. Since the anterior maxillary segment is slightly larger than the corresponding mandibular segment (due to the unequal sizes of the maxillary and mandibular central incisors), each maxillary tooth will contact its corresponding mandibular antagonist and its distal neighbour. Thus, the maxillary first permanent molar will contact the distal part of the mandibular first permanent molar and the mesial part of the mandibular second permanent molar. The only exceptions are the mandibular central incisor and the maxillary third molar (see **86**).

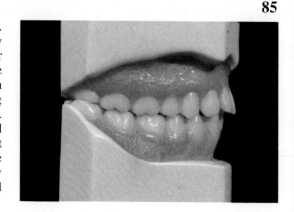

85

86 The relationships between maxillary and mandibular permanent teeth in anatomical centric occlusal position. The teeth are identified according to the Zsigmondy System.

86

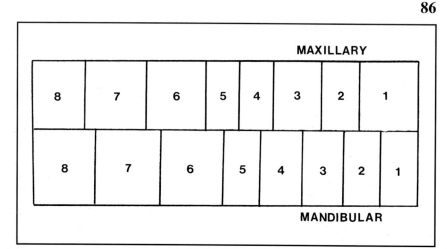

								MAXILLARY
8	7	6	5	4	3	2	1
8	7	6	5	4	3	2	1
							MANDIBULAR

87

87 The relationships between the maxillary and mandibular permanent teeth in anatomical centric occlusion shown by the superimposition of the occlusal surfaces of the teeth in the maxillary arch (**red**) on those of the mandibular arch (**black**). This diagram not only illustrates the general anteroposterior relationships of the maxillary teeth and their antagonists, but also the buccolingual relationships of the arches. Since the maxillary arch is a little larger and broader than the mandibular arch, there is a slight overlap of the mandibular arch by the maxillary arch such that the buccal cusps of the maxillary teeth extend a few millimetres beyond the buccal occlusal edge of the mandibular teeth. This overlap is termed overjet.

48

88 & 89 The buccolingual incisor relationships in anatomical centric occlusion. The maxillary incisors overlap the mandibular incisors in two planes. The overlap in the horizontal plane (overjet) is approximately 2–3mm. The vertical overlap, peculiar to the incisors and canines, is termed overbite. The overbite in anatomical centric occlusion is such that the palatal surfaces of the maxillary incisors overlap the incisal third of the labial surfaces of the mandibular incisors.

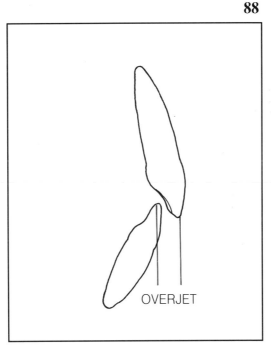

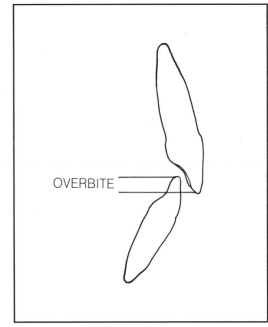

90 The occlusal surfaces of the permanent dentition marked to show the positions of hard contact in anatomical centric occlusion (centric stops). The black marks represent the intercuspal contact positions. While the major markings register on the occlusal surfaces of the posterior teeth, note the labioincisal and palatoincisal markings of the mandibular and maxillary incisors. As befits the anatomical overjet relationships, the tips of the maxillary buccal cusps and the mandibular lingual cusps remain relatively unmarked. Similar marks can be made *in vivo* by interposing articulating paper between the teeth and then instructing the patient to go into centric position.

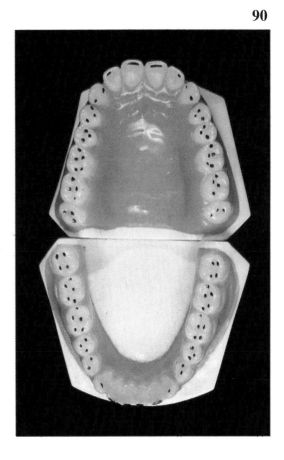

Variations in the relationships of the dental arches in centric position

Malocclusions should be regarded as anatomical variations rather than as abnormalities, for while they may be aesthetically displeasing they are rarely involved in masticatory dysfunction. Our lack of understanding of the relationships between masticatory efficiency and tooth and arch form is responsible for the classification of malocclusion in terms of variations in the anatomical centric position and not in more functional terms.

Malocclusions result from malposition of individual teeth, malrelationship of the dental arches and/or variation in skeletal morphology of the jaws. Techniques for determining the skeletal relationships of the jaws are described on page 60. Two classifications describing malposition of teeth and malrelationship of the arches are in general use. One, Angle's classification, relies upon the relationship of the arches in the anteroposterior plane using the first permanent molars as key teeth. The other classification relates malocclusion to the position of the incisors.

91

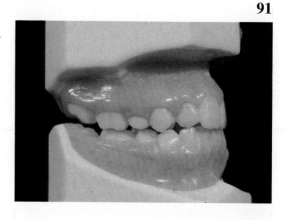

91 Angle's Class I malocclusion. Though one or more of the teeth are malpositioned, this does not affect the standard anatomical relationship of the first permanent molars (see **85** and **86**). In the models shown, the maxillary canine is missing and the premolars are malaligned.

92

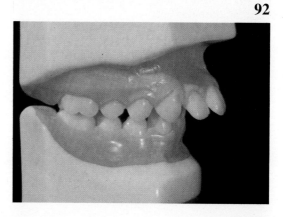

92 Angle's Class II malocclusion (Division 1). Angle's Class II malocclusion is characterised by a 'prenormal' maxillary arch relationship, the maxillary first permanent molars occluding at least half a cusp more mesial to the mandibular first permanent molars than the standard anatomical position. 'Division 1' indicates that the maxillary incisors are proclined.

93

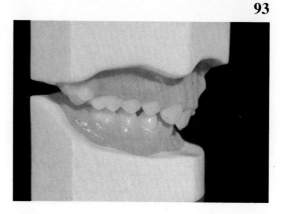

93 Angle's Class II malocclusion (Division 2). The molar relationship is 'prenormal'; 'Division 2' indicates that the maxillary incisors are retroclined. Frequently, however, only the central incisors are retroclined, the lateral incisors being proclined.

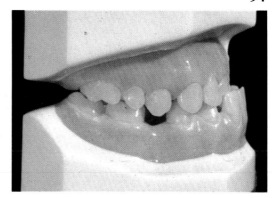

94 Angle's Class III malocclusion. This malocclusion is characterised by a 'postnormal' maxillary arch relationship, the maxillary first permanent molars occluding at least half a cusp more distal to the mandibular first permanent molars than the standard anatomical position. The incisor relationship varies from 'normal' overjet to an edge-to-edge bite to reverse overjet.

Since the permanent molars do not have a fixed relationship in the arch and may migrate following early loss of deciduous teeth, the classification of malocclusion based upon incisor relationships is often preferred to the Angle's classification. Furthermore, a classification of malocclusion related to the incisors is seen by many clinicians to be more appropriate since a major objective of orthodontic treatment is to establish an anatomical incisor relationship (patients being more concerned and aware of the aesthetics of the incisor relationship than they are of the molar relationship).

95 Classification of malocclusion using incisor relationships.

Class I. This represents the relationship where the incisors do not show any malposition. The incisal margins of the mandibular incisors occlude with, or lie directly below, the middle of the palatal surfaces of the maxillary incisors (i.e. on the cingulum shelf).

Class II. The incisal margins of the mandibular incisors lie behind the middle part of the palatal surfaces of the maxillary incisors. Division 1 indicates that the maxillary central incisors are proclined; Division 2 indicates that the maxillary central incisors are retroclined.

Class III. The incisal margins of the mandibular incisors lie in front of the middle part of the palatal surfaces of the maxillary incisors.

It must be emphasised that although terms similar to those used in Angle's classification are also used in classifying malocclusions using incisor relationships, they are not the same.

I   II₁   II₂   III

Some other malalignment problems

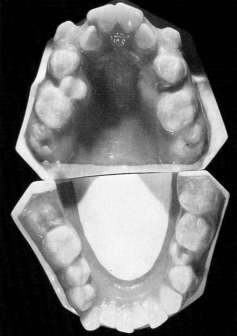

96 Crowding is the term used to describe the condition where teeth are markedly out of the line of the dental arch because there is disproportion between the size of the arch and the size of the teeth. The severe crowding illustrated here reflects the developmental positions of the teeth before eruption (note that the second incisors develop inside the dental arch and the canines develop outside the arch). Spacing within an arch occurs where the teeth are small in relation to the size of the arch (or where there are missing teeth).

97 Anterior open bite occurs where there is no incisor contact and no incisor overbite. It may be caused by thumb sucking habits, by abnormal swallowing patterns or because of skeletal deformities. Skeletal anterior open bites sometimes result from lack of development of the anterior alveolar region, but more often are associated with an increase in anterior intermaxillary height (i.e. the distance between the maxillary and mandibular dental bases; see **108**).

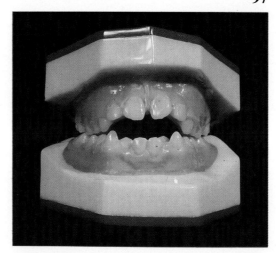

98 Crossbite. This is a transverse abnormality of the dental arches where there is an asymmetrical bite. It may be unilateral or bilateral, as illustrated here. Crossbites are frequently related to discrepancies in the widths of the dental bases and may involve the displacement of the mandible to one side to obtain maximal intercuspation.

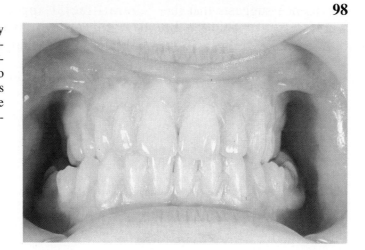

Table 5: Severity and type of malocclusions in the population.

	Distribution (%)	
	Age 6–11	Age 12–17
A. Severity		
Near-ideal occlusion	23	10
Mild malocclusion	40	35
Moderate malocclusion	23	26
Severe or very severe	14	29
B. Type		
Crowding/malalignment problems		
Ideal	57	13
Moderate	39	44
Severe	4	43
Anteroposterior problems		
Overjet (6mm or more)	17	15
Reverse overjet (1mm or more)	1	
Vertical problems		
Open bite (2mm or more)	1	1
Overbite (6mm or more)	8	12
Transverse problems		
Lingual crossbite (two or more teeth)	5	6
Buccal crossbite (two or more teeth)	1	2

Approximately 80% of children and adolescents (USA data) show some degree of malocclusion. Most commonly there are problems of crowding (for about 40% of children and 80% of adolescents). The second most common type of malocclusion is excessive overjet of the maxillary incisors (about 15% of children and of adolescents).

Mandibular posture

When the mandible is at rest, a gap of a few millimetres remains between the occlusal surfaces of the teeth — the so-called freeway space. The opinion has long been held that the position of rest is innate and unalterable throughout life. However, the concept of a fixed mandibular resting posture is an over-simplification. Indeed, psychological state, body posture and fatigue are well known short-term influences that can change the resting interocclusal distance. Furthermore, research shows that, following speech, mastication or swallowing, the mandible appears to return to whatever position of rest it can find. In the long term, ageing and the removal of occlusal contacts affect the resting position. Although the physiological mechanisms responsible for maintaining a rest position are not fully understood, evidence suggests that the physical properties of the soft tissues are responsible for the rest position, not tonic activity of the elevator muscles of the jaw.

Several instruments and techniques have been devised to measure freeway space – some elaborate, some relatively simple. All suffer from inaccuracies produced by examiner bias, and to misconceptions of the nature of the mandibular resting posture. The use of measuring techniques relies upon the concept that the mandibular resting position is innate and unalterable. Consequently, the removal of teeth is deemed not to affect the rest position. Thus, when a patient has lost all natural occlusal contacts, it is considered necessary only to put a prosthesis into the mouth at a level which reproduces the freeway space to restore the original occlusal vertical dimension.

Although most clinicians would prefer objective criteria for determining vertical jaw relationships, it is realised by many that, because of the relative instability of such relationships, at best one has to rely upon such subjective assessments as overall facial appearance, mandibular position during deglutition, jaw posture giving greatest comfort, position allowing the development of maximum biting force, and lip and tongue posture. Nevertheless, however one gauges the mandibular resting position, if one is to place prosthetic appliances into the mouth, it is necessary to ensure that the vertical dimensions of the jaws are not adversely affected.

99a **99b**

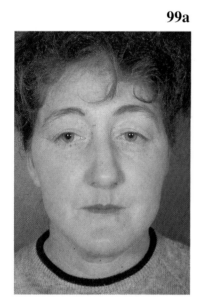 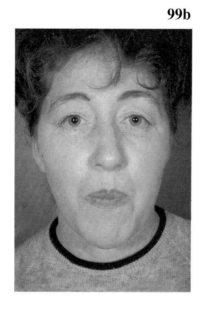

100a **100b**

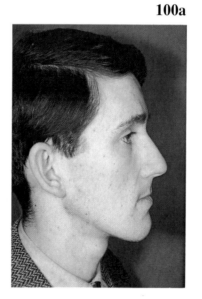 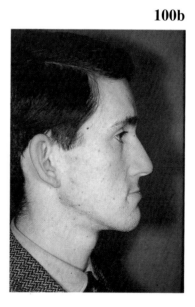

99 The appearance produced as a result of over-opening.
99a Normal resting position for patient without dentures.
99b Over-opened appearance produced typically by the wearing of dentures without the provision of adequate freeway space. Note that the result of over-opening is an elongation of the face, a parting of the lips at rest, and a 'strained' facial appearance.

100 The appearance produced by over-closure.
100a Normal resting position.
100b Over-closed appearance. The general effect of over-closure on facial appearance is to produce features of increased age. There is a closer approximation of the nose and chin than normal. The greater the degree of over-closure, the more the soft tissues of the face appear to sag and fall in, and the more pronounced are the lines on the face.

The radiographic appearance of jaws and teeth

Dental radiography and radiology are concerned with the techniques of producing and interpreting photographic images of oro-dental tissues taken with X-rays (see Table 6). X-rays, being part of the spectrum of electromagnetic radiation, have a wavelength of approximately 10^{-8}cm compared with wavelengths around 10^{-4}cm for visible light. It is the short wavelengths that allow X-rays to penetrate materials which would otherwise absorb or reflect light. X-rays do not pass through all matter with similar ease. Materials composed of elements with low atomic numbers are readily penetrated by X-rays and are described as being radiolucent, whereas elements with high atomic numbers absorb X-rays and are termed radio-opaque. Thus, gases and soft tissues are radiolucent while calcified materials such as bone and teeth are radio-opaque. X-rays produce a photosensitisation reaction when they strike a silver–salt emulsion. When a radio-opaque structure is placed between a beam of X-rays and a photographic plate which is subsequently developed, the radio-opaque structure is 'mapped out' as a white area on the negative. It is because of the properties of tissue penetration and photosensitisation that X-rays can be used in dentistry to provide valuable information concerning underlying hard tissue structures not otherwise visible.

X-rays produce a shadow picture without a focus; therefore a large object such as a skull does not show all its features equally distinctly on a radiograph. As a general rule, structures nearest the photographic plate appear clearer than those some distance from the plate. Superimposition may also make interpretation of radiographs difficult, for most radiographs are two-dimensional representations of three-dimensional objects. Care must be taken not to overinterpret radiographs by diagnosing pathological conditions without recourse to other diagnostic aids or clinical findings. The prime use of a radiograph is, therefore, to describe gross topographic features.

Table 6: Radiographic projections describing jaws and teeth.

Projection/technique	Purpose	Projection/technique	Purpose
A. Extra-oral			
Posteroanterior skull (PA)	Survey of facial bones and mandible.	Transcranial temporo-mandibular joint	Movement of mandibular condyles in mandibular fossae.
Anteroposterior skull (AP)	Survey of posterior part of cranium, mandible and temporomandibular articulation.	Sialography	Infusion of radio-opaque material into the main salivary ducts to study their structure and distribution.
Reverse Towne's	Anatomy of mandibular condyles and temporomandibular articulation.	Tomography	Technique for the radiography of selected areas which under standard radiographic technique are obscured by superimposition of other structures e.g. temporomandibular joint and air sinuses.
Occipitomental skull	Survey of facial bones and air sinuses.		
Lateral skull	Survey of lateral regions of face, cranium and mandible. View of facial profile and covering soft tissues.		
Lateral skull with cephalostat	Recording of relationships between teeth, jaws and cranial base.	**B. Intra-oral**	
Lateral oblique view of mandible	Survey of posterior regions of body and ramus of mandible.	Maxillary and mandibular occlusal views of teeth	Relationship of structures in buccolingual plane.
Orthopantomogram	A tomogram to display the whole of maxilla, mandible and the dentition on a single film.	Periapical view of teeth	Examination of apices of teeth. Relationships of structures in mesiodistal plane.
		Bitewing examination of teeth	Survey of crowns of the teeth and the alveolar crests.

Extra-oral radiographic projections of jaws and related structures

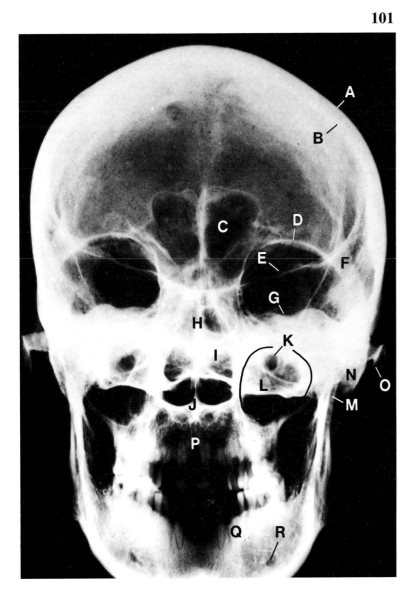

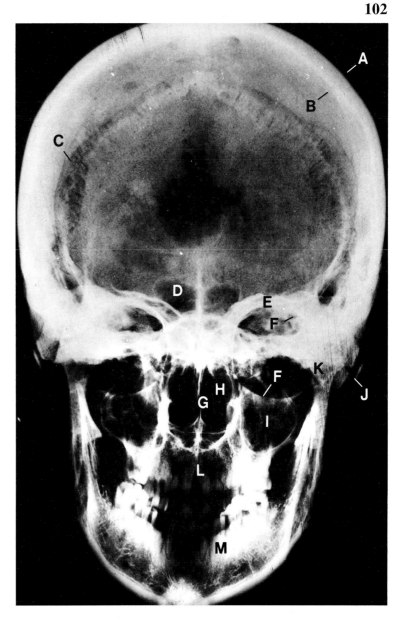

101 Posteroanterior (PA) view of skull.

A Outer table of cranium.
B Inner table of cranium.
C Frontal air sinus.
D Superior rim of orbit.
E Sphenoid ridge in middle cranial fossa.
F Zygomatic process of frontal bone.
G Petrous ridge.
H Nasal septum.
I Nasal fossa.
J Anterior nasal spine.
K Infra-orbital foramen.
L Maxillary air sinus.
M Neck of mandibular condyle.
N Mastoid process of temporal bone.
O Zygomatic arch.
P Maxilla and teeth.
Q Body of mandible and teeth.
R Mental foramen.

102 Anteroposterior (AP) view of skull.

A Outer table of cranium.
B Inner table of cranium.
C Lambdoid suture.
D Frontal air sinus.
E Superimposed sphenoid, petrous and supra-orbital ridges.
F Rim of orbit.
G Nasal septum.
H Nasal fossa.
I Maxillary air sinus.
J Zygoma.
K Condyle of mandible.
L Maxilla and teeth.
M Body of mandible and teeth.

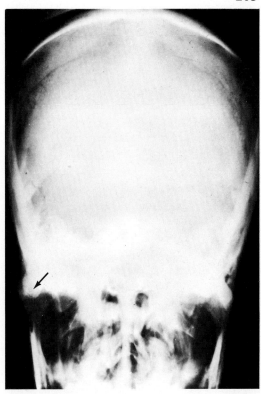

103 Reverse Towne's view showing position of mandibular condyle (*arrowed*).

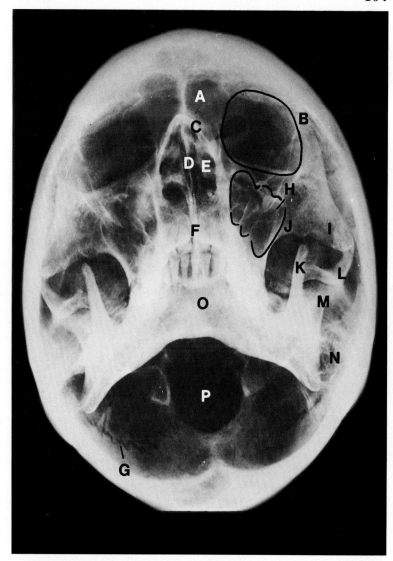

104 Occipitomental view of skull (OM 30°).

A Frontal air sinus.
B Outline of orbit.
C Nasal bones.
D Nasal septum.
E Nasal fossa with superimposed shadows of ethmoidal air cells.
F Maxilla and teeth.
G Lambdoid suture.
H Malar (zygomatic) extension of maxillary sinus.
I Zygoma.
J Outline of maxillary air sinus.
K Coronoid process of mandible.
L Zygomatic process of temporal bone.
M Condyle of mandible.
N Mastoid air cells.
O Body of mandible and teeth.
P Foramen magnum.

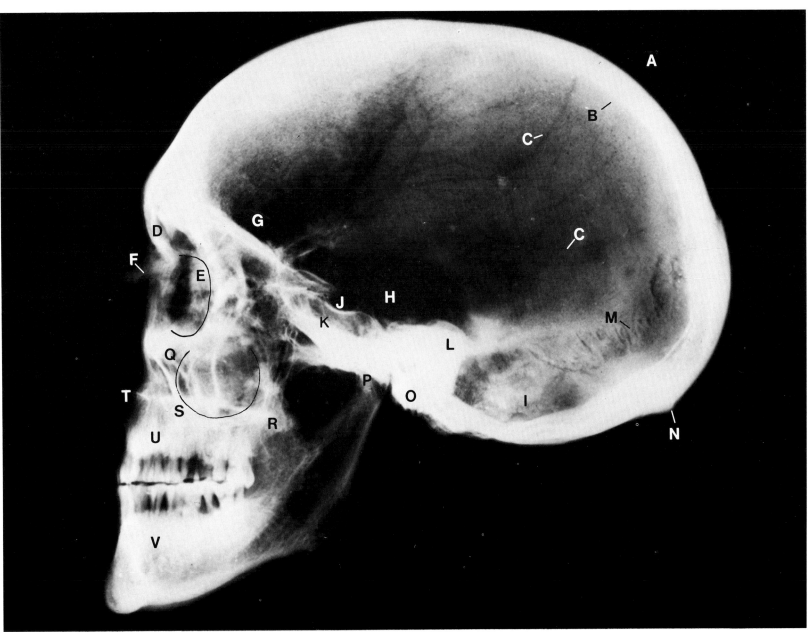

105 Lateral skull radiograph.

A Outer table of cranium.
B Inner table of cranium.
C Depressions in cranium related to middle meningeal vessels.
D Frontal air sinus.
E Margins of orbit.
F Nasal bone.
G Anterior cranial fossa.
H Middle cranial fossa.
I Posterior cranial fossa.
J Hypophyseal (pituitary) fossa.
K Sphenoid air sinus.
L Petrous ridge.
M Lambdoid suture.
N External occipital protuberance.
O Mastoid process.
P Condyle of mandible.
Q Margin of maxillary air sinuses.
R Coronoid process of mandible.
S Hard palate.
T Anterior nasal spine.
U Maxilla and teeth.
V Body of mandible and teeth.

Cephalometric analysis of lateral skull radiographs

Lateral skull radiographs are often used in dentistry to assess by measurement general skeletal morphology, particularly for recording relationships between the jaws and the cranial base. They are also of value for the evaluation of the direction and the amount of growth, for determining dento-skeletal relationships, and even for soft tissue analysis. In order to provide the most meaningful measurements, cephalometric radiographs are taken under standard conditions to enable comparisons between patients, and for the same patient at different times. Thus, the position of the head must be standardised using a cephalostat (head holder) such that the beam of X-rays is shot in a predetermined plane to the head from a standard distance. This necessitates that the Frankfort plane (between the ear and orbit; see **108**) is horizontal, that the dentition is in centric occlusion (see page 48) and that the lips are in their habitual position. Lateral skull radiographs are preferred for dental cephalometry primarily because the facial variations of greatest importance are located in the sagittal plane. Normal values for cephalometric measurements are given in Table 7 (page 62).

106

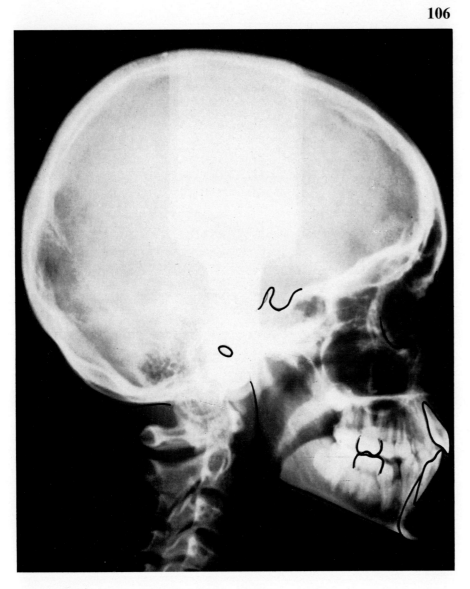

106 Lateral skull radiograph taken using a cephalostat.

107 Lateral view of skull (107a) and tracing taken from a lateral skull radiograph (107b) illustrating the most common cephalometric landmarks used in dentistry.

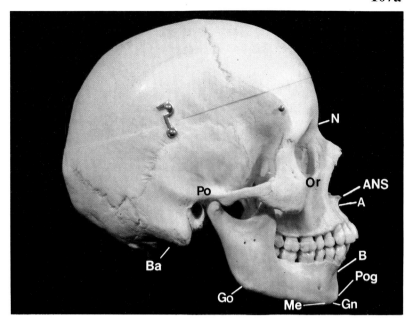

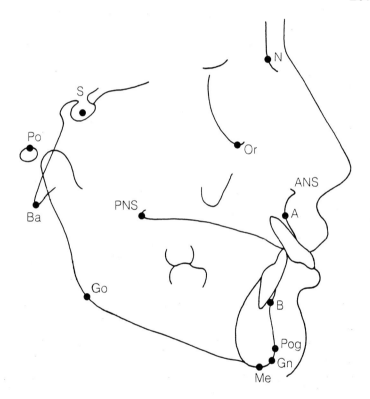

Basion (Ba) — The most inferior and posterior point on the basiocciput, lying on the anterior margin of the foramen magnum.

Sella point (S) — Centre of shadow of sella turcica (pituitary fossa).

Nasion (N) — Junction between frontal and nasal bones in midline on the frontonasal suture.

Porion (Po) — Highest bony point of margin of external acoustic meatus.

Orbitale (Or) — Lowest point of the infra-orbital margin.

Anterior nasal spine (ANS)

Posterior nasal spine (PNS)

Subspinale (A point) — Position of greatest concavity of maxillary alveolus in the midline.

Supramentale (B point) — Position of greatest concavity of mandibular alveolus in the midline.

Pogonion (Pog) — Most anterior point on the chin.

Menton (Me) — Lowest point of the chin.

Gnathion (Gn) — Point between the most anterior and inferior points of chin established by bisecting the angle formed between the N-Pog and mandibular planes.

Gonion (Go) — Most inferior and posterior point at the angle of the mandible established by bisecting the angle formed between the planes through the lower border of the mandible and posterior border of ramus.

59

108 Cephalometric analysis of jaw relationships and facial form. The mandibular plane passes through the menton and gonion. It is used in conjunction with the Frankfort, maxillary and Ba–N planes to assess the vertical development of the anterior part of the face. The Frankfort plane extends from the orbitale to the porion. The Frankfort–mandibular angle in 'normal' subjects is said to be approximately 27°. The maxillary plane extends through the anterior and posterior nasal spines (ANS, PNS) and is easier to identify on a lateral skull radiograph than the Frankfort plane. Both the maxillary–mandibular plane angle and the mandibular–cranial base (Ba–N) angle are of the same order as the Frankfort–mandibular plane angle. A plane termed the facial line can be drawn between the nasion and the pogonion. This plane aids the assessment of facial profile and the angle it makes with the Frankfort plane indicates whether the profile is orthognathic, prognathic or retrognathic.

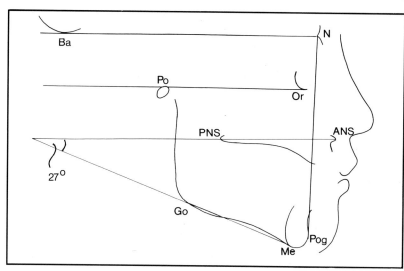

109 The use of SNA and SNB angles to record maxillary–mandibular skeletal relationships. SNA measures the degree of prognathism of the maxillary alveolar base. Its average value is 82°. SNB assesses the degree of prognathism of the mandibular alveolar base. SNA–SNB (i.e. ANB) is frequently used to determine the skeletal pattern for the jaws since the cranial base (SN plane) is thought to undergo very little change from the later years of childhood. Where ANB is 2–5°, the skeletal pattern is designated to be Class I. Where ANB is greater than 5°, the jaws show a Class II relationship with maxillary prognathism. Where ANB is less than 2°, the jaws show a Class III relationship with mandibular prognathism. Should SNA be significantly different from its normal value, a correction must be made before assigning an ANB value to a specific skeletal class.

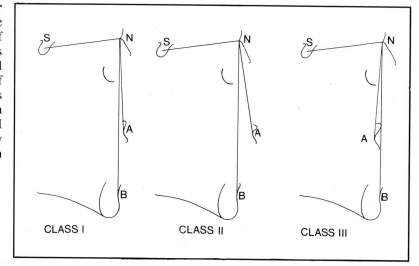

110 Cephalometric landmarks used for assessing dentoskeletal relationships.

Centroid of the maxillary incisor root (**C**)	The midpoint along the root axis of the most prominent maxillary incisor.
Incision superius (**IS**)	The incisal tip of the most prominent maxillary incisor.
Incision inferius (**II**)	The incisal tip of the most prominent mandibular incisor.
Infradentale (**Id**)	The junction of alveolar crest with the outline of the most prominent mandibular incisor.

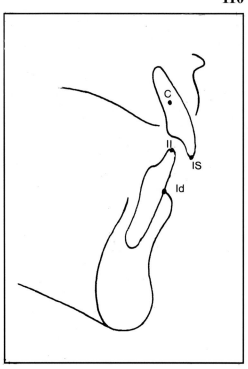

111 The inclinations of the incisors to the planes of the jaws. The inclination of the maxillary incisor can be determined by measuring the angle between a line drawn through its root axis and the Frankfort (or maxillary) plane. On average, this angle is 109°. The inclination of the mandibular incisor is assessed by the angle formed between its root axis and the mandibular plane. It is approximately a right angle.

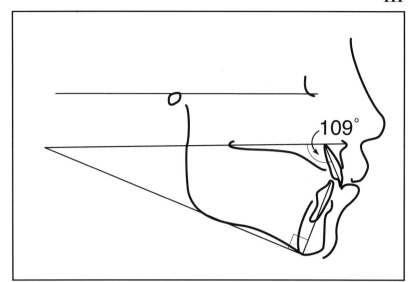

112 Interincisor relationships. The intercisal angle formed by the junction of the longitudinal axes of the maxillary and mandibular central incisors is of the order of 135°. However, its clinical usefulness is limited since of greater importance are the anteroposterior relationships of the incisal edges. This is assessed by analysing the distance between the mandibular incisal edge and the centroid (**C**) of the maxillary incisor root. Two examples are shown. In both, the maxillary and mandibular incisors meet at the same angle of approximately 135°. However, they differ markedly in terms of the distances between the mandibular incisal edges and the centroids.

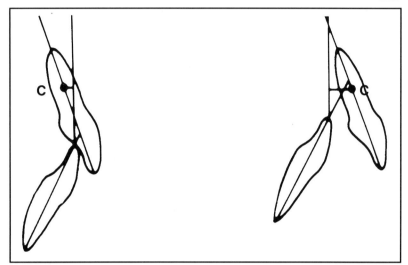

113a Cephalometric growth studies. Every bone of the skull in the growing child shows some degree of growth and consequently no point can be considered 'fixed'. For analytical convenience, however, several landmarks and strategies are defined and/or adopted to study the degree and direction of cranial growth. The Y-axis is a line from the sella point to the gnathion, and is used to describe the general direction of facial growth relative to the cranial base. The angle between the Y-axis and the Ba–N plane is used to assess changes in growth direction.

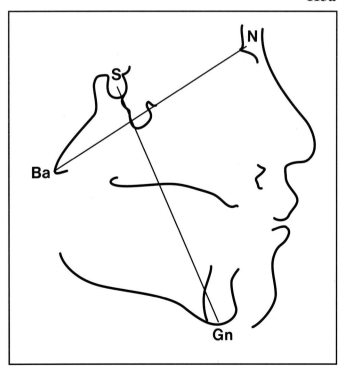

113b Cephalometric growth studies. A frequently employed strategy to assess growth relies upon the superimposition of successive cephalometric tracings of the same individual at different ages. A reasonably reliable picture of growth of the facial skeleton can be obtained by superimposition at the S–N planes with registration of the sella point. Growth at the maxillary region is notoriously difficult to assess but can be analysed by superimposition at the maxillary plane with registration of the anterior surface of the zygomatic process of the maxilla. For the mandibular region it is necessary to superimpose at the mandibular canal and at the inner surface of the mandible behind the chin.

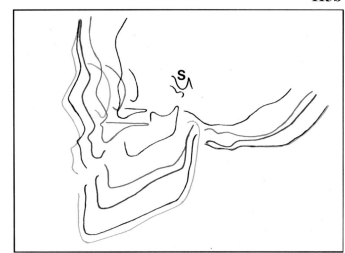

114 Soft tissue analysis is possible from cephalometric radiographs provided that the soft tissue outlines are sufficiently clear and that the lips are in their habitual posture. To undertake such analysis, reference is often made to the following three planes:

The H line (the Harmony line of Holdaway, **H**) is drawn between the chin and the vermilion border of the upper lip. It can be used to assess the degree of lower lip pout. The vermilion border of the lower lip should be within 1mm of the **H** line.

The upper lip tangent (**ULT**) describes the plane perpendicular to the Frankfort plane and tangential to the vermilion border of the upper lip. It is used to assess the amount of upper lip curl, the concavity of the upper lip profile normally being 1–4mm behind the upper lip tangent.

The aesthetic line (**AL**) extends from the tip of the nose to the chin. The vermilion borders of both upper and lower lips usually lie close to the aesthetic line.

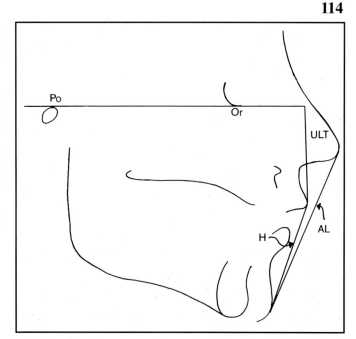

Table 7: Normal values for cephalometric measurements.

Maxillary–mandibular plane angle	27° ±5°
SNA angle	82° ±3°
ANB angle	3° ±1°
Maxillary incisor/maxillary plane angle	109° ±5°
Mandibular incisor/mandibular plane angle	90° ±5°
Maxillary incisor/mandibular incisor angle	135° ±9°
N–S–Ba angle	130° (150° at birth)

115 Lateral oblique view of mandible.

A   Mastoid process of temporal bone.
B   Condyle of mandible lying in mandibular fossa of temporomandibular joint.
C   Zygomatic arch.
D   Shadow of mandibular coronoid process on maxillary tuberosity.
E   Body of mandible showing teeth posterior to premolars.
F   Mental foramen.

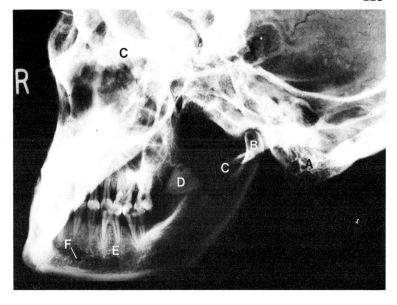

116 Orthopantomogram (OPG). A panoramic radiographic survey of the jaws and teeth. Dentition is radiographed at 6 years of age.

A   External auditory meatus.
B   Mandibular condyle.
C   Coronoid process of mandible.
D   Maxillary air sinus.
E   Nasal cavity.
F   Vertebral column.

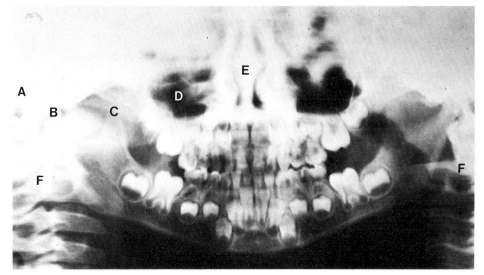

117 Transcranial temporomandibular articulation (117a, mouth closed and 117b, mouth open).

A   Mandibular condyle.
B   Temporomandibular joint cavity space.
C   Articular tubercle.
D   External auditory meatus.
E   Mastoid air cells.
F   Zygomatic arch.
G   Coronoid process.

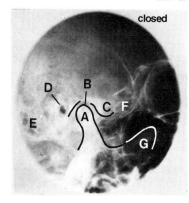

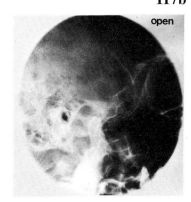

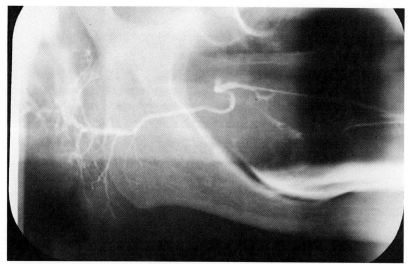

118 Sialogram. Parotid gland, lateral view. A radio-opaque oil suspension of iodine-containing compounds has been introduced into a parotid duct.

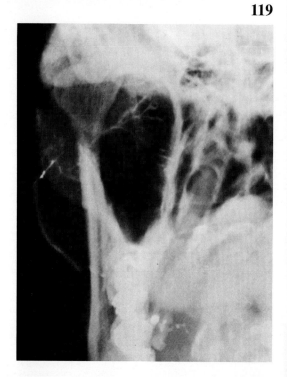

119 Sialogram. Right parotid gland, antero-posterior view.

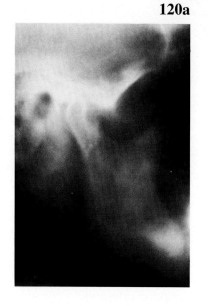
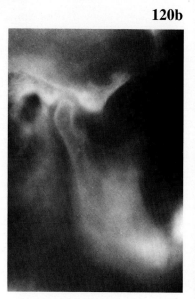

120 Tomographic examination of the temporomandibular articulation. Tomography is a radiographic technique used to study layers within a volume of tissue, in a way analogous to the examination of a single portion of bread within a whole loaf without physically slicing it. The two pictures of the temporomandibular joint illustrated here represent two layers in this region approximately 0.5cm apart.

Intra-oral radiographic projections of jaws and teeth

121 Maxillary occlusal view — vertex approach (121a) and nasal approach (121b). As the names suggest, the vertex and nasal occlusal views of the maxilla essentially differ in the positioning of the X-ray tube, which is either to the vertex of the skull or to the nasion. Differences in the radiographic pictures obtained relate to the degree of superimposition (greater in the vertex occlusal) and the direction and proportions of the longitudinal axes of the teeth (more vertical and less distorted roots with the vertex occlusal). In addition to surveying the maxillary dentition, the maxillary occlusal views may also be used to define the nasal fossae and maxillary air sinuses.

121a

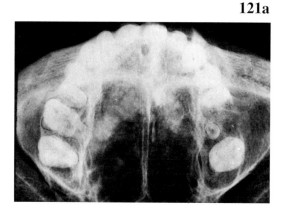

121b

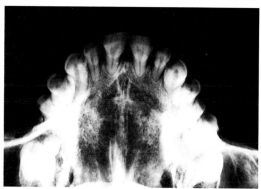

122

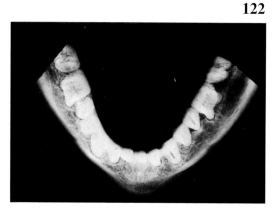

122 Mandibular occlusal view.

123

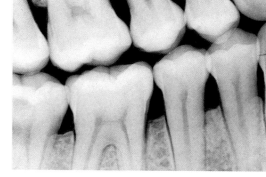

123 Examination of the crowns of the permanent molars and associated alveolar crests using bitewing radiographs.

124 Intra-oral survey of the permanent dentition with peri-apical views of the teeth.

124

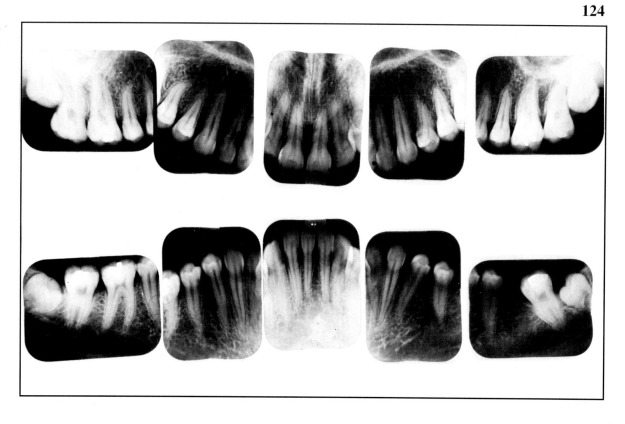

Anatomical features seen on intra-oral radiographs

The importance of appreciating the radiographic appearance of the teeth and their supporting tissues need hardly be emphasised. However, equally essential for the interpretation of an apparent divergence from the normal is an awareness of non-dental anatomical structures which, to the unwary, may simulate pathological lesions on intra-oral radiographs. The radio-opacity of normal anatomical structures seen on intra-oral radiographs is given in Table 8.

Table 8:   Radio-opacity of normal anatomical structures seen on intra-oral radiographs.

Radiolucent	Radio-opaque
Dental Pulp	Enamel
Gingiva and periodontal ligament	Dentine
Bone marrow	Cementum
	Cortical bony plates
	Lamina dura
Maxillary sinus	Bony walls of maxillary sinus
Naval cavity	Bony walls of nasal cavity
Incisive foramen	Nasal septum
Median palatine suture	Anterior nasal spine
Intermaxillary suture	Maxillary tuberosity
Nasolacrimal canal	Zygomatic arch
	Coronoid process
Mandibular canal	Pterygoid hamulus
	Internal and external oblique lines of mandible
Mental foramen	Borders of mandibular canal
Mandibular symphysis	Mental and canine prominences
	Genial tubercles
Bony depressions e.g. mental and submandibular fossa	
Nutrient canals	

125

125 Radiographic image of a tooth. Tooth substance absorbs more X-rays than any other tissue of comparable size and thickness. Enamel is the most radio-opaque and is easily distinguished, covering the anatomical crown of the tooth. In normal teeth the enamel is of uniform density, though in some areas where the enamel is thin (e.g. the cervical regions) it may appear relatively radiolucent. Such an appearance may easily be misinterpreted as dental caries. Dentine and cementum cannot be readily distinguished from each other radiographically because of their similar capacity to absorb X-rays. Owing to the lower radio-opacity of dentine, it appears comparatively 'greyer' than the enamel and thus the enamel–dentine junction is clearly demarcated. The pulp of a tooth, being soft tissue, is readily penetrated by X-rays and consequently, on a radiograph, the pulp cavity is clearly defined as the central radiolucent region of the tooth. However, because of distortion, foreshortening and superimposition, care should be taken in assessing the pulpal anatomy from radiographs. The tooth is supported in the bony alveolus. In this text, the alveolus refers to the whole of the bony supporting tissue of the tooth, and the lamina dura refers to the compact bone lining the tooth socket. The morphology of the margins of the alveolus (alveolar crest) is important in the diagnosis of periodontal disease. As a general rule, the width of the crest depends upon the distance the teeth are separated. Consequently, between the molars the crests are flat and horizontal, while between the incisors the crests rise only as points or spines. In the healthy situation, the crest rises to the level of the cement–enamel junction. The lamina dura is considered to be a very important structure in the radiographic interpretation of periodontal and periapical pathologies. It appears as a continuous, radio-opaque lining of the socket and usually is continuous over the alveolar crests. However, the radio-opacity of the lamina dura does not indicate any hypermineralisation, but is a consequence of superimposition. Discontinuity of the lamina dura in the root region is usually indicative of abnormality or disease. Between the root of the tooth and the lamina dura of the socket is the connective tissue of the periodontal ligament, which appears as a thin radiolucent region.

126 Radiolucent, anatomical features seen on an intra-oral, maxillary occlusal oblique view.

A Maxillary antrum.
B Incisive foramen.
C Nasolacrimal canal.
D Nasal fossa.

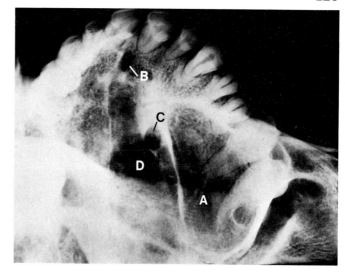

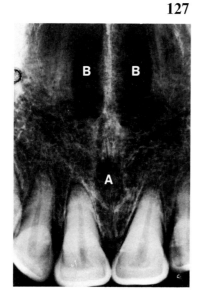

127 The incisive foramen (A) and nasal fossae (B) seen on an intra-oral periapical view of the maxillary central incisors.

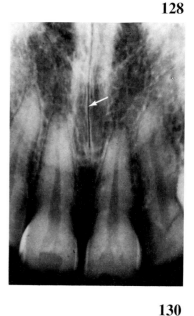

128 The median palatine suture (*arrowed*) seen on an intra-oral periapical view of the maxillary central incisors.

129 The floor of the maxillary antrum seen on an intra-oral periapical view of the maxillary premolars and molars. The maxillary antrum or sinus is an air-filled cavity of varying dimensions; it appears radiographically as a dark, radiolucent shadow bounded by radio-opaque lines representing the lining layers of cortical bone. The radiolucency is not usually uniform because of superimposition of the zygomatic process and the soft tissues of the cheek. The antrum often presents not as a single sinus but as several compartments due to bony septation. It is said that the cortical lining of the antrum is not continuous but exhibits numerous, small, linear interruptions associated with nutrient canals (**135**). This radiographic characteristic may be important in avoiding misinterpretation of the sinus as a pathological lesion. The floor of the antrum is closely related to the root apices of the maxillary teeth. It is generally stated that the sinus extends from the premolars to the tuberosity, though variations are frequent. Because of the close relationship of the teeth to the antrum, communication between the antrum and the oral cavity (oro-antral fistula) following tooth extractions is unfortunately all too frequent. Because of the problems of interpreting three-dimensional situations on a two-dimensional radiograph, care must be taken to avoid misreading the relationship of the teeth to the antrum.

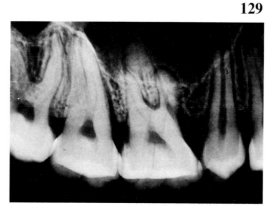

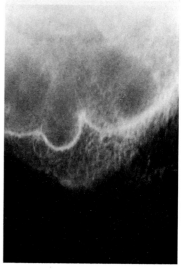

130 The maxillary antrum seen on an intra-oral view of an edentulous maxillary tuberosity.

131 The configuration termed the Y-of-Ennis is formed by the abutment of the anterior wall of the antrum and the floor of the nasal fossa.

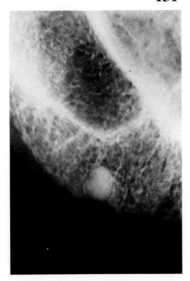

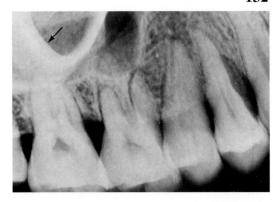

132 **Malar (zygomatic) shadow.** The shadow (*arrowed*) is seen on an intra-oral periapical view of the maxillary molars.

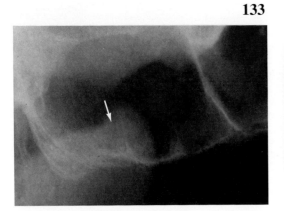

133 **Radio-opaque shadow cast by a coronoid process.** The shadow (*arrowed*) is superimposed on a maxillary tuberosity.

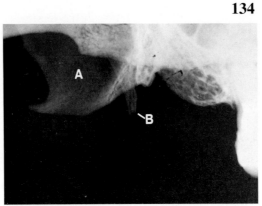

134 **Shadows of the pterygoid plates (A) and pterygoid hamulus (B) near the maxillary tuberosity.**

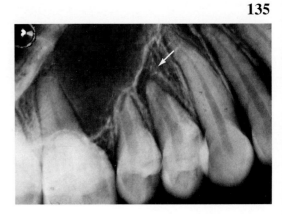

135 **Nutrient canals** (*arrowed*) in the walls of the maxillary antrum.

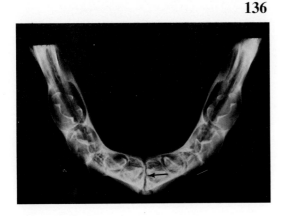

136 **The mandibular symphysis at birth** (*arrowed*) shown on an intra-oral mandibular occlusal radiograph.

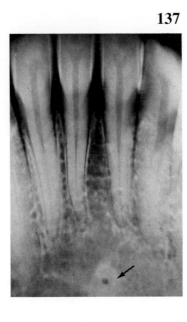

137 The genial tubercles (*arrowed*) seen on an intra-oral periapical view of the mandibular central incisors. Note the characteristic radiographic appearance of the tubercles, i.e. a radiolucent dot surrounded by a distinct radio-opaque region.

138 Mandibular canal in the region of the mandibular third molar tooth.

The mandibular canal commences at the mandibular foramen and passes downwards and forwards from the ramus into the body of the mandible where, near the root apices of the premolars, it terminates by dividing into the mental and incisive canals. The radiographic appearance of the mandibular canal is generally that of a radiolucent shadow bounded superiorly and inferiorly by radio-opaque lines.

The width and position of the canal varies considerably. Most commonly, it is closely related to the roots of the molars, though it lies some distance from the roots of the premolars. Generally, the canal lies buccal to the root apices, a feature which should be remembered when interpreting the relationship of the root apices to the canal. The precise relationship of the teeth to the canal is difficult to determine from radiographs, though some hint of a very close relationship can be obtained by reference to the densities of shadows cast by the roots and canal, the position and densities of the lamina dura and the radio-opaque margins of the canal, and the dimensions of the lumen of the canal.

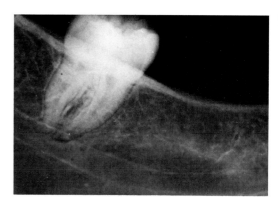

138

139

139 Mental foramen (*arrowed*) near the apices of the mandibular premolars.

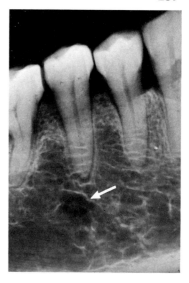

140

141

140 Internal (A) and external (B) oblique lines of the mandible. Occlusal view of an edentulous mandible demonstrating the prominent radio-opacities associated with these lines.

141 Radiograph of developing and erupting molars and premolars. Note the radiolucent regions around the emerging crowns and the developing root apices of the second premolar and second permanent molar.

The regional topography of the mouth and related areas

The temporomandibular joint

142 The temporomandibular joint (TMJ) is the synovial articulation between the mandible and the cranium. For this reason, the joint is sometimes referred to as the craniomandibular joint. The specimen shown is a sagittal section through the joint illustrating the articulation of the head of the mandibular condyle (**A**) into the mandibular fossa (glenoid fossa) of the temporal bone (**B**), with an articular disc (**C**) intervening. The TMJ, although basically a hinge joint, also allows some gliding movements. Movement of the condylar head occurs within the mandibular fossa and down a bony prominence immediately anterior to the mandibular fossa, the articular eminence (**D**).

Since the joints develop in membrane, the articular surfaces are covered with fibrous tissue. The articular disc is also fibrous and is moulded to the bony joint surfaces. **E**, external acoustic meatus. **F**, floor of middle cranial fossa.

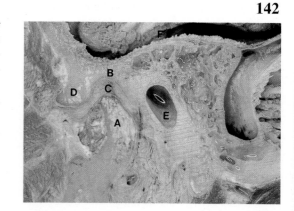

143

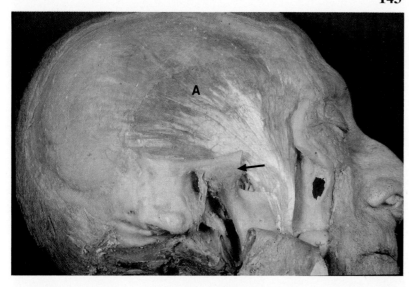

144

143 The capsule of the TMJ (*arrowed*) is a thin, slack cuff which consequently does not limit mandibular movements and is too weak to provide much support for the joint. It is attached to the neck of the condyle of the mandible and to the margins of the mandibular fossa of the temporal bone. Posteriorly, the capsule forms a thick, vascular, but loosely arranged connective tissue (the retrodiscal pad). Internally, it is attached to the articular disc and it is lined by synovial membrane. The capsule is richly innervated. Laterally, the capsule of the TMJ becomes organised to form the temporomandibular ligament. This ligament provides the main means of joint support, restricting distal and inferior movements of the mandible and resisting dislocation during functional movements. It takes origin from the lateral surface of the articular eminence of the temporal bone and inserts onto the posterior surface of the condyle. The temporomandibular ligament is reinforced by a horizontal band of fibres running from the articular eminence to the lateral surface of the condyle. These horizontal fibres restrict posterior movement of the condyle (**192**). All these ligaments are well-innervated and, if excessively stressed, may become inflamed and cause much pain. **A**, temporalis muscle.

144 The articular disc (meniscus) of the TMJ is closely adapted to the joint space between the articular surfaces of the condyle (**A**) and the mandibular fossa (**B**) when the teeth are in centric position (see page 48). It is of variable thickness, being thinnest centrally (**C**) over the articular surface of the condyle and thickest posteriorly (**D**) in the region above and behind the condyle. Anteriorly, the disc covers the slope of the articular eminence (**E**). The shape of the disc is thought to provide a self-centering mechanism to maintain its relationship to the articular surface of the condyle. The articular disc is attached anteriorly to the crest of the articular eminence and to the anterior margin of the mandibular condyle (**F**). The disc is also attached to the lateral pterygoid muscle (**G**) (see **150**). Medially and laterally, the disc is attached to the joint capsule and thus forms upper and lower joint spaces. Posteriorly, the disc becomes bilaminar and folds/unfolds as the condyle and disc move. The upper part of the bilaminar zone is attached onto the anterior margin of the squamotympanic fissure (**H**) (and can extend into the middle ear to become continuous with the anterior malleolar ligament), the lower part to the posterior margin of the condyle (**I**). Functionally, the disc enables gliding movements of the condyle down the slope of the articular eminence and stabilises the joint by maintaining good contact between the joint surfaces.

145 The mandibular fossa (**A**) is an oval depression in the temporal bone lying immediately anterior to the external acoustic meatus (**B**). It is bounded anteriorly by the articular eminence (**C**), laterally by the zygomatic process of the temporal bone (**D**) and posteriorly by the tympanic plate of the temporal bone (**E**). The petrotympanic fissure (**F**) separates the mandibular fossa from the petrous part of the temporal bone and is the site at which the chorda tympani nerve exits from the cranium into the infratemporal fossa. Occasionally, a ridge of bone, the postglenoid process, forms a prominence at the posterior boundary of the mandibular fossa immediately anterior to the external acoustic meatus. The shape of the mandibular fossa does not exactly conform to the shape of the mandibular condyle, the articular disc moulding together the joint surfaces. The bone of the central part of the mandibular fossa is extremely thin and may be translucent. Masticatory loads are not dissipated through the mandibular fossa but through the teeth and thence the facial bones and base of the cranium.

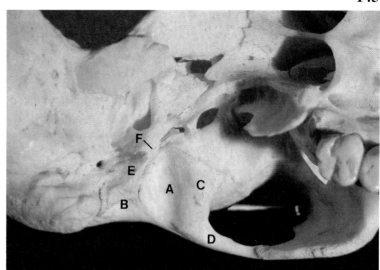

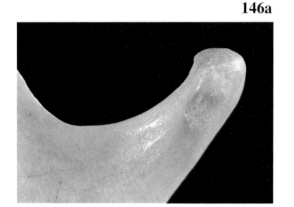

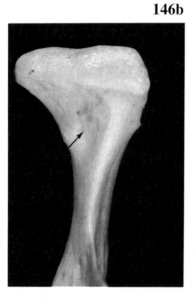

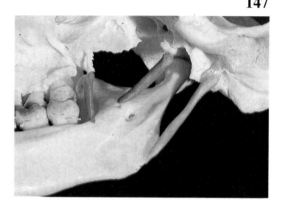

146a   **146b**   **147**

146a & 146b The mandibular condyle. The size and shape of the condyle varies considerably. The broad articular head of the condyle joins the ramus through a thin bony projection termed the neck of the condyle. The anteroposterior dimension of the condylar head is approximately half the mediolateral dimension. The long axis of the condyle is not, however, at right angles to the ramus but diverges posteriorly from a strictly coronal plane such that the long axes of the two condyles, if extended, would meet, forming an obtuse angle of approximately 150° at the anterior border of the foramen magnum. The convex anterior and superior surfaces of the head of the condyle are the articular surfaces. The posterior surface of the head of the condyle is, however, broad and flat. A small depression, the pterygoid fossa (*arrow*), marks part of the attachment of the lateral pterygoid muscle and is situated on the anterior part of the neck below the articular surface of the condyle.

147 The accessory ligaments of the temporomandibular joint. The stylomandibular and sphenomandibular ligaments are described as accessory ligaments of the temporomandibular joint, though neither has any significant influence upon mandibular movements. The stylomandibular ligament (yellow) is a reinforced lamina of the deep cervical fascia as it passes medial to the parotid salivary gland. It extends from the top of the styloid process of the temporal bone and the stylohyoid ligament to the angle of the mandible. The sphenomandibular ligament (green) is a remnant of the perichondrium of Meckel's cartilage (the cartilage of the embryonic first branchial arch) and extends from the spine of the sphenoid bone to the lingula near the mandibular foramen. Also shown is the pterygomandibular raphe (brown) from which the buccinator and superior constrictor muscles arise. It extends from the pterygoid hamulus to the posterior end of the mylohyoid line in the retromolar region of the mandible.

See page 100 for the functional anatomy of the joints, including masticatory movement, and pages 217–219 for histology.

The muscles of mastication

Although many muscles, both in the head and neck, are involved in mastication, the muscles of mastication is a collective term reserved for the masseter, temporalis and medial and lateral pterygoid muscles. All the muscles of mastication develop from the mesenchyme of the first branchial arch. They therefore receive their innervation from the mandibular branch of the trigeminal nerve (cranial nerve V). Closely associated functionally and developmentally with the muscles of mastication is the digastric muscle.

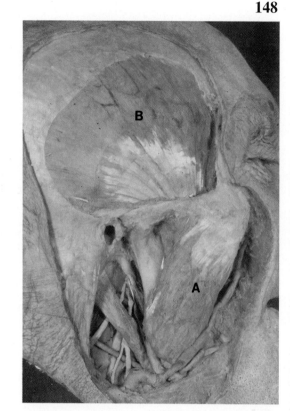

148 The masseter (A) and temporalis (B) muscles lie respectively in the face over the ramus of the mandible and in the temple. They are important elevators of the mandible.

The masseter muscle consists of two overlapping heads. The superficial head arises from the zygomatic process of the maxilla and from the anterior two-thirds of the lower border of the zygomatic arch. The deep head arises from the deep surface of the zygomatic arch. Internally, the muscle has many tendinous septa which greatly increase the area for muscle attachment and which provide a multipennate arrangement, thereby increasing its power. The superficial head passes downwards and backwards to insert into the lower half of the lateral surface of the ramus. The deep head, whose posterior fibres are more vertically orientated, inserts into the upper half of the lateral surface of the ramus, particularly over the coronoid process. The muscle elevates the mandible and is primarily active when grinding tough food. Indeed, the muscle exerts considerable power when the mandible is close to the centric occlusal position. On the basis of its fibre orientation the posterior fibres of the deep head may have some retrusive capability for the mandible.

The temporalis muscle is the largest muscle of mastication. It takes origin from the floor of the temporal fossa of the lateral surface of the skull and from the overlying temporal fascia, and should thus be regarded as a bipennate muscle. The attachment of the muscle is limited above by the inferior temporal line. From this wide origin, the fibres converge towards their insertion on the apex, the anterior and posterior borders, and the medial surface of the coronoid process. Indeed, the insertion extends down the anterior border of the ramus almost as far as the third molar tooth. The posterior fibres of the temporalis muscle pass horizontally forwards while the anterior fibres pass vertically downwards onto the coronoid process. To reach the coronoid process, the muscle runs beneath the zygomatic arch. The lowermost fibres, closely related to the superior head of the lateral pterygoid muscle (see **150**), are said to insert into the capsule and disc of the temporomandibular joint. The anterior (vertical) part of the temporalis muscle elevates the mandible, while the posterior (horizontal) part retracts the protruded mandible. By its attachments into the temporomandibular joint, it may influence the position of the articular disc.

In certain sites, the masseter and temporalis muscles are joined. This is particularly so for the deep fibres of the deep head of the masseter and the overlying temporalis muscle. The functional significance of this 'zygomatico-mandibular mass' is unclear.

Both the masseter muscle and the temporalis muscles are innervated by branches of the anterior division of the mandibular nerve (see **178**). Both muscles receive their blood supply from the maxillary artery (masseteric and deep temporal branches), the superficial temporal artery (transverse facial and middle temporal branches) and, for the masseter muscle, the facial artery.

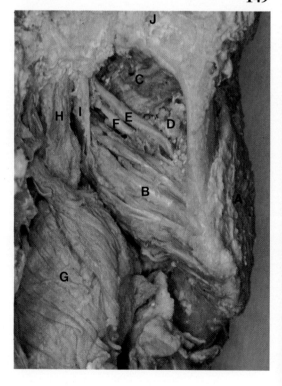

149 Dissection of the masseter (A), medial pterygoid (B) and lateral pterygoid (C) muscles viewed from behind the posterior border of the mandibular ramus. The pterygomandibular space (D) lies between the ramus and the medial pterygoid muscle, the two nerves passing through it being the inferior alveolar (E) and lingual (F) nerves. Also shown are the constrictor muscles of the pharynx (G) (the infratemporal fossa being the space between the superior constrictor and the ramus); the levator veli palatini (H) and tensor veli palatini (I) muscles, and the posterior aspect of the temporomandibular joint (J).

150 **The pterygoid muscles** are situated deep in the face in the infra-temporal fossa (i.e. medial to the ramus of the mandible).

The medial pterygoid muscle consists of two heads. The bulk of the muscle arises as a deep head (**A**) from the medial surface of the lateral pterygoid plate of the sphenoid bone. The smaller superficial head (**B**) arises from the maxillary tuberosity and the neighbouring part of the palatine bone (pyramidal process). From these sites of origin, the fibres of the medial pterygoid pass downwards, backwards and laterally to insert into the roughened surface of the medial aspect of the angle of the mandible (see **24**). Tendinous septa within the muscle increase the surface area for muscle attachment, providing a multipennate arrangement and therefore increasing the power the muscle can exert. The main action of the muscle is to elevate the mandible but it also assists in lateral and protrusive movements. The accessory medial pterygoid muscle is a separate slip of muscle close to the deep surface of the medial pterygoid. This takes origin from the base of the skull close to the foramen ovale and merges with the deep head of the medial pterygoid. Its function is unknown. The masseter and medial pterygoid muscles together form a muscular sling which supports the mandible on the cranium.

The lateral pterygoid muscle lies in the roof of the infratemporal fossa and, in contrast to the vertical orientation of the medial pterygoid, has a more horizontal alignment. It has two heads, superior and inferior. The superior head (**C**) is the smaller and arises from the infratemporal surface of the greater wing of the sphenoid bone. The inferior head (**D**) forms the bulk of the muscle and takes origin from the lateral surface of the lateral pterygoid plate of the sphenoid bone. Both heads pass backwards and outwards towards the temporomandibular joint and merge before inserting into the pterygoid fossa of the mandibular condyle (see **146b**), and into the articular disc and capsule of the temporomandibular joint. In particular, it is the superior head which continues into the articular disc (medial side). Functionally, the superior and inferior heads should be considered as two separate muscles. The inferior head is concerned with mandibular protrusion, depression and lateral excursions. The superior head is activated during mandibular retrusion (providing controlled movements) and during clenching of the mandible.

The medial pterygoid muscle is innervated by a branch of the mandibular nerve that arises proximal to the division of the mandibular nerve into anterior and posterior trunks. The lateral pterygoid receives its nerve supply from the anterior trunk. Both muscles receive their blood supply from the maxillary artery.

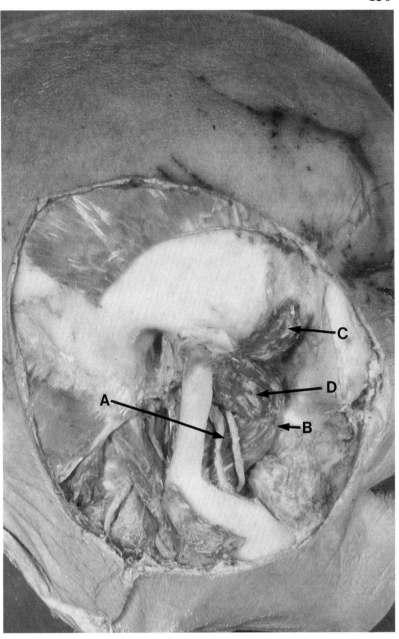

151 **The digastric muscle** is located below the inferior border of the mandible. it consists of an anterior and a posterior belly connected by an intermediate tendon. The posterior belly (**A**) arises from the mastoid notch immediately behind the mastoid process of the temporal bone; it passes downwards and forwards towards the hyoid bone, where it becomes the digastric tendon(**B**). This muscle passes through the insertion of the stylo-hyoid muscle (**C**) and is attached to the greater horn of the hyoid bone by a fibrous loop. The anterior belly of the digastric muscle (**D**) is attached to the digastric fossa on the inferior border of the mandible (see **24**) and runs downwards and backwards to the digastric tendon. The digastric muscle depresses and retrudes the mandible, and is also involved in stabilising the position of the hyoid bone and in elevation of the hyoid during swallowing.

The anterior belly of the digastric muscle is innervated by the mylohyoid branch of the mandibular nerve, the posterior belly by the digastric branch of the facial nerve. This reflects different embryological origins, from first and second branchial arch mesenchyme respectively. The anterior belly receives its blood supply from the facial artery, the posterior belly from the posterior auricular and occipital arteries.

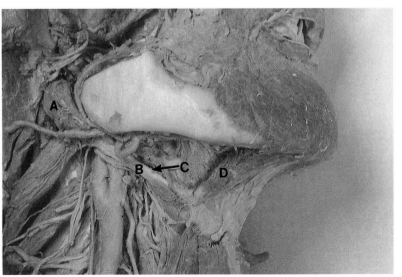

The palate

152 Dissection of the palate — inferior view.

A   Greater palatine nerves and vessels crossing lateral margin of hard palate.
B   Palatoglossus muscle.
C   Palatopharyngeus muscle.
D   Aponeurosis from tensor veli palatini.
E   Muscle fibres in the uvula (musculus uvulae).
F   Pterygoid hamulus.

The levator and tensor veli palatini muscles are also shown in **153**.

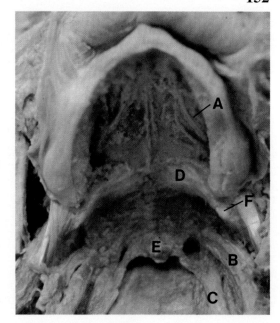

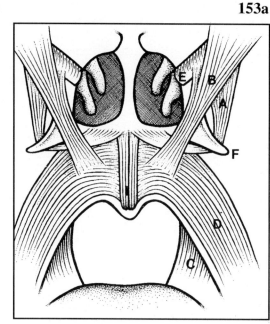

153 The palatal muscles — posterior view (153b) and viewed from the side of the oropharynx (153b).

Functionally, the soft palate is a fibrous aponeurosis whose shape and position is altered by the tensor veli palatini (**A**), the levator veli palatini (**B**), the palatoglossus (**C**) and the palatopharyngeus muscles (**D**).

The tensor veli palatini muscle arises from the scaphoid fossa of the sphenoid bone at the root of the pterygoid plates and from the lateral side of the cartilaginous part of the auditory (pharyngotympanic) tube (**E**). From its origin, the fibres converge towards the pterygoid hamulus (**F**), whence the muscle becomes tendinous, the tendon bending at right angles around the hamulus to become the palatine aponeurosis. The anterior border of the aponeurosis is attached to the posterior border of the hard palate. Medially, it merges with the aponeurosis of the other side. Posteriorly, it becomes indistinct, merging with submucosa at the posterior edge of the soft palate. When the tensor veli palatini muscle contracts, the aponeurosis becomes a taut, horizontal plate of tissue upon which other palatine muscles may act to change its position. The motor innervation of tensor veli palatini is derived from the mandibular branch of the trigeminal nerve via the nerve to the medial pterygoid muscle and the otic ganglion. Levator veli palatini originates from the base of the skull at the apex of the petrous part of the temporal bone, anterior to the opening of the carotid canal, and from the medial side of the cartilaginous part of the auditory tube. The muscle curves downwards, medially and forwards to enter the palate immediately below the opening of the auditory tube.

The levator muscles of the palate form a U-shaped muscular sling. When the palatine aponeurosis is stiffened by the tensor muscles, contraction of the levator muscles produces an upwards and backwards movement of the soft palate. In this way, the nasopharynx is shut off from the oropharynx by the apposition of the soft palate onto the posterior wall of the pharynx. The nerve supply to levator veli palatini is derived from the cranial part of the accessory nerve via the pharyngeal plexus.

The palatopharyngeus muscle arises from two heads, one from the posterior border of the hard palate, the other from the upper surface of the palatine aponeurosis. The two heads unite after arching over the lateral edge of the palatine aponeurosis, where the muscle passes downwards beneath the mucous membrane of the lateral wall of the oropharynx as the posterior pillar of the fauces (palatopharyngeal arch). The muscle is inserted into the posterior border of the thyroid cartilage of the larynx. The main action of the palatopharyngeus muscle is to elevate the larynx and pharynx, but it may also arch the relaxed palate and depress the tensed palate. Its nerve supply is derived from the accessory nerve via the pharyngeal plexus.

Passavant's muscle is a sphincter-like muscle which encircles the pharynx at the level of the palate, inside the fibres of the superior constrictor muscles (**G**). It is formed by fibres arising from the anterior and lateral part of the upper surface of the palatine aponeurosis. Contraction of this muscle forms a ridge (Passavant's ridge) against which the soft palate is elevated.

The salpingopharyngeus muscle (**H**) is a slip of muscle which arises from the cartilage of the auditory tube and passes downwards to converge with the palatopharyngeus muscle.

The palatoglossus muscle is described with the tongue (see **158**). The musculus uvulae (**I**) arises from the posterior nasal spine and the palatine aponeurosis. It inserts into the mucosa of the uvula and moves the uvula upwards and laterally.

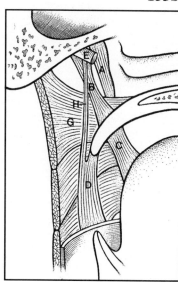

The floor of the mouth and the tongue

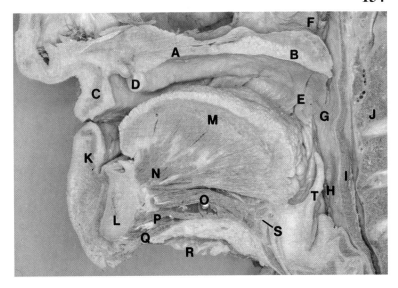

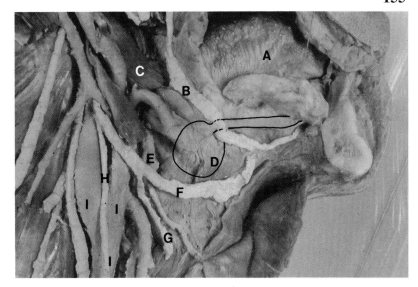

154 Median sagittal section through the head to show the tongue and floor of mouth.

A   Hard palate.
B   Soft palate.
C   Upper lip and superior part of orbicularis oris muscle.
D   Edentulous maxillary alveolar ridge.
E   Pillars of fauces.
F   Nasopharynx.
G   Oropharynx.
H   Laryngopharynx.
I   Constrictor muscles of pharynx.
J   Vertebral column.
K   Lower lip with inferior part of orbicularis oris muscle.
L   Body of mandible.
M   Tongue.
N   Genioglossus muscle.
O   Geniohyoid muscle.
P   Mylohyoid muscle.
Q   Anterior belly of digastric muscle.
R   Platysma muscle.
S   Hyoid bone.
T   Epiglottis.

155 Dissection of deep submandibular region. The body of the mandible has been removed and the position occupied by the deep part of the submandibular salivary gland and by its duct is indicated by the black outline.

A   Tongue.
B   Lingual nerve.
C   Styloglossus muscle.
D   Hyoglossus muscle.
E   Lingual artery.
F   Hypoglossal nerve.
G   Nerve to thyrohyoid muscle.
H   Descendens hypoglossi.
I   Carotid system of arteries.

156 The mylohyoid muscle (A) contributes to a muscular diaphragm for the floor of the mouth. It arises from the mylohyoid line on the medial surface of the body of the mandible (see **24**). Its fibres slope downwards, forwards and inwards. The anterior fibres of the mylohyoid muscle interdigitate with the corresponding fibres on the opposite side to form a median raphe. This raphe is attached above to the chin and below to the hyoid bone. The posterior fibres are inserted onto the anterior surface of the body of the hyoid bone. The muscle raises the floor of the mouth during the early stages of swallowing. It also helps to depress the mandible when the hyoid bone is fixed. The mylohyoid muscle is supplied by the mylohyoid branch of the inferior alveolar branch of the mandibular nerve. **B**, sublingual gland; **C**, deep part of submandibular gland; **D**, submandibular duct (green).

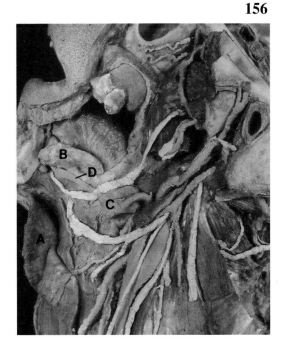

Muscles of the tongue

The intrinsic muscles of the tongue can be divided into three fibre groups: transverse, longitudinal and vertical. Rarely can these three groups be distinguished in dissections, but their interlacing gives the tongue its characteristic appearance in cross-section. The transverse fibres arise from a sheet of connective tissue, called the lingual septum, running longitudinally through the midline of the tongue. These transverse fibres pass laterally from the septum to intercalate with fibres of the other groups of intrinsic muscles. The longitudinal fibres may be subdivided into upper and lower groups, the superior and inferior longitudinal muscles of the tongue. The vertical fibres pass directly between the upper and lower surfaces, particularly at the lateral borders of the tongue. The function of the intrinsic muscles is to change the shape of the tongue. They receive their motor innervation from the hypoglossal cranial nerve.

157

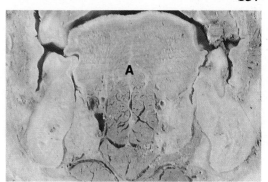

157 Cross-section through tongue illustrating the interlacing of the fibres of the intrinsic muscles. A, lingual septum.

The extrinsic muscles of the tongue arise from the skull and hyoid bone and thence spread into the body of the tongue. The extrinsic musculature is composed of four groups of muscles: genioglossus, hyoglossus, styloglossus, and palatoglossus. The function of the extrinsic muscles is to change the position of the tongue.

158a

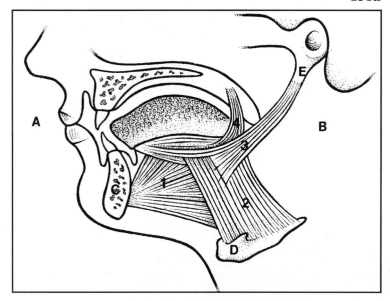

158b

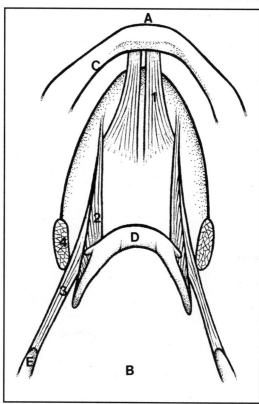

158 The relationships of the extrinsic muscles to the tongue — lateral view (158a) and medial view (158b). A, anterior; **B**, posterior; **C**, mandible; **D**, hyoid bone; **E**, styloid process. The genioglossus muscles (**1**) arise from the superior genial tubercles on the medial surface of the body of the mandible. At this level, the two muscles cannot be readily separated. As the muscles enter the tongue, a thin strip of connective tissue intervenes between the right and left genioglossus muscles. The bulk of the fibres fan out into the body of the tongue, but its superior fibres pass upwards and anteriorly to the tip of the tongue, and some of its inferior fibres insert onto the body of the hyoid bone. The genioglossus is mainly a protractor and depressor of the tongue.

The hyoglossus muscles (**2**) originate from the superior border of the greater horns of the hyoid bone and pass vertically upwards into the tongue. Their function is to depress the tongue. Each styloglossus muscle (**3**) arises from the anterior surface of the styloid process of the temporal bone, from which the muscle runs downwards and forwards to enter the tongue below the insertion of the palatoglossus muscle. At this point, its fibres intercalate with the fibres of the hyoglossus before continuing forwards towards the tip of the tongue. The styloglossus muscle is a retractor of the tongue. Each palatoglossus muscle (**4**) arises from the aponeurosis of the soft palate and descends to the tongue in the anterior pillar of the fauces, whence its fibres intercalate with the transverse fibres of the tongue. The action of the palatoglossus muscles is to raise the tongue in order to narrow the transverse diameter of the oropharyngeal isthmus. The extrinsic muscles of the tongue are innervated by the hypoglossal nerve (except for the palatoglossus, which is innervated by the cranial part of the accessory nerve via the pharyngeal plexus).

The salivary glands

159 The parotid gland (**A**) is the largest of the major salivary glands and secretes a serous saliva. It occupies the region between the ramus of the mandible and the mastoid process. The parotid is pyramidal in shape; its apex extends beyond the angle of the mandible and the base is closely related to the external acoustic meatus (**B**). A deep surface of the gland rests anteriorly on the ramus and masseter muscle and extends around the posterior border of the mandible where it can reach the pharynx. The gland is surrounded by an unyielding capsule which is derived from the investing layer of deep cervical fascia. The parotid duct (Stensen's duct) (**C**) appears at the anterior border of the gland and passes horizontally across the masseter muscle (**D**) before piercing the buccinator to terminate in the oral cavity opposite the maxillary second molar. Lying with the duct on the masseter may be an accessory parotid gland.

Within the parotid gland are found the external carotid artery, the retromandibular vein, and the facial nerve. Branches of the facial nerve (**E**) are seen emerging from the anterior and inferior margins of the gland.

The parotid gland is innervated via the otic ganglion (see **174**), and the parotid capsule by the great auricular nerve (**F**). **G**, facial vessels coursing through muscles of facial expression; **H**, superficial part of the submandibular gland.

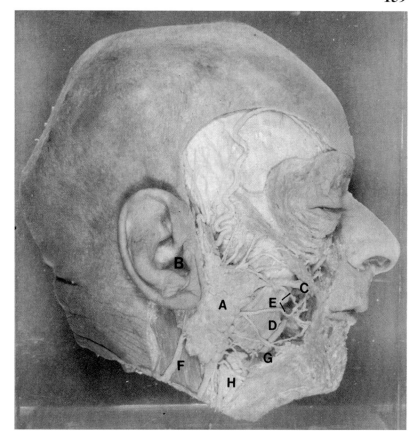

160 The submandibular and sublingual salivary glands. The submandibular gland produces both serous and mucous saliva (in a 3:2 ratio). It is located close to the lower border of the mandible (superficial part of gland; see **159**) and, after turning around the posterior border of the mylohyoid muscle comes to lie in the floor of the mouth (deep part of gland, **A**). The submandibular duct (green — Wharton's duct, **B**) appears from the deep part of the gland and crosses the hyoglossus muscle (**C**) to terminate on the sublingual papilla in the floor of the mouth (see **10**). The sublingual gland (**D**) also produces serous and mucous saliva, but in the ratio 1:3. It is located on the hyoglossus muscle in the floor of the mouth adjacent to the sublingual fossa of the mandible. The gland is associated with the sublingual folds beneath the tongue (see **10**). It may be joined to the deep part of the submandibular gland to form a single sublingual–submandibular complex. The sublingual gland is subdivided into anterior and posterior parts. The ducts of the anterior part may unite to form a large main duct (Bartholin's duct) which either joins the submandibular duct or drains directly onto the sublingual papilla. The ducts from the posterior part of the sublingual gland drain through the sublingual fold.

Both the submandibular and sublingual glands are innervated via the submandibular ganglion (see **175**).

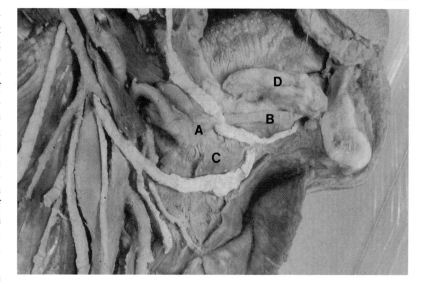

The superficial muscles of the face

The muscles of facial expression are characterised by their superficial arrangement in the face, by their activities on the skin (brought about directly by their attachment to the facial integument), and by their common motor innervation, the facial nerve. They are all derived embryologically from mesenchyme of the second branchial arch. Functionally, the muscles of facial expression are grouped around the orifices of the face (i.e. the orbit, nose, ear and mouth) and should be considered primarily as muscles controlling the degree of opening and closing of these apertures. The expressive functions of the muscles have developed secondarily. The muscles of facial expression vary considerably between individuals in terms of size, shape and strength.

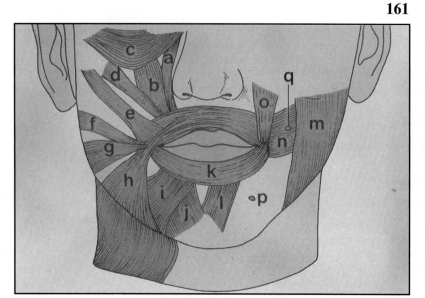

161 & 162 The superficial muscles around the lips and cheeks may be subdivided into two groups: the various parts of the orbicularis oris muscle, and muscles which are radially arranged from the orbicularis oris muscle. The fibres of the orbicularis oris muscle (**k**) pass around the lips. The muscle is divided into four parts, each part corresponding to a quadrant of the lips. Its muscle fibres do not gain attachment directly to bone but occupy a central part of the lip. Muscle fibres in the philtrum insert onto the nasal septum. The range of movement produced by the orbicularis oris muscle includes lip closure, protrusion and pursing. The radial muscles can be divided into superficial and deep muscles of the upper and lower lips. The levator labii superioris (**b**), levator labii superioris alaeque nasi (**a**), and zygomaticus major (**e**) and minor (**d**) are superficial muscles of the upper lip. The levator anguli oris (**o**) is a deep muscle of the upper lip. The depressor anguli oris (**h**) is a superficial muscle of the lower lip, and the depressor labii inferioris (**i**), and mentalis muscles (**j**) are deep muscles of the lower lip. As their names suggest, the levator labii superioris elevates the upper lip, the depressor labii inferioris depresses the lower lip, and the corners of the mouth are raised and lowered by the levator and depressor anguli oris muscles.

Two muscles extend to the corner of the mouth, the risorius (**f**) and buccinator (**n**) muscles. The risorius muscle lies superficial to the buccinator muscle. The risorius muscle stretches the angles of the mouth laterally. The buccinator arises from the pterygomandibular raphe, and from the buccal side of the maxillary and mandibular alveoli above the molar teeth. Most of its fibres insert into mucous membrane covering the cheek; other fibres intercalate with the orbicularis oris muscle in the lips. As the fibres of the buccinator converge towards the angle of the mouth, the central fibres decussate. The main function of the buccinator muscle is to maintain the tension of the cheek against the teeth during mastication.

Also shown on the diagram are the inferior fibres of the orbicularis oculi (**c**), the platysma (**g**), and the masseter (**m**) muscles, the mental foramen (**p**) and the passage of the parotid duct through the buccinator muscle (**q**).

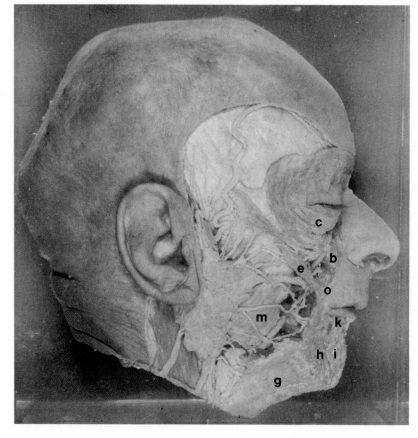

The deep face — the infratemporal fossa

163 The infratemporal fossa is the region located deep to the ramus of the mandible (**A**). It is bounded anteriorly by the posterior surface of the maxilla (**B**), posteriorly by the styloid apparatus (**C**), carotid sheath, and deep part of the parotid gland. Medially lie the lateral pterygoid plate and the superior constrictor of the pharynx. The roof is formed by the infratemporal surface of the greater wing of the sphenoid. The infratemporal fossa has no floor, being continuous with the neck. The fossa contains the lateral pterygoid (**D**) and medial pterygoid (**E**) muscles, branches of the mandibular nerve (including the inferior alveolar (**F**) and lingual (**G**) nerves), the chorda tympani branch of the facial nerve, the otic ganglion, the maxillary artery and the pterygoid venous plexus.

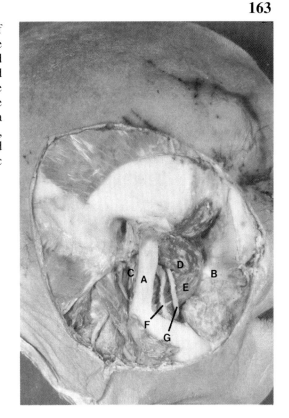

164 The maxillary air sinus (or antrum, A) is the largest of the paranasal air sinuses. It is situated in the body of the maxilla. The sinus is pyramidal in shape. The base (medial wall) forms part of the lateral wall of the nose. The apex extends into the zygomatic process of the maxilla. The roof of the sinus is part of the floor of the orbit, and the floor of the sinus is formed by the alveolar process, and part of the palatine process, of the maxilla. The anterior wall of the sinus is the facial surface of the maxilla, and the posterior wall is the infratemporal surface of the maxilla. The maxillary sinus may be partially divided by incomplete bony septa. Running in the roof of the sinus is the infra-orbital nerve and vessels. Within the floor of the sinus are the roots of the maxillary cheek teeth (see **21**). The anterior superior alveolar nerve and vessels run in the anterior wall of the sinus. The posterior superior alveolar nerve and vessels pass through canals in the posterior surface of the sinus.

The medial wall of the maxillary air sinus contains the opening (ostium) of the sinus (see **184a**). This ostium lies high up, being unfavourably situated for drainage. It opens into the hiatus semilunaris of the middle meatus of the lateral wall of the nose. The osteology of the ostium has been described previously (see **19**).

The maxillary air sinus is lined by ciliated columnar epithelium and is innervated by the infra-orbital and superior alveolar branches of the maxillary nerve.

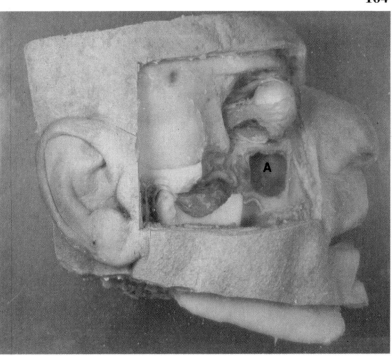

Tissue spaces around the jaws

The dissemination of infection in soft tissues is influenced by the natural barriers presented by bone, muscle and fascia. Around the jaws are body compartments, the so-called tissue spaces, whose boundaries are primarily defined by the mylohyoid, buccinator, masseter, medial pterygoid, superior constrictor and orbicularis oris muscles. The fascial layers of the neck are less important in influencing the spread of infection around the jaws. None of the 'spaces' are actually empty; they are potential spaces normally occupied by loose connective tissue. It is only when inflammatory products destroy the loose connective tissue that an anatomically defined space is produced.

The most important potential spaces are:

Lower jaw	Upper jaw
1. Submental.	10. Palatal.
2. Submandibular.	11. Canine fossa.
3. Sublingual.	12. Infratemporal.
4. Buccal.	
5. Submasseteric.	
6. Parotid.	The spaces are paired except for the submental, submandibular and palatal spaces.
7. Pterygomandibular.	
8. Parapharyngeal.	
9. Peritonsillar.	

165 The relationships of tissue spaces around the mandibular ramus.

1. Body of mandible bearing the molar teeth.
2. Ramus of mandible.
3. Buccinator muscle.
4. Mylohyoid muscle.
5. Buccal pad of fat.
6. Superior constrictor muscle.
7. Mucosa overlying palatal tonsil.
8. Medial pterygoid muscle.
9. Masseter muscle.
10. Parotid gland.
11. Stylomandibular ligament.
12. Base of skull.
A Sublingual space in the floor of the mouth above the mylohyoid muscle which, over its posterior margin, leads to:
B Submandibular space.
C Buccal vestibule, delineated by the buccinator from:
D Buccal space.
E Submasseteric spaces formed by the multiple insertion of the masseter muscle on the lateral surface of the ramus.
F Pterygomandibular space bounded by the lateral surface of the medial pterygoid muscle and the medial surface of the ramus.
G Parapharyngeal space bounded by the superior constrictor of the pharynx and the medial surface of the medial pterygoid muscle.
H Peritonsillar space bounded by the medial surface of the superior constrictor of the pharynx and its mucosa.
I Parotid space (in and around the parotid gland).

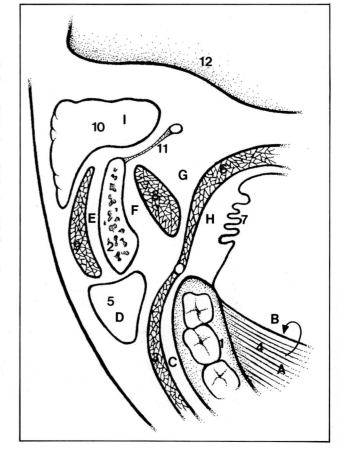

The parapharyngeal space is particularly prone to infections from the jaws and teeth. This space is restricted to the suprahyoid region of the neck and the infratemporal region. For infection to spread inferiorly from the parapharyngeal space, it must first pass into the retropharyngeal region, since suprahyoid structures (particularly the sheath around the submandibular gland formed by the investing layer of deep cervical fascia) provide a restrictive inferior boundary.

166 Inferior view of the submental and submandibular tissue spaces.

1. Body of mandible.
2. Hyoid bone.
3. Anterior belly of digastric muscle.
4. Posterior belly of digastric muscle.
5. Mylohyoid muscle.
6. Masseter muscle.
7. Medial pterygoid muscle.

A The submental space lying between the mylohyoid muscle and the investing layer of deep cervical fascia. Laterally, it is bounded by the two anterior bellies of the digastric muscles. The submental space communicates posteriorly with:
B The submandibular space.

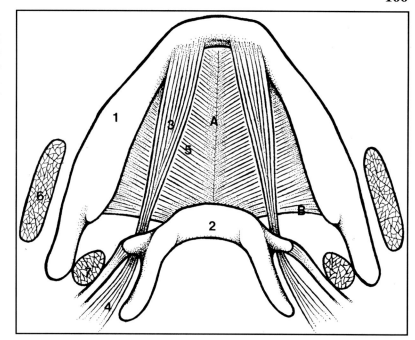

167 The relationships of a number of tissue spaces to the tongue.

1. Tongue.
2. Body of mandible.
3. Hyoid bone.
4. Mylohyoid muscle.
5. Hyoglossus.
6. Genioglossus.
7. Sublingual salivary gland.
8. Submandibular salivary gland.

A Cleft between genioglossus and hyoglossus muscles which communicates directly with the parapharyngeal space.
B Sublingual space between the mylohyoid and hyoglossus muscles.
C Submandibular space below the mylohyoid muscle.

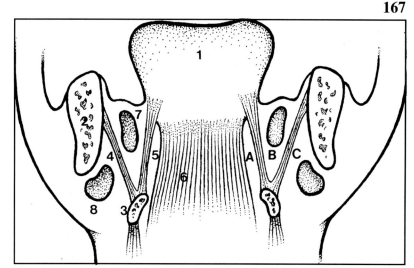

In the anterior region of both the upper and lower jaws, the orbicularis oris muscle presents a barrier to pus between the vestibule on the oral side and the skin of the lip on the facial side.

In the upper jaw, pus may accumulate between the muscles of facial expression, particularly in the canine fossa between the levator labii superioris and zygomaticus muscles.

The palatal space only exists when pus strips the mucoperiosteum from the underlying bone of the hard palate.

The infratemporal space is the upper extremity of the pterygomandibular space and is closely related to the maxillary tuberosity and, therefore, the maxillary molars.

The way in which infections of dental origin spread through the bone of the jaws into the tissue spaces naturally depends upon the site at which the pus escapes the bone. Thus, a periapical abscess in a mandibular incisor which escapes inferior to the mylohyoid muscle will enter the submental space, while pus escaping superior to this muscle will enter the sublingual space. It should also be borne in mind that the tissue spaces are not discrete regions; they intercommunicate. Thus, a sublingual abscess may spread from the sublingual space over the posterior margin of the mylohyoid muscle into the submandibular space (see **165**). Furthermore, none of the muscle or fascial barriers defining the spaces are impenetrable.

The vasculature and innervation of the mouth

Blood supply to oro-dental tissues

The face is supplied mainly through the facial artery (see **159**). This artery first appears on the face as it hooks round the lower border of the mandible, at the anterior edge of the masseter. It then runs a tortuous course between the facial muscles towards the medial angle of the eye. There is a rich anastomosis with the artery of the opposite side and with additional vessels supplying the face (transverse facial branch of the superficial temporal artery; infra-orbital and mental branches of the maxillary artery; and the dorsal nasal branch of the ophthalmic artery).

The main arteries to the teeth and jaws are derived from the maxillary artery, a terminal branch of the external carotid. The alveolar arteries follow roughly the same course as the alveolar nerves.

Mandibular teeth and periodontium. The inferior alveolar artery which supplies the mandibular teeth is derived from the maxillary artery before it crosses the lateral pterygoid muscle in the infratemporal fossa. A mylohyoid branch is given off before the inferior alveolar artery enters the mandibular foramen. The inferior alveolar artery passes through the mandibular foramen to enter the mandibular canal and terminates as the mental and incisive arteries.

Posteriorly, the buccal gingiva is supplied by the buccal artery (a branch of the maxillary artery as it crosses the lateral pterygoid muscle) and by perforating branches from the inferior alveolar artery. Anteriorly, the labial gingiva is supplied by the mental artery and by perforating branches of the incisive artery. The lingual gingiva is supplied by perforating branches from the inferior alveolar artery and by the lingual artery of the external carotid.

Maxillary teeth and periodontium. The posterior superior alveolar artery arises from the maxillary artery in the pterygopalatine fossa. Occasionally, it is derived from the buccal artery. It courses tortuously over the maxillary tuberosity before entering bony canals to supply molar and premolar teeth. The artery also gives off branches to the adjacent buccal gingiva, maxillary sinus and cheek.

The middle superior alveolar artery, when present, arises from the infra-orbital artery (which is itself a branch of the third part of the maxillary artery in the pterygopalatine fossa). The middle superior alveolar artery runs in the lateral wall of the maxillary sinus, terminating near the canine tooth where it anastomoses with the anterior and posterior superior alveolar arteries. The anterior superior alveolar artery also arises from the infra-orbital artery and runs downwards in the anterior wall of the maxillary sinus to supply the anterior teeth. Like the superior alveolar nerves, the superior alveolar arteries form plexuses.

The buccal gingiva around the posterior maxillary teeth is supplied by gingival and perforating branches from the posterior superior alveolar artery and by the buccal artery. The labial gingiva of anterior teeth is supplied by labial branches of the infra-orbital artery and by perforating branches of the anterior superior alveolar artery.

The palatal gingiva is supplied primarily by branches of the greater palatine artery, a branch of the third part of the maxillary artery in the pterygopalatine fossa.

The palate, cheek, tongue and lips. The palate derives its blood supply from the greater and lesser palatine branches of the maxillary artery. The greater palatine artery passes through the incisive foramen, where it anastomoses with the nasopalatine artery.

The cheek is supplied by the buccal branch of the maxillary artery, and the floor of the mouth and the tongue by the lingual arteries. The lips are mainly supplied by the superior and inferior labial branches of the facial arteries.

Venous drainage of oro-dental tissues

The venous drainage of this region is extremely variable. The facial vein is the main vein draining the face. It begins at the medial corner of the eye by confluence of the supra-orbital and supratrochlear veins and passes across the face behind the facial artery. Below the mandible it joins with the anterior branch of the retromandibular vein to form the common facial vein.

Teeth and periodontium. Small veins from the teeth and alveolar bone pass into larger veins surrounding the apex of each tooth, or into veins running in the interdental septa. In the mandible, the veins are then collected into one or more inferior alveolar veins, which themselves may drain anteriorly through the mental foramen to join the facial veins or posteriorly through the mandibular foramen to join the pterygoid plexus of veins in the infratemporal fossa. In the maxilla, the veins may drain anteriorly into the facial vein or posteriorly into the pterygoid plexus. No accurate description is available concerning the venous drainage of the gingiva, though it may be assumed that the buccal, lingual, greater palatine and nasopalatine veins are involved; apart from the lingual veins which pass directly into the internal jugular veins, these veins run into the pterygoid plexuses.

The palate, cheek, tongue and lips. The veins of the palate are rather diffuse and variable. However, those of the hard palate generally pass into the pterygoid plexus, those of the soft palate into the pharyngeal plexus. The buccal vein of the cheek drains into the pterygoid venous plexus. Venous blood from the lips drains into the facial veins via superior and inferior labial veins. The veins of the tongue follow two different routes. Those of the dorsum and sides of the tongue form the lingual veins which, accompanying the lingual arteries, empty into the internal jugular veins. Those of the ventral surface form the deep lingual veins, which ultimately join the facial, internal jugular or lingual veins.

Lymphatic drainage of oro-dental tissues

As with the venous system, the lymphatic drainage is extremely variable. Lymphatics from the lower part of the face generally pass through or around buccal lymph nodes to reach submandibular lymph nodes. However, lymphatics from the medial portion of the lower lip drain into the submental nodes.

168 Lymphatic drainage of oral structures. A, submental nodes; **B**, submandibular nodes; **C**, jugulodigastric nodes.

The lymph vessels from the teeth usually run directly into the submandibular nodes on the same side. However, lymph from the mandibular incisors drains into the submental nodes. Occasionally, lymph from the molars passes directly into the jugulodigastric group of nodes.

The lymph vessels of the labial and buccal gingivae of the maxillary and mandibular teeth unite to drain into the submandibular nodes, though in the labial region of the mandibular incisors they may drain into the submental nodes. The lingual and palatal gingivae drain into the jugulodigastric group of nodes either directly or indirectly through the submandibular nodes.

Lymphatics from most areas of the palate terminate in the jugulodigastric group of nodes. Vessels from the posterior part of the soft palate terminate in pharyngeal lymph nodes.

Lymphatics from the anterior two-thirds of the tongue may be subdivided into two groups: marginal and central vessels. The marginal lymphatic vessels drain the lateral third of the dorsal surface of the tongue and the lateral margin of its ventral surface. The remaining regions drain into the central vessels. The marginal vessels pass to the submandibular lymph nodes of the same side. The central vessels at the tip of the tongue pass to the submental lymph nodes. Central vessels behind the tip drain into ipsilateral and contralateral submandibular lymph nodes. Some marginal and central lymph vessels pass directly to the jugulodigastric group of nodes (or even the juguloomohyoid nodes). Lymphatics from the posterior third of the tongue drain into the deep cervical group of nodes, vessels centrally draining both ipsilaterally and contralaterally.

At the oropharyngeal isthmus lie the palatine tonsils between the pillars of the fauces and the lingual tonsils on the pharyngeal surface of the tongue. These tonsils form part of a ring of lymphoid tissue known as Waldeyer's tonsillar ring. The other components are the tubal tonsils and adenoid tissue (pharyngeal tonsils) located in the nasopharynx.

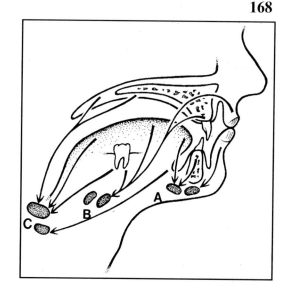

Innervation of oro-dental tissues

Excepting regions around the oropharyngeal isthmus, the oral mucosa receives sensory innervation from the maxillary and mandibular divisions of the trigeminal nerve. The trigeminal nerve also supplies the teeth and their supporting tissues (Table 9). Both the major and minor salivary glands are supplied by secretomotor parasympathetic fibres from the facial and glossopharyngeal nerves. The motor innervation of the muscles related to the jaws and oral cavity is from the trigeminal, facial, accessory and hypoglossal nerves.

169 Cutaneous innervation of the face.

A Supra-orbital nerve.
B Supratrochlear nerve.
C Infratrochlear nerve.
D External nasal nerve.
E Lacrimal nerve.
F Zygomaticotemporal nerve.
G Zygomaticofacial nerve.
H Infra-orbital nerve.
I Auriculotemporal nerve.
J Buccal nerve.
K Mental nerve.
L Great auricular nerve.

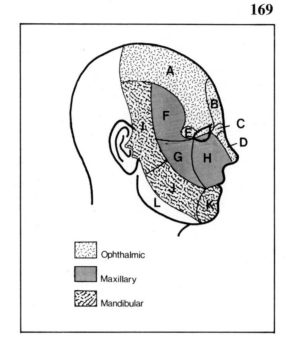

Ophthalmic

Maxillary

Mandibular

Table 9: Nerve supply to the teeth and gingivae.

Maxilla	Nasopalatine nerve	Greater palatine nerve		Palatal gingiva
	Anterior superior alveolar nerve	Middle superior alveolar nerve	Posterior superior alveolar nerve	Teeth
	Infra-orbital nerve	Posterior superior alveolar nerve and buccal nerve		Buccal gingiva
	1 2 3 4 5 6 7 8			Tooth position (Zsigmondy system)
Mandible	Mental nerve	Buccal nerve and perforating branches of inferior alveolar nerve		Buccal gingiva
	Incisive nerve	Inferior alveolar nerve		Teeth
	Lingual nerve and perforating branches of inferior alveolar nerve			Lingual gingiva

170 The course of the inferior alveolar nerve through the mandible. The distribution of nerves to the premolars and molars is variable, dental branches either coming directly from the inferior alveolar nerve by short (**A**) or long (**B**) branches or indirectly through several alveolar branches (**C**). In rare instances, the nerve to the mandibular third molar may arise from the inferior alveolar nerve before it enters the mandibular canal. Communications between the inferior alveolar nerve and nerves from the temporalis and lateral pterygoid muscles have been described, the nerves penetrating the mandible through foraminae in the region of muscle attachments. It has been suggested that such nerve connections might explain why, in approximately 5% of patients, the teeth need not be anaesthetised after the main trunk of the inferior alveolar nerve has been blocked at the mandibular foramen by the injection of local anaesthetic solution.

It is said that, in any one individual, the mandibular canal remains in a relatively fixed position with respect to the lower border of the mandible. The canal is often closely related to the roots of the mandibular molars. Indeed, the roots of lower third molars may even be perforated by the mandibular canal.

In the premolar region, the main trunk of the inferior alveolar nerve divides into mental and incisive nerves. The mental nerve runs for a short distance in a mental canal before leaving the body of the mandible at the mental foramen to emerge onto the face. In about 50% of cases, the mental foramen lies on a vertical line passing through the mandibular second premolar. However, in negroid races the mental foramen may be situated slightly more posteriorly, midway between the roots of the second premolar and first permanent molar. In an adult with a full dentition, the mental foramen usually lies midway between the upper and lower borders of the mandible. During the first and second years of life, as the prominence of the chin develops, the opening of the mental foramen alters in direction from facing forwards to facing upwards and backwards. As well as supplying the skin of the lower lip, the mental nerve provides fibres to an incisor plexus which innervates the labial periodontium of the mandibular incisors. The incisive nerve runs forwards in an intraosseous incisive canal. This nerve primarily supplies the incisors and canine teeth but may also supply the first premolar. In some instances, the canine may be supplied directly from the inferior alveolar nerve.

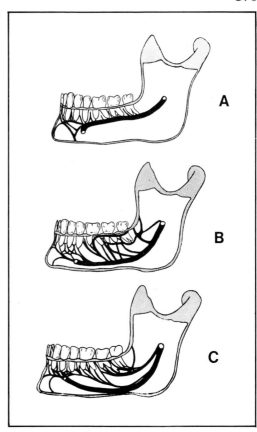

171 The superior alveolar nerves and associated dental plexuses. A, maxillary nerve; **B**, infra-orbital nerve; **C**, pterygopalatine fossa; **D**, **E**, and **F**, posterior, middle and anterior superior alveolar nerves respectively.

The posterior superior alveolar nerve arises from the maxillary nerve in the pterygopalatine fossa whence it descends to the posterior wall of the maxilla. The dental branches of the nerve enter the maxilla and run in narrow posterior superior alveolar canals above the roots of the molar teeth. The gingival branch does not enter the bone, however, but runs downwards and forwards along the outer surface of the maxillary tuberosity.

The middle superior alveolar nerve is found in about 70% of subjects. The nerve generally arises from the infra-orbital nerve in the floor of the orbit, though alternatively it may arise from the maxillary nerve in the pterygopalatine fossa. The nerve may run in the posterior, lateral or anterior walls of the maxillary sinus. It terminates above the roots of the premolar teeth.

The anterior superior alveolar nerve arises from the infra-orbital nerve within the infra-orbital canal, generally as a single nerve but occasionally as two or three small branches. The nerve leaves the infra-orbital canal near its termination and then, diverging laterally from the infra-orbital nerve, runs in the anterior wall of the maxillary sinus. It terminates near the anterior nasal spine after giving off a small nasal branch.

The superior alveolar nerve forms a plexus above the root apices of the maxillary teeth. From this plexus nerves pass to the teeth, though it is difficult to trace the precise innervation of the teeth from specific superior alveolar nerves. As a general rule, however, the incisors and canine are supplied by the anterior nerve, the molars by the posterior nerve and intermediate areas by the middle nerve.

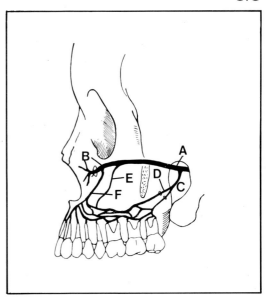

172 The sensory nerve supply to the palate is derived from the branches of the pterygopalatine ganglion. A small area behind the incisor teeth is supplied by terminal branches of the nasopalatine nerves (**A**). These nerves emerge onto the palate at the incisive foramen. The remainder of the hard palate is supplied by the greater palatine nerves (**B**), emerging onto the palate at the greater palatine foraminae. The soft palate is supplied by the lesser palatine nerves (**C**), emerging onto the palate via the lesser palatine foraminae. Thus, the maxillary division of the trigeminal nerve supplies most of the palate. However, there is evidence to suggest that some areas supplied by the lesser palatine nerves may also be innervated by fibres from the facial nerve. The posterior part of the soft palate and the uvula may be supplied by the glossopharyngeal nerve.

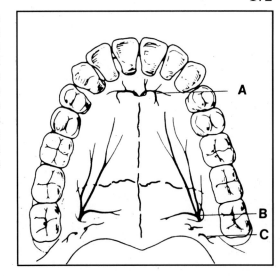

173 Sensory innervation of the tongue. Three distinct nerve fields can be recognised on the dorsum of the tongue. The anterior part of the tongue, in front of the circumvallate papillae, is supplied by the lingual nerve (although its accompanying chorda tympani fibres are those associated with the perception of taste). Behind and including the circumvallate papillae, the tongue is supplied primarily by the glossopharyngeal nerve (providing both general sensation and taste). A small area on the posterior part of the tongue around the epiglottis is supplied by the vagus nerve via its superior laryngeal branch. The mucosa on the ventral surface of the tongue is supplied by the lingual nerve.

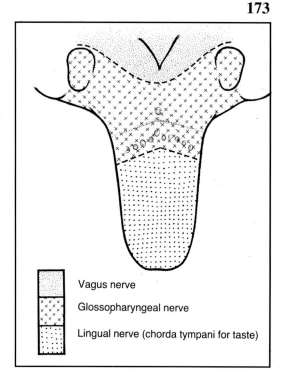

Vagus nerve

Glossopharyngeal nerve

Lingual nerve (chorda tympani for taste)

The mucosa of the upper lip is supplied by the infra-orbital branch of the maxillary division of the trigeminal nerve. That of the lower lip is supplied by the mental branch of the mandibular division of the trigeminal nerve. The mucosa of the cheeks is supplied by the buccal branch of the mandibular division of the trigeminal. The mucosa on the floor of the mouth is innervated by the lingual nerve. The mucosa over the pillars of the fauces is supplied by the glossopharyngeal nerve.

The secretomotor innervation of the salivary glands

174 The secretomotor supply of the parotid gland is derived through the otic parasympathetic ganglion (**A**). This ganglion is situated in the roof of the infratemporal fossa, close to the foramen ovale and the mandibular nerve. Like other parasympathetic ganglia in the head, three types of nerve fibre are associated with it: parasympathetic, sympathetic and sensory. However, only the parasympathetic fibres synapse in the ganglion. The preganglionic parasympathetic fibres to the otic ganglion originate from the inferior salivatory nucleus (**B**) in the brainstem and pass with the glosso-pharyngeal nerve via its lesser petrosal branch (**C**). The sympathetic root of the otic ganglion is derived from postganglionic fibres from the superior cervical ganglion (**D**) and reach the otic ganglion via the plexus around the middle meningeal artery (**E**) in the infratemporal fossa. The sensory root is derived from the auriculo-temporal branch (**F**) of the mandibular division of the trigeminal nerve. The postganglionic parasympathetic fibres (with sensory and sympathetic fibres) reach the parotid gland (**G**) through the auriculotemporal nerve.

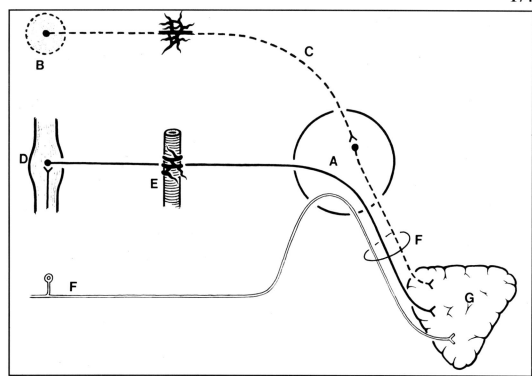

175 The secretomotor supply of the sub-mandibular and sublingual glands is derived through the submandibular parasympathetic ganglion (**A**). This ganglion is situated, with the lingual nerve, on the hyoglossus muscle in the floor of the mouth above the deep part of the submandibular gland (see **155**). The pregan-glionic parasympathetic fibres to the ganglion originate from the superior salivatory nucleus (**B**) in the brainstem and pass with the nervus intermedius of the facial nerve, and subsequent-ly its chorda tympani branch (**C**), to reach the lingual nerve in the infratemporal fossa. It is via the lingual nerve that the preganglionic fibres are conveyed to the submandibular ganglion. The sympathetic root of the ganglion is derived from postganglionic fibres from the superior cervical ganglion (**D**) and reach the submandib-ular ganglion via the plexus around the facial artery (**E**). The sensory root is derived from the lingual nerve (**F**). The postganglionic para-sympathetic fibres (with sensory and sympa-thetic fibres) pass directly to the adjacent sub-mandibular gland (**G**) but reach the sublingual gland (**H**) after re-entering the lingual nerve.

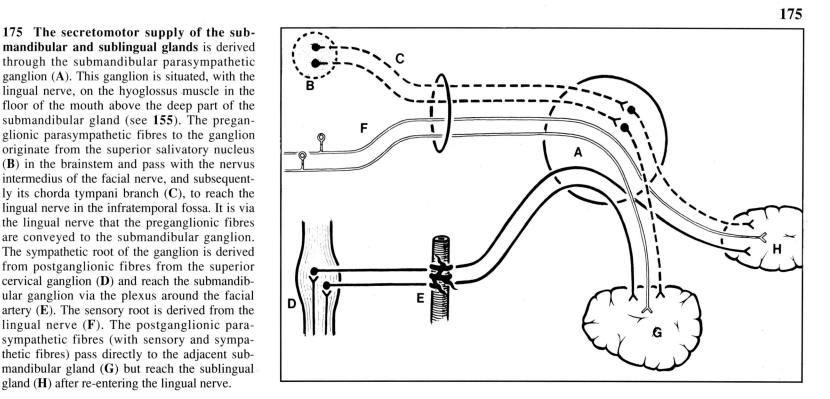

The innervation of the oral musculature

Table 10: Innervation of the oral musculature.

Region	Muscle	Nerve
Lips	Orbicularis oris	Facial
Cheeks	Buccinator	Facial
Tongue (intrinsic musculature)	Transverse Longitudinal Vertical	Hypoglossal
Tongue (extrinsic musculature)	Genioglossus Hyoglossus Styloglossus	Hypoglossal
	Palatoglossus	Accessory (cranial part)
Floor of mouth	Mylohyoid	Mandibular division of trigeminal
	Geniohyoid	Hypoglossal (C1 fibres)
Palate	Tensor veli palatini	Mandibular division of trigeminal
	Levator veli palatini Palatoglossus Palatopharyngeus Salpingopharyngeus Muscululus uvulae	Accessory (cranial part)

The trigeminal nerve (maxillary and mandibular divisions)

176 The maxillary nerve is a division of the trigeminal nerve and contains only sensory fibres. It supplies the maxillary teeth and their supporting structures, the palate, the maxillary air sinus, much of the nasal cavity, and skin overlying the middle part of the face. The nerve emerges into the pterygopalatine fossa through the foramen rotundum (**A**) of the sphenoid bone. Its subsequent branches can be subdivided into branches from the main nerve trunk and branches from the pterygopalatine ganglion (see **177**). From the main trunk are the meningeal (**B**), ganglionic (**C**), zygomatic (**D**), posterior superior alveolar (**E**) and infra-orbital nerves (**F**). The infra-orbital nerve gives rise to the middle (**G**) and anterior (**H**) superior alveolar nerves.

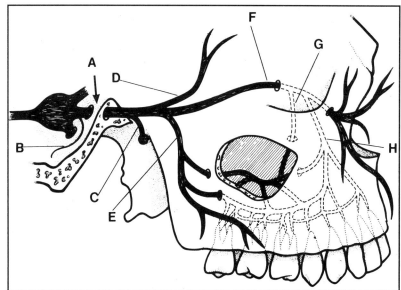

177 The branches of the maxillary nerve via the pterygopalatine ganglion (**A**) contain a mixture of sensory, parasympathetic (secretomotor) and sympathetic (vasomotor) fibres. The branches arising from the ganglion are the orbital, nasopalatine (**B**), posterior superior nasal (**C**), greater (**D**) and lesser palatine (**E**), and pharyngeal nerves (**F**).

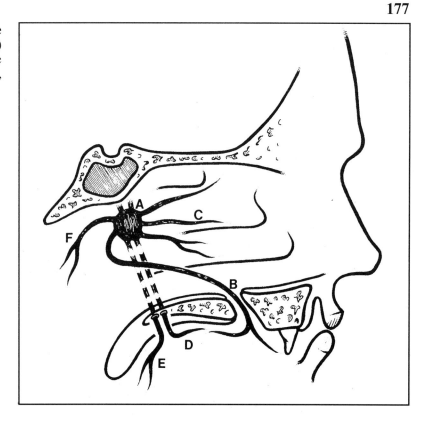

178 The mandibular nerve is the largest division of the trigeminal nerve. It is the only division that contains motor fibres as well as sensory fibres. Its sensory fibres supply the mandibular teeth (and their supporting structures), the mucosa of the anterior two-thirds of the tongue and the floor of the mouth, the skin of the lower part of the face, and parts of the temple and auricle. Its motor fibres supply the muscles of mastication, the mylohyoid, anterior belly of the digastric, and the tensor veli palatini and tensor tympani muscles. The mandibular nerve emerges into the infratemporal fossa through the foramen ovale of the sphenoid bone. It lies deep to the lateral pterygoid muscle, where it gives off all its branches, dividing into anterior (mainly motor) and posterior (mainly sensory) trunks. Proximal to this division, it gives off the meningeal branch (**A**) and the nerve to the medial pterygoid (**B**). The anterior trunk (**C**) gives motor branches to the masseter, temporalis and lateral pterygoid, and the sensory buccal nerve (**D**). The posterior trunk gives off the sensory auriculotemporal (**E**), lingual (**F**) and inferior alveolar (**G**) nerves, and the motor mylohyoid nerve (**H**). Note that the chorda tympani branch (**I**) of the facial nerve joins the lingual nerve.

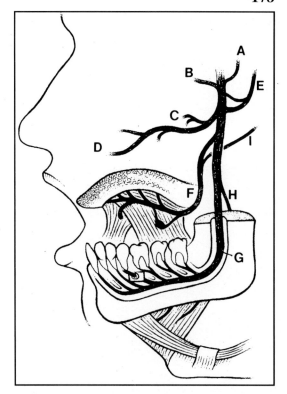

179 Central connections of the trigeminal nerve. The trigeminal nerve conveys discriminative tactile information from the ipsilateral half of the face and the top of the head; the axons of the trigeminal ganglion cells pass to the principal sensory nucleus and to the pars oralis of the spinal tract of the trigeminal nerve. Proprioceptive information from the ipsilateral muscles of mastication and the temporomandibular joint reach the mesencephalic nucleus of the trigeminal. However, recent evidence suggests that proprioceptive information from the teeth also pass to the principal sensory nucleus. Direct and indirect connections of these nuclei form the basis of cranial nerve reflexes. Signals from the principal sensory and mesencephalic nuclei are transmitted mainly via the contralateral ventral trigeminothalamic tract (trigeminal lemniscus) and the ipsilateral dorsal trigeminothalamic tract to the nucleus ventralis posterior medialis of the thalamus. Axons from this nucleus pass through the posterior limb of the internal capsule to the inferior part of the postcentral gyrus and frontoparietal operculum. The nucleus of the spinal tract of the trigeminal is subdivided into the pars oralis, pars interpolaris and pars caudalis. The pars oralis deals mainly with tactile signals. The pars interpolaris receives cutaneous and proprioceptive information and sends fibres to the cerebellum. The pars caudalis deals particularly with nociceptive signals (but also with tactile and thermal information). Fibres from the nucleus of the spinal tract pass to the reticular formation (for cranial nerve reflexes). Some fibres run near the medial lemniscus in the contralateral ventral trigeminothalamic tract to reach the various thalamic nuclei. The motor nucleus of the trigeminal nerve lies close to the principal central nucleus in the central part of the pons. It receives fibres from the other sensory trigeminal nuclei, the reticular formation, the cerebellum and the cerebral cortex via bilateral corticonuclear fibres.

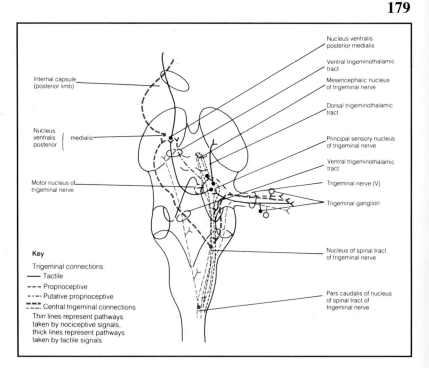

Sectional anatomy of the oral cavity and related areas

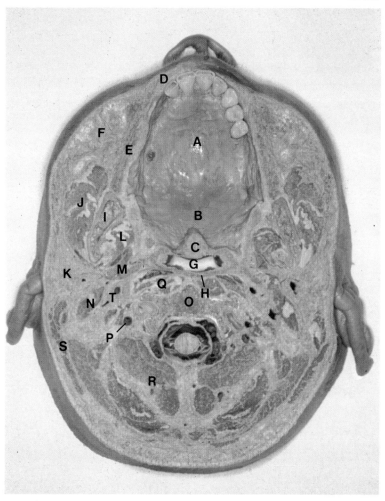

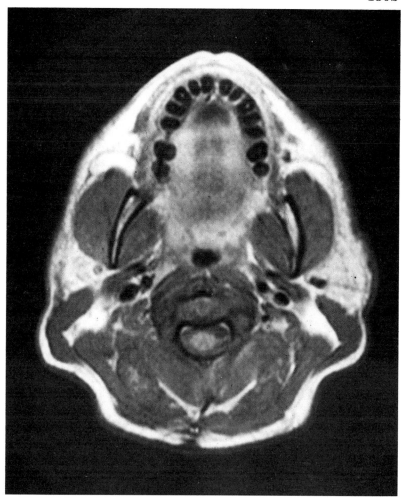

180a Transverse section through the head to show the palate and its topographic relationships

180b NMR scan of the head at the level of the palate.

A	Hard palate.	M	Styloid group of muscles: stylopharyngeus, stylohyoid, styloglossus.
B	Soft palate.		
C	Uvula.		
D	Upper lip.	N	Posterior belly of digastric muscle.
E	Buccinator muscle.		
F	Buccal pad of fat.	O	Axis (second cervical vertebra).
G	Nasopharynx.		
H	Superior constrictor muscle of pharynx.	P	Vertebral artery.
		Q	Prevertebral muscles.
I	Ramus of mandible.	R	Postvertebral muscles.
J	Masseter muscle.	S	Sternocleidomastoid muscle.
K	Parotid gland.	T	Internal carotid artery and internal jugular vein.
L	Medial pterygoid muscle.		

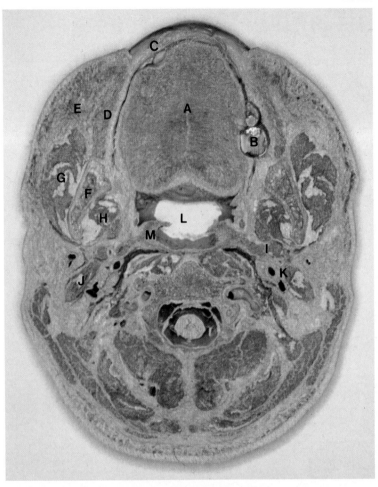

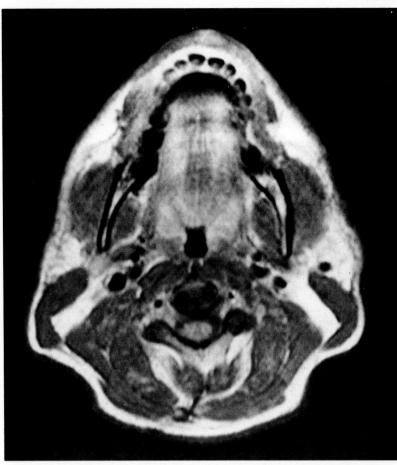

181a Transverse section through the head at the level of the palatine tonsil to show the tongue and its topographic relationships.

181b NMR scan of the head at the level of the tongue and palatine tonsil.

A   Tongue.
B   Mandibular molar.
C   Lower lip.
D   Buccinator muscle.
E   Buccal pad of fat.
F   Ramus of mandible.
G   Masseter muscle.
H   Medial pterygoid muscle.
I   Styloid group of muscles.

J   Posterior belly of digastric muscle.
K   Carotid sheath containing internal carotid artery, internal jugular vein and vagus nerve.
L   Oropharynx.
M   Palatopharyngeus muscle.

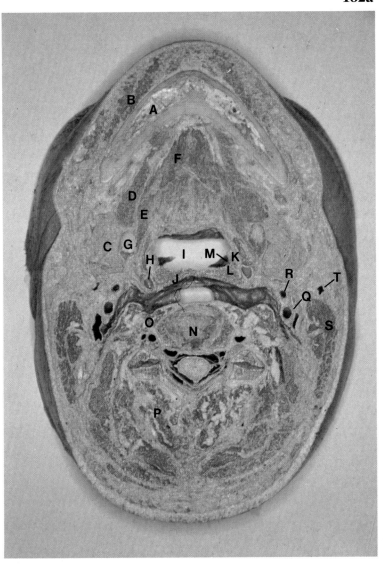

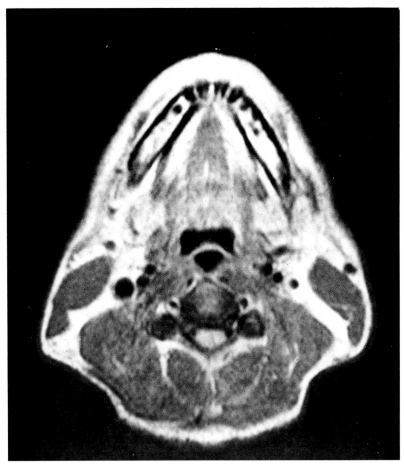

182b   NMR scan of the head at the level of the floor of the mouth.

182a   Transverse section through the head to show the floor of the mouth and its topographic relationships.

A   Body of mandible.
B   Depressor labii superioris and depressor anguli oris muscles.
C   Submandibular gland.
D   Mylohyoid muscle.
E   Hyoglossus muscle.
F   Genioglossus muscle.
G   Tendon of digastric muscle.
H   Tip of greater horn of hyoid bone.
I   Oropharynx.
J   Middle constrictor muscle of pharynx.
K   Palatoglossal fold ⎱
L   Palatopharyngeal fold ⎰ Pillars of the fauces.
M   Tonsillar crypt.
N   Cervical vertebra.
O   Prevertebral group of muscles.
P   Postvertebral group of muscles.
Q   Carotid sheath containing internal carotid artery, internal jugular vein and vagus nerve.
R   External carotid artery.
S   Sternocleidomastoid muscle.
T   External jugular vein.

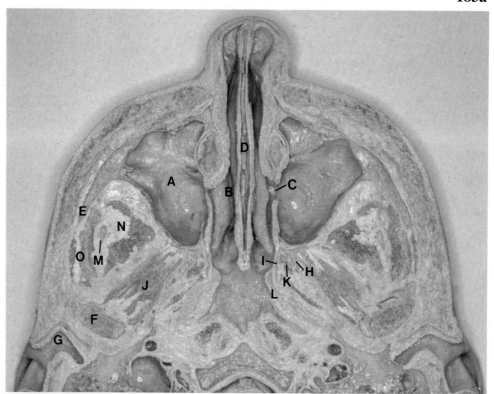

183a Transverse section through head to show the maxillary air sinuses and their topographic relationships.

A Floor of maxillary air sinus.
B Nasal fossa.
C Ostium — opening of maxillary sinus into middle meatus on the lateral wall of the nose.
D Nasal septum.
E Zygomatic arch.
F Condyle of mandible.
G External acoustic meatus.
H Lateral pterygoid plate of sphenoid bone.
I Medial pterygoid plate of sphenoid bone.
J Lateral pterygoid muscle.
K Medial pterygoid muscle.
L Superior constrictor of pharynx.
M Coronoid process of mandible.
N Temporalis muscle.
O Masseter muscle.

183b NMR scan of the head to show maxillary air sinuses.

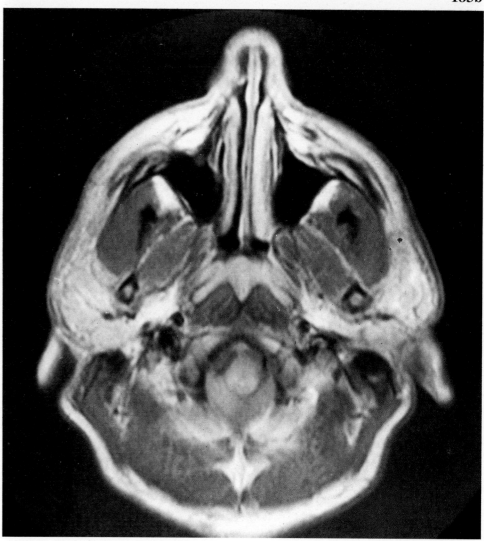

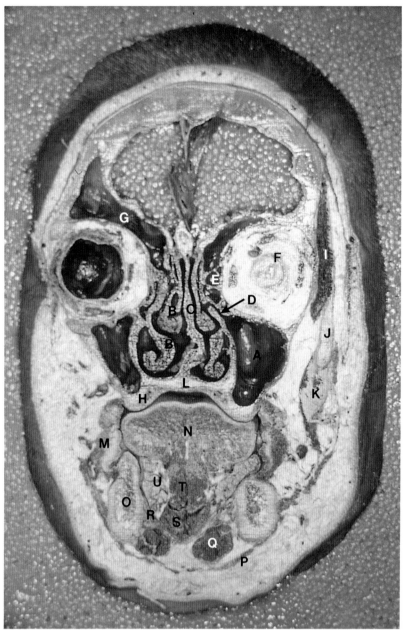

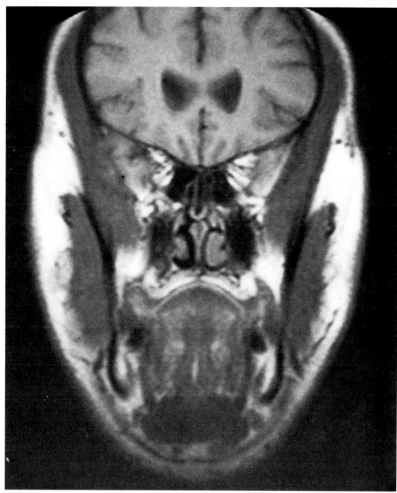

184b NMR scan of the head in coronal section to show topographical relationships around the maxillary air sinuses and the mouth.

184a Coronal section through the head to show the maxillary air sinus and the tongue and their topographical relationships.

A Maxillary air sinus.
B Conchae on lateral wall of nose.
C Nasal septum.
D Ostium of maxillary air sinus.
E Ethmoidal air cells.
F Orbital structures.
G Frontal air sinus.
H Maxillary alveolus.
I Temporalis muscle.
J Zygomatic arch.
K Masseter muscle.
L Hard palate.
M Buccinator muscle.
N Tongue.
O Body of mandible.
P Platysma muscle.
Q Anterior belly of digastric muscle.
R Mylohyoid muscle.
S Geniohyoid muscle.
T Genioglossus muscle.
U Sublingual salivary gland.

Functional anatomy

Mastication

Mastication is the process whereby ingested food is cut or crushed into small pieces, mixed with saliva, and formed into a bolus in preparation for swallowing. It is characteristic of mammals, which possess teeth of different forms (heterodonty) adapted to the comminution of food. In non-mammalians, the teeth are used mainly for prehension, the prey generally being seized head first and swallowed whole.

Various functions have been ascribed to mastication, it:

1. Enables the food bolus to be easily swallowed.
2. Enhances the digestibility of food by:
   i) decreasing the size of particles to increase the surface area for enzyme activity.
   ii) reflexively stimulating the secretion of digestive juices (e.g. saliva and gastric juice).
3. Mixes the food with saliva, initiating digestion by the activity of salivary amylase.
4. Prevents irritation of the gastro-intestinal system by large food masses.
5. Ensures healthy growth and development of the oral tissues.

Of all these, the increase in digestive efficiency is usually considered to be the primary purpose of mastication. Indeed, it has been suggested that there is an enormous gain in digestive efficiency without which the high rate of metabolism associated with homothermy in mammals could not be sustained. However, some experimental evidence indicates that mastication produces little gain in digestive efficiency in man.

185

185 Table classifying different foods according to the value of mastication in their digestion. This table summarises research in which 1g of either premasticated or unmasticated food was placed in cotton net bags, swallowed and subsequently collected from the faeces. Category 1 foods were those which left some large residues if swallowed with or without mastication. Category 2 foods left some residues when unchewed but were usually completely digested when chewed. Category 3 foods were likely to be fully digested, with or without mastication. Thus, it is only for the few types of food in Category 2 that mastication improves digestion.

Category 1	Category 2	Category 3
Roast and fried pork	Roast chicken	Fried and stewed beef fat
Fried bacon	Stewed lamb	Fried and boiled cod
Roast, fried and stewed beef		Fried kipper
Roast and stewed mutton		Hard-boiled egg
Roast and fried lamb		Boiled rice
Fried and boiled potatoes		White and wholemeal bread
Boiled garden peas		Cheddar cheese
Boiled carrots		

Mastication occurs by the convergent movements of maxillary and mandibular teeth. Most foods are first crushed by vertical movements of the mandible before being sheared to make a bolus. The initial crushing of the food does not require full occlusion of the teeth. Indeed, it is only after the food has been well softened that the maxillary and mandibular teeth eventually contact. Once the cusps can interdigitate, the ridges on the slopes of the cusps shear the food as the mandibular teeth move across the maxillary teeth. As the cusps cross the depressions within the opposing occlusal surfaces, there is grinding of food which has been likened to the action of a pestle and mortar.

186 Morphology of the cheek teeth in relation to the displacement of food (arrows). A, buccal view; B, interproximal view. Several features common to all the cheek teeth provide protection for the adjacent gingiva during chewing. The marginal ridges bounding the interproximal edges of the occlusal surfaces of the teeth are important protective features. These ridges deflect most of the food, potentially driven between adjacent teeth by their opponents, onto the occlusal surfaces. The contact points beneath the marginal ridges should abut firmly to prevent food being wedged between the teeth and above the interdental papillae. These contacts are maintained by the process of mesial drift (see page 294), despite the constant attrition of interproximal dental tissue. The buccal cusps of the mandibular cheek teeth bite between the buccal and palatal cusps of the maxillary cheek teeth with the result that food trapped between them is forced up over the palatal sides of the maxillary teeth and down over the buccal sides of the mandibular teeth. The palatal gingiva for the maxillary teeth is thus protected by the marked curvature of these teeth. In addition, it is the buccal surfaces of the mandibular cheek teeth which are the most curved.

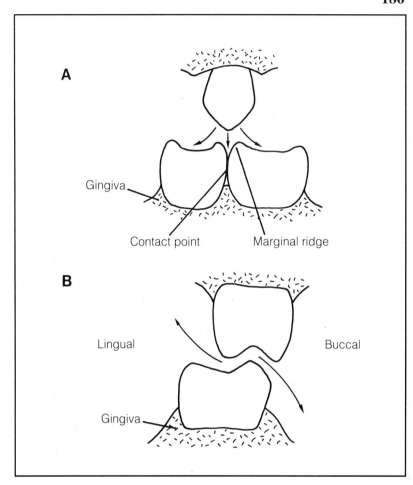

Mastication does not rely merely upon the form and activity of the teeth. Other features associated with mastication which are peculiar to mammals include:

Temporomandibular jaw articulation.
Serous salivary glands.
Prismatic enamel.
Diphyodonty.
Secondary palate.
Significant muscle development associated with lips, cheeks, tongue and muscles of mastication.
Gomphosis type of tooth attachment.

The development of a temporomandibular articulation and the muscles of mastication allow the force of the bite and the range of movement for chewing to be increased. Saliva moistens and lubricates the food during mastication. Additionally, its enzymes allow digestion to commence at an early stage in the mouth. The prismatic arrangement of dental enamel (see page 113) and its greater thickness in mammals are said to be more efficient in resisting masticatory loads and attrition than non-prismatic enamel. The development of a secondary palate is thought to be related to the necessity of maintaining ventilation during prolonged masticatory periods. The development of muscles within the lips, cheeks and tongue is associated with manipulation of the bolus within the mouth. The change from polyphyodonty (i.e. multiple tooth succession) to diphyodonty (two dentitions: deciduous and permanent) may be related to a 'grinding-in' period necessary to produce an efficient cutting or grinding tooth surface; it seems inefficient to replace such teeth too frequently. The gomphosis type of attachment (with a periodontal ligament; see pages 188 and 189) may be associated with the increased stresses and strains brought to bear on the tooth during mastication and allows for tooth movement.

Mastication is dependent upon a complex chain of events, which produce rhythmic opening and closing movements of the jaws and significant tongue movement. It is also significant physiologically for the very large forces which are exerted on the teeth.

187 A diagrammatic representation of the way jaw movements are thought to operate. An oral rhthym/pattern generator is situated in the brain stem and is activated by drive from the higher centres and from peripheral sensory input. The pattern of activity is then distributed to the motor neuron pools, which also receive excitatory or inhibitory sensory inputs from a variety of peripheral structures. The hypothesis is that the sensory input generated by closing on hard food supports the generation of rhthymic activity, whereas closure on a softened bolus elicits a swallow, and may consequently terminate the rhthymic activity. **EL**, jaw elevator musculature; **H**, hyoid and associated musculature; **T**, tongue and associated musculature; **CH**, cheek and associated musculature.

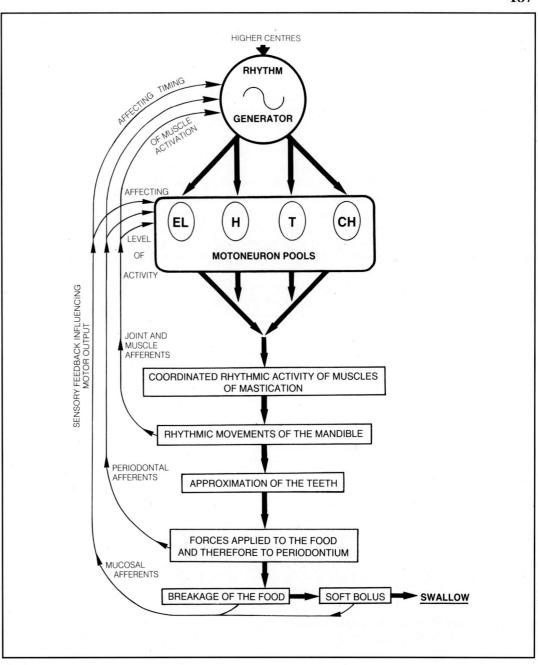

The bite pressure. Experiments involving the implantation of force transducers into the occlusal surfaces of teeth have shown that the force exerted on the food during mastication is in the order of 5–15kg. This force varies according to the texture of the food. When bite pressure is measured with a gnathodynamometer, maximum pressures in the order of 50kg can be readily recorded.

The chewing cycle

Mammals generally chew on one side at a time. Two methods of chewing have been distinguished, depending upon the texture of the food:

1. Puncture/crushing. Hard food is first crushed and pierced between the teeth without direct tooth-to-tooth contact.

This results in wear (attrition) of the teeth, especially at the tips of the cusps.

2. Shearing stroke. This method involves tooth contacts that only take place after the food has been sufficiently reduced. This type of movement produces attrition facets with characteristic directional scratch lines.

The action of the teeth during mastication depends on their morphology, the movements of the mandible, and the nature of the forces generated by the muscles of mastication. The chewing cycle involves three basic movements (or strokes) of the mandible in relation to the maxilla. From a position in which the jaw is open, the closing stroke results in the teeth being brought into initial contact with the food. This is followed by the power stroke when the food undergoes reduction. Movement of the mandible in this phase is slower than that in the closing stroke because of the resistance caused by the food. Finally, there is the opening stroke, when the mandible is lowered, with an initial slower stage followed by a faster stage.

188

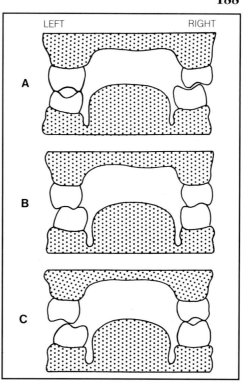

188 Occlusal relationships of the cheek teeth during chewing on the left side. From an open position, the mandible is moved upwards and outwards, bringing the buccal cusps of the maxillary and mandibular teeth on the working (left) side in contact (**A**). Note that, as mentioned previously, the teeth may not initially contact each other during the initial masticatory cycles. In the power stroke, the mandibualr teeth then slide upwards and medially against the maxillary teeth to momentarily attain intercuspal position (**B**). Following attainment of the intercuspal position, the mandibular teeth continue downwards and inwards against the maxillary teeth (the lingual phase, **C**). The opening stroke then follows and the cycle is repeated. The relationships of the teeth on the balancing side are also illustrated. Note that, while the teeth on the working side are moving through the buccal phase (**A**), those on the balancing (right) side are in the lingual phase, but in the reverse direction. Although the diagram shows tooth contact, it is probable that any contact on the balancing side is only transient.

189

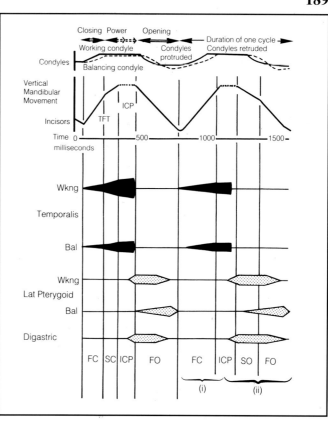

189 Two non-identical cycles of jaw movement. Note that the vertical component of condylar movement is due to its movement up and down the slope of the articular eminence (see page 100).

The first cycle has a profile that is commonly found when solid food is chewed. After a previous opening, the jaw accelerates into relatively fast closing (**FC**). At this stage the food is only being accelerated against gravity, and the electromyographic (EMG) activity in the jaw-closing muscles is of low amplitude. As tooth-food-tooth (TFT) contact is made, activity in the jaw-closing muscles increases and force is exerted on the food. The food resistance slows the jaw closing (**SC**). As the cusps continue to interdigitate, closing velocity slows to zero. The duration of this stationary phase is a matter of dispute. Because of uncertainty, the intercuspal phase (**ICP**) is shown as a dashed line. The jaw subsequently opens with a relatively constant velocity.

The second cycle is more diagrammatic in that it consists of closing and opening profiles of movement that are not necessarily found together:

i) closing characteristic of closure on soft or well-masticated food — mainly a fast closing
ii) occasionally, there is found a two phase opening (slow and fast) of uncertain significance.

The main point is that cycle form is variable, depending upon the sensory feedback (see **187**).

190 The envelope of motion of the contact point between the mandibular incisors. This demonstrates the symmetrical mandibular movements produced during opening and closing of the jaw. The envelope of motion is the volume of space within which all movements of (a point on) the mandible occur. It is limited by anatomical considerations such as ligaments. Most natural movements do not utilise this maximum volume but occur well within the 'envelope'. The yellow trajectory depicts a two-phased, conscious movement from the rest position to the fully opened position. The first phase is a hinge-like movement during which the condyles are maximally retruded within the mandibular fossae. When the teeth are opened by approximately 25mm, the second phase of opening occurs by anterior movement or protrusion of the condyles down the articular eminences. The blue and red trajectories describe a biphasic path of closure from the fully opened mandibular position, which can only be performed with conscious effort. The first phase (the blue trajectory) takes the mandible up to a protruded closed position, while the second phase (the red trajectory) takes the mandible from this protruded contact position to a retruded contact position. The green trajectory describes the free, habitual, unconscious movement during both mandibular opening and closing. The points on the ramus represent the centres of rotation during opening and closure. Point A is the fulcrum associated with simple hinge movements. The path described between points A and B represent the shifting fulcrum of movement during opening and closure involving hinge movements and protrusion or retrusion of the mandible.

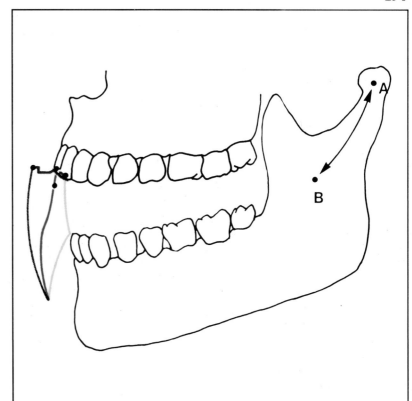

191 Profile showing the average incisal movements in the frontal plane during a masticatory cycle. This figure shows that the opening movement rarely goes straight down but deviates to one side. There is a wide variation in profiles between individuals and also continuous variation between consecutive chewing cycles in the same individual. For example, the initial deviation may be either towards the chewing side or away from it (as shown here). Furthermore, the profiles differ according to the type of occlusion and the texture of the food.

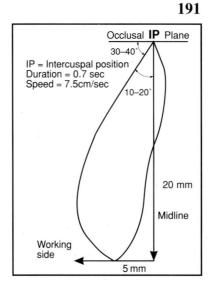

192 Transverse movements of the lower jaw (lateral excursions or side-to-side movements). These movements involve bilaterally asymmetric movements of the mandible. They are produced by protrusion of the condyle down the articular eminence on one side with reactive movements of the other condyle (rotation around a laterally shifting axis). The solid outline indicates the position of the mandible in centric position; the broken outline indicates the position associated with lateral movement of the mandible to the left. Additional drawings of the condyles illustrate the changing positions of the long axes of the condyles during this lateral movement. The red line represents the horizontal band of fibres of the temporomandibular ligament, passing from the articular eminence (**A**) to the lateral surface of the condyle (see **143**). Tension generated in the horizontal band produces a slight lateral shift in the condyle (Bennett shift).

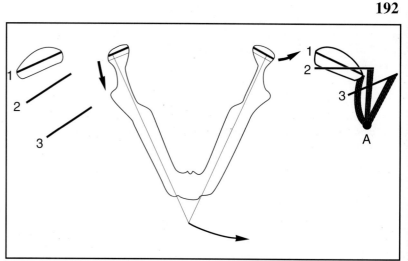

The control of mastication

There has been much controversy concerning the origin and control of the rhythmic activity of the jaws during mastication. One view, the cerebral hemispheres theory, holds that mastication is a conscious act, a patterned set of instructions originating in the higher centres of the central nervous system (in particular the motor cortex) and descending to directly drive the motoneurones within the brainstem (trigeminal, facial and hypoglossal motoneurones). Another idea, the reflex chain theory, holds that mastication involves a series of interacting chains of reflexes. Accordingly, sensory input from the region of the mouth (e.g. pressure on the teeth) triggers the motoneurones in the brainstem to elicit a jaw opening movement. In turn, this movement produces another sensory input (e.g. from stretch receptors in the jaw muscles) which results in a jaw closing reflex. Such a theory could explain the rhythmic jaw movements seen in decerebrate animals. Although there are several, well-recognised types of jaw reflexes (see figures below for examples), objections to the reflex chain theory have been raised on the basis that mastication involves prolonged bursts of muscle activity and not the brief and abrupt behaviour usually associated with reflex activation of muscle. A third theory, the rhythm (pattern) generator theory, has more recently been proposed to explain rhythmic jaw functioning. This theory is based upon the proposition that there are pattern generators within the brainstem which, on being stimulated from either higher centres or from sensory inputs in the region of the mouth, are driven into rhythmic activity. This idea could account for rhythmic activity obtained by stimulating either the motor cortex or the oral cavity in decerebrate animals. It is this latter theory, supported mainly by comparisons with other physiological systems that require pattern generators (e.g. respiration), which appears to be gaining most credence. However, the neural mechanisms underlying rhythmicity are still unknown.

193

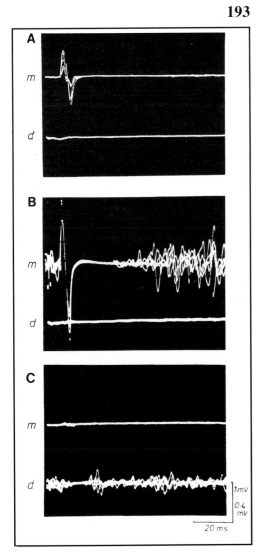

194

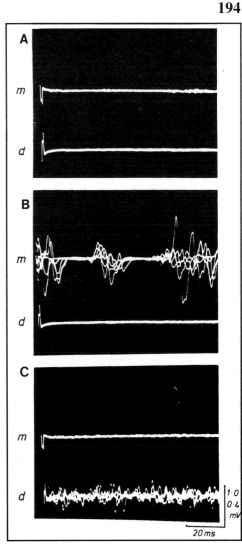

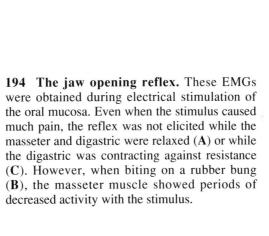

193 The jaw jerk reflex. The EMGs shown were obtained by placing electrodes from the skin covering the masseter (**m**) and anterior belly of digastric (**d**) muscles of a human subject. The reflex was then elicited by tapping the chin to obtain a sudden downward movement of the mandible. The jaw jerk reflex was obtained when the subject was relaxed (**A**), biting on a rubber bung (**B**), or contracting the digastric against resistance (**C**). Note that the reflex was exaggerated if either muscle was active.

194 The jaw opening reflex. These EMGs were obtained during electrical stimulation of the oral mucosa. Even when the stimulus caused much pain, the reflex was not elicited while the masseter and digastric were relaxed (**A**) or while the digastric was contracting against resistance (**C**). However, when biting on a rubber bung (**B**), the masseter muscle showed periods of decreased activity with the stimulus.

Swallowing

Swallowing (deglutition) involves an ordered sequence of reflex events that carry food (or saliva) from the mouth into the stomach. Although a continuous activity, swallowing is subdivided into stages for descriptive convenience. It is important to appreciate that, alongside muscle activity required to move the bolus, there must be mechanisms to protect the airway (e.g. closure of the nasopharynx by the soft palate, elevation of the larynx, closure of the laryngeal inlet by the epiglottis).

The first stage of swallowing involves the passage of the bolus of food onto the tongue and towards the oropharyngeal isthmus. It is essentially voluntary, although there may be some reflex involvement associated with the sensory inputs signalling an appropriate food consistency. The airway remains patent during this phase. When the bolus reaches the oropharyngeal isthmus during the second stage of swallowing, the process becomes involuntary. The soft palate and larynx are elevated and a wave of muscular activity of the pharyngeal constrictor muscles carries the bolus through the pharynx. This stage ends when the bolus passes into the oesophagus.

Table 11 summarises the main events during swallowing.

Table 11: Main events during swallowing.

Stage	Mechanisms associated with passage of bolus	Mechanisms associated with protecting airway
1. VOLUNTARY **Bolus in mouth**	Mouth closed (temporalis, masseter, medial pterygoid)	**Airway open**
	Lips closed (orbicularis oris)	Pillars of fauces contracted against posterior surface of tongue (palatoglossus, palatopharyngeus)
	Tongue grooved, anterior part raised against palate (intrinsic tongue muscles, genioglossus)	
2. INVOLUNTARY **Bolus passes into oropharynx**	Posterior part of tongue moves upwards and backwards (styloglossus, mylohyoid)	**Nasopharynx closed off**
	Groove in tongue flattened out (intrinsic tongue muscles)	Soft palate tensed and elevated (tensor veli palatini, levator veli palatini, Passavant's muscle)
	Pillars of fauces contract behind bolus	
Bolus passes over epiglottis to lateral food channels	Pharynx elevated (stylopharyngeus, salpingopharyngeus, palatopharyngeus)	**Inlet of larynx closed off**
		Larynx elevated beneath epiglottis and posterior part of tongue (stylopharyngeus, salpingopharyngeus, palatopharyngeus, thyrohyoid)
		Laryngeal inlet reduced by approximation (interarytenoid, thyroarytenoid) and tension (lateral cricoarytenoid, interarytenoid) of aryepiglottic folds
Bolus passes into oesophagus	Relaxation of cricopharyngeus	**Airway re-established** Soft palate and larynx return to original positions

195 The stages of swallowing. Although the act of swallowing is not discontinuous, for descriptive convenience it can be divided into four stages. At each stage it is necessary to consider not only the movement of the bolus of food in the upper digestive tract but also the mechanisms required to protect the airway.

Stage 1 – bolus in the mouth (A & B). The mouth is closed by the action of the masseter and temporalis muscles, and the lips are approximated (anterior oral seal) by the circumoral facial musculature. The upper surface of the tongue is grooved by the vertical fibres of the intrinsic musculature, and the anterior part of the tongue is raised against the palate by the genioglossus muscles. The pillars of the fauces at the oropharyngeal isthmus are contracted against the posterior surface of the tongue by the palatoglossus and palatopharyngeus muscles. The airway remains open at this stage, with the soft palate lying away from the posterior wall of the pharnyx.

Stage 2 – bolus passes through the oropharyngeal isthmus into the oropharnyx (C–E). The tongue is elevated against the palate by the action of the mylohyoid muscles and, by means of the styloglossus, the posterior part moves backwards with the food bolus. The groove in the tongue is 'ironed' out by relaxation of the vertical intrinsic muscles, and the palatoglossal folds contract behind the bolus as it leaves the oral cavity. To protect the nasopharnyx, the soft palate is tensed and elevated (via the tensor veli palatini and the levator veli palatini muscles) to contact the posterior wall of the pharnyx.

Stage 3 – bolus passes over the epiglottis to the lateral food channels (E–G). The pharnyx is elevated (by means of the stylo-, salpingo- and palatopharyngeal muscles) along with the larnyx, which consequently is protected by descending beneath the epiglottis and the posterior part of the tongue. The laryngeal inlet is reduced by the 'passive' closing of the epiglottis (which is depressed by the weight of the bolus and by the movement of the tongue and the larnyx) and by approximation of the aryepiglottic folds.

Stage 4 – bolus passes through the laryngopharnyx, through the cricopharyngeal sphincter and into the oesophagus (G–J). Both gravity and a wave of contraction within the pharyngeal constrictor muscles propel the food through the pharnyx. Relaxation of the cricopharyngeal part of the inferior constrictor allows the food into the oesophagus, whereupon peristalsis takes it towards the stomach. Once the bolus is in the oesophagus, the cricopharyngeal sphincter closes to prevent reflux. The airway is re-established during this phase; the soft palate, tongue and epiglottis return to their normal positions.

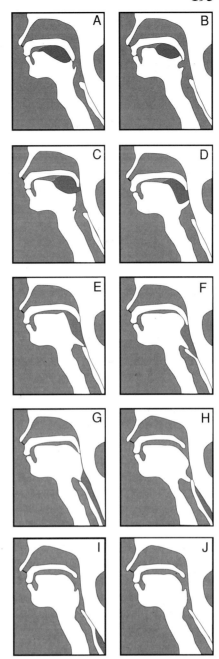

Speech

The acquisition of language is probably the most complex sensorimotor developmental process in a person's life. Sounds are produced initially in the larynx (phonation) by the coordinated movements of abdominal, thoracic and laryngeal muscles. Subsequent modification of this laryngeal sound to produce meaningful speech (articulation) occurs principally within the pharyngeal, oral and nasal cavities.

196 The principal sensory and motor mechanisms in speech. The main speech area of the brain is located within the temporoparietal region of the dominant cerebral hemisphere (i.e. the left cerebral hemisphere for a right-handed person). The diagram indicates the many monitoring systems which are involved in the control of speech (e.g. hearing, proprioceptive information from the various muscles involved). Note that there has to be coordinated activity of respiration, laryngeal behaviour and oral structures to produce effective speech.

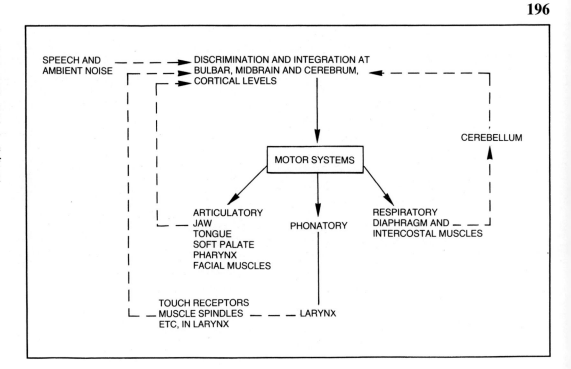

The fundamental laryngeal note has a thin and reedy quality. This sound therefore contains a limited amount of speech information and so it is modified within resonating chambers and by the activity of organs such as the lips, tongue and soft palate. By a process of sympathetic vibration, the resonators act as acoustic filters, amplifying selected frequencies and attenuating others.

Table 12: The vocal resonators.

The following spaces are present in the vocal apparatus, any or all of which might be available as variable resonating chambers:

1. The vestibule between the true and false vocal cords.
2. Between the larynx and the root of the tongue, possibly involving the epiglottis.
3. Between the pharyngeal wall and the soft palate and uvula.
4. Between the dorsum of the tongue and the posterior surface of the hard palate.
5. Between the dorsum of the tongue and the anterior surface of the hard palate.
6. Between the tip of the tongue and the teeth.
7. Between the teeth and the lips.
8. The nasal passages.

The classification of sounds

Sounds may be voiced (i.e. the vocal folds in the larynx vibrate for sound production) or breathed (i.e. the vocal folds do not vibrate). The two main groups of speech sounds are vowels and consonants. Vowel sounds are modified by resonance and voiced consonants are modified by resonance and air flow obstruction. All vowel sounds are voiced. They are produced without interruption of the air flow, the air being channelled or restricted by the position of the tongue and lips.

197 Lip postures during the production of vowel sounds. The diagrams show the short vowel sounds on the left side and the long vowel sounds on the right.

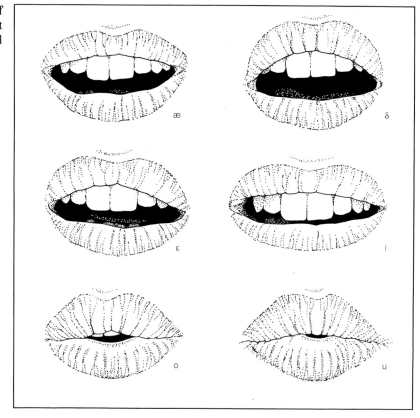

A consonant is produced when the air flow is impeded before it is released. Consonants may be voiced (e.g. b, d, z) or breathed (e.g. p, t, s). Consonant sounds are of low amplitude (vowels are created by high amplitude waves) and are classified in two ways: according to the place of articulation or according to the manner of articulation.

For the classification based upon the place of articulation, consonants are categorised into bilabial, labiodental, linguodental, linguopalatal and glottal sounds. In bilabial sounds, the two lips are used (e.g. b, p, m). In labiodental sounds, the lower lip meets the maxillary incisors (e.g. f, v).

Linguodental sounds involve the tip of the tongue contacting the maxillary incisors and the adjacent hard palate (e.g. d, t). For linguopalatal sounds, the tongue meets the palate away from the region of the maxillary incisors (g, k).

For the classification of consonant sounds based upon the manner of articulation, the degree of stoppage of the air flow is an important criterion, as shown in Table 13.

Table 13: Classification of consonant sounds based upon manner of articulation.

Plosives	(p, b, t, d, g, k)	Require a complete stoppage of air
Fricatives	(f, v, th)	Require only a partial stoppage
Affricatives	(ch, j)	Although involving only a partial stoppage of the air, require a rapid release of this air
Nasals	(m, n)	Require obstruction of the mouth with the the nasal passages open
Laterals	(l)	Air forced to leave sides of mouth
Rolled	(r)	

Both systems for classifying consonant sounds can be linked as in Table 14.

Table 14: Classification of consonant sounds based upon place *and* manner of articulation.

	Place of articulation						
			Linguodentals		*Linguopalatals*		
Manner of articulation	*Bilabial*	*Labiodental*	*Dental*	*Alveolar*	*Alveolar*	*Palatal*	*Glottal*
Voicing	− +	− +	− +	− +	− +	− +	− +
Plosives	p b			t d		k g	
Fricatives		f v	θ ð	s z	ʃ ʒ		h
Affricatives				tʃ			
				tr dr		j	
Nasals	m			n		ng	
Laterals				l			
Semi-vowels	w						

106

198 Configuration of the oral structures during consonant articulations.

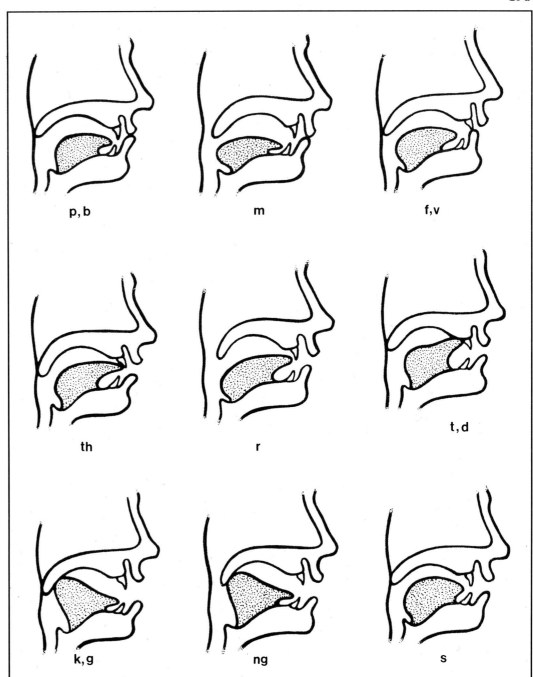

Although one may describe the position of articulators for a particular vowel or consonant, it must be remembered that there are no fixed positions during speech, only continuous movement.

Microscopic anatomy
of oro-dental tissues

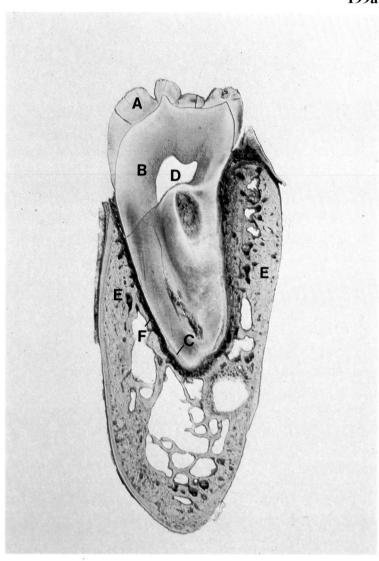

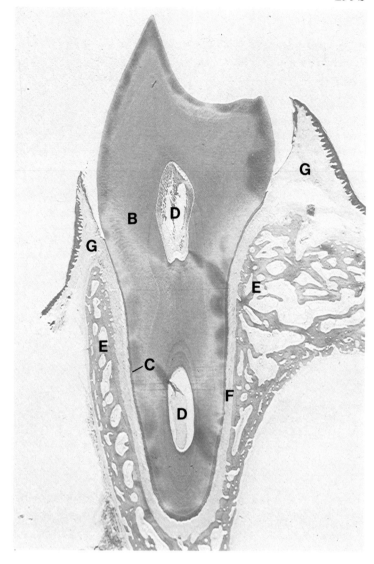

199 Ground (199a) and decalcified (199b) sections of a tooth *in situ.*
The teeth are composed of three calcified tissues — enamel (**A**), dentine (**B**) and cementum (**C**) — surrounding an inner core of connective tissue, the dental pulp (**D**). Dentine forms the bulk of the tooth, being covered in the crown by enamel and in the root by cementum. The dental pulp is the sensitive, nutritive portion of the tooth, protected from external noxious stimuli by the overlying hard tissues. Dentine, cementum and pulp are of mesenchymal origin, while enamel is of epithelial origin.

The tissues which support the teeth in the jaws are collectively termed the periodontium and comprise the alveolar bone (**E**), which houses the sockets for the roots of the teeth, the periodontal ligament (**F**), a con-

nective tissue which attaches the cementum to the alveolar bone, and the gingiva (**G**).

The appearance of the dental tissues is dependent upon the method used to prepare the specimen. Thus, in ground section the soft connective tissues of the pulp, periodontal ligament and gingiva will be removed by the act of wearing away the tissues to obtain a thin section. In the ground section shown in **199a**, however, the periodontal ligament has been retained due to the specimen being embedded in plastic prior to sectioning. In decalcified material, the soft connective tissues and the organic matrix of the calcified tissues are retained but, unless the decalcifying procedure is carried out under special conditions, decalcification generally results in loss of the highly mineralised enamel, as seen in **199b**. (**199a**, × 4. **199b**, H & E; × 6)

Enamel

200 The distribution of enamel. Dental enamel (**A**) covers the anatomical crown of the tooth. It meets the dentine (**B**) at the enamel–dentine junction (amelodentinal junction), and the cementum at the cervical margin or cement–enamel junction (**C**). The thickness of enamel varies according to location. It is thickest over the incisal edge and cusps (up to 2.3mm) and thins to a knife-edge at the cervical margin. On lateral surfaces, the enamel is intermediate in thickness (up to 1.3mm). (Ground, longitudinal section; ×3).

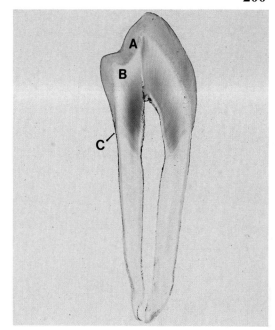

Physical properties of enamel. Enamel has a bluish-white colouration and is semitranslucent. However, the bluish tinge is only seen on the intact tooth at the biting edges of unworn incisors. Elsewhere, the crowns of healthy teeth appear yellowish-white, the colour of the enamel being modified by the underlying dentine. The enamel on deciduous teeth, being more opaque, appears much whiter. Enamel is a crystalline material and is birefringent, the crystals refracting light differently in different directions. The tissue has an average refractive index of 1.62. These optical properties considerably influence the histological appearance of enamel (for example explaining why there are differences with various mounting media).

Enamel is the hardest tissue in the body. This property enables enamel to withstand the heavy loads of mastication and limit the amount of wear. Although enamel has a low tensile strength and is brittle, it has a high modulus of elasticity (in other words, it is rigid) and this, together with the flexible support of the underlying dentine, minimises the possibility of fracture. Enamel has a high specific gravity (2.8–3.1). This fact has been useful when separating enamel from dentine for analytical purposes.

The properties of enamel vary at different regions within the tissue. Surface enamel is harder, denser and less porous than subsurface enamel. Hardness and density also decrease from the surface towards the interior, and from the cuspal/incisal tip towards the cervical margin.

Chemical composition of enamel. Mature enamel is highly mineralised. It contains by weight 96% inorganic material, 1% organic material and 3% water (89%, 2%, and 9% by volume). The inorganic component is mainly calcium phosphate in the form of hydroxyapatite crystals. Small amounts of carbonate, magnesium, potassium, sodium and fluoride are also present. The exact composition varies between teeth, within different parts of the same tooth, and even between the core and periphery of the same prism. Two groups of proteins are found in developing enamel: the unique amelogenins (which are well characterised), and much smaller amounts of non-amelogenins (often collectively known as enamelins). The amelogenins are removed during the enamel's development, although small amounts persist in the fully formed tissue. Mature enamel contains degradation products of amelogenins as well as non-amelogenin proteins. The amino acid composition of the enamel proteins are described in relation to the development of the tissue (amelogenesis) on page 263. The enamel proteins do not appear to be fibrous and they may form a relatively structureless gel. The presence of other organic elements such as lipids is controversial. The functions of the organic matrix are unclear, but it is probably implicated in the mineralisation of the enamel.

Enamel prisms and crystals

Our understanding of the structure and composition of enamel is complicated by technical difficulties encountered in preparing the tissue for examination. Procedures such as sectioning, decalcification and mounting alter its appearance, and some features discernible by one preparation are absent or different in another.

The basic histological unit of mammalian enamel is the prism and each prism is comprised of large numbers of hydroxyapatite crystals.

201

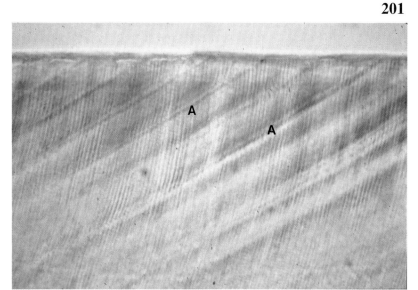

201 Enamel prisms in longitudinal section. A ground section of enamel is seen to be made up of prisms (or rods) 3–6µm in diameter. Most of the prisms appear to cross the full thickness of the tissue, their direction following the path of the ameloblasts during development. In cuspal and incisal regions, the prisms run perpendicular to the tooth surface. On lateral surfaces, they slope upwards from the enamel–dentine junction towards the surface. In inner enamel, the prisms follow a wavy course. The obliquely running lines (**A**) crossing the prisms are called the striae of Retzius (see pages 118–119). (Ground, longitudinal section through enamel; × 300)

202

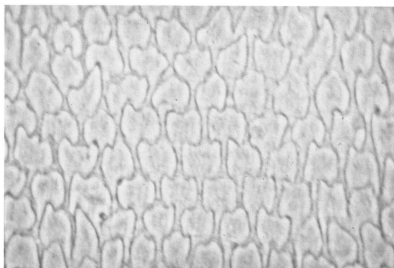

202 Enamel prisms in transverse section. The shape of the prisms in transverse section varies according to the techniques employed to prepare the tissue and to the orientation of the section or surface observed. In most areas of human enamel, prisms appear keyhole-shaped; the tail of one prism lies between the heads of two lower prisms. (Ground, transverse section through enamel viewed by phase contrast microscopy; × 1,800)

203

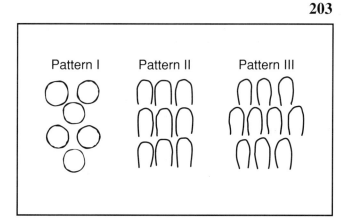

203 Different prism patterns seen in transverse section. Not all prismatic enamel in the human tooth shows the keyhole pattern. Indeed, three shapes are commonly seen. In pattern 1 enamel, the prisms appear completely circular. This pattern is most often found near the enamel–dentine junction. In pattern 2 enamel, the prisms are arranged in longitudinal rows (see **215**). In pattern 3 enamel, the prisms are also arranged in rows but are staggered to give the keyhole shapes.

204

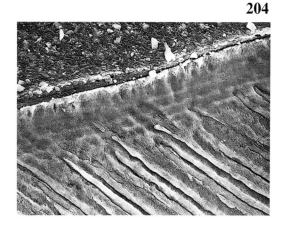

204 Prismless enamel. Surface enamel is often prismless. There may also be a very thin, prismless layer immediately adjacent to the enamel–dentine junction. Prismless enamel differs from prismatic enamel in that the former has its crystals aligned parallel, and the latter shows abrupt changes in orientation at the prism boundaries. Prismless enamel occurs because of the absence of Tomes' processes on the cells (ameloblasts) responsible for the development of enamel (see pages 260 and 261). (SEM; × 63)

113

205

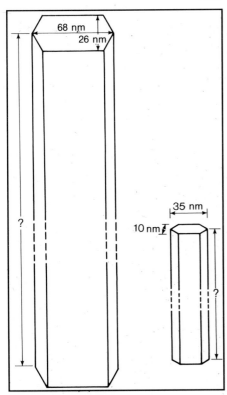

206

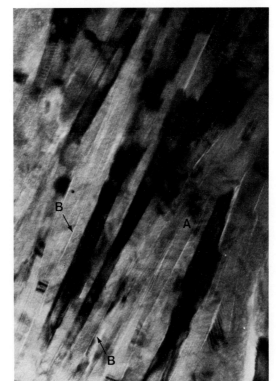

206 Enamel crystals in longitudinal section prepared by ion-beam thinning. A detailed examination of prisms and crystal structure requires the use of electron microscopy at high magnifications and high resolution. Only very thin sections (50–100nm) can be examined in the transmission electron microscope, because of the limited penetrating power of the electron beam. Although ultrathin sections of enamel can be prepared, the procedures fracture the crystals and consequently there is an underestimate of their lengths. Thin ground sections of enamel, in which the crystals are more complete, can be reduced to ultrathin dimensions (at least in parts) by the technique of ion-beam thinning. For this technique, a beam of ionised argon is directed obliquely onto the section so that it is etched. In such specimens, crystals (**A**) up to 100μm long are seen and it is possible that some crystals cross the full thickness of the enamel. **B**, pores between crystals. (TEM; × 100,000).

205 Enamel crystals consist of impure hydroxyapatite. In the pure form, this has an empirical formula of $Ca_5(PO_4)_3(OH)$. Indeed, hydroxyapatite is the main mineral found in all mammalian calcified tissues and can take a variety of crystalline forms. In enamel, the crystals are large, elongated, and irregularly hexagonal in section. The dimensions shown for enamel are those usually quoted (the smaller hydroxyapatite crystal from dentine is shown for comparison). However, evidence from ion-beam thinned sections (see **206**) suggests that the crystal may be 100μm or more in length.

207 Enamel crystals in cross-section prepared by ion-beam thinning. The hexagonal pattern of the enamel crystal is clearly seen both *in situ* (**207a**) and in isolation (**207b**). The core of the crystal is said to differ slightly in composition from the periphery (being richer in magnesium and carbonate). Indeed, there is evidence that the core of the crystal is more soluble than the periphery. It is not known, however, whether this reflects chemical or physical differences. Small gaps or pores (**A**), which may contain water and organic material, occur between crystals. The isolated crystals shown in **207b** contain many hydroxyapatite molecules organised in a repeating pattern or lattice. It is thought by some that the hexagonal images seen in thin sections result from viewing parallel piped segments of these crystals as two-dimensional shadows (**207a**, TEM; × 120,000. **207b**, TEM; × 800,000)

207a

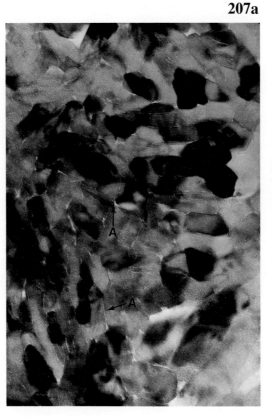

207b

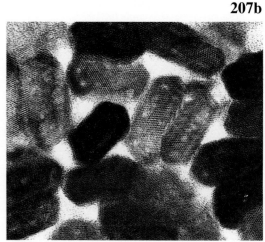

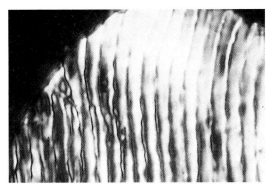

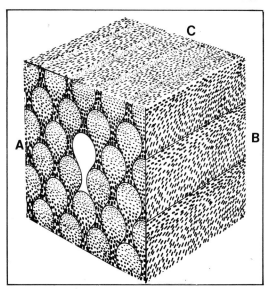

208 Crystal orientation within prisms assessed by polarised light. In polarised light, enamel cut longitudinal to the prisms shows a series of light and dark lines which distinguish the prism cores from the prism boundaries. This appearance is due to the abrupt change in orientation of the crystals at the prism boundary and not to different degrees of mineralisation. Indeed, the presence of the enamel prism as a subunit of enamel is entirely due to these changes in crystal orientation. (Ground, longitudinal section of enamel; × 600)

209 The relationship between crystal orientation and prism structure. This diagram represents a block of enamel, the cross-sectional view (**A**), revealing the characteristic keyhole arrangement of enamel prisms with the tails pointing cervically and the heads occlusally. In the head of the prism, the crystals run parallel to the long axis of the prism. In the tail, the crystals gradually diverge from this to become angled 65–70° to the long axis. The change within a single prism is gradual, such that no clear division between head and tail of the same prism is seen. However, the crystals in the tail of one prism show a sudden divergence from the crystals in the head of an adjacent prism. The sudden change in crystal orientation at the prism boundary can be seen most clearly in the lateral surface of the block (**B**). On this surface, where the prisms have been cut exactly centrally through the head–tail axis, there are produced rows of equal, but wide, prisms. On the top surface (**C**), where the plane of section has passed through adjacent heads and tails, there is the appearance of broad prisms separated by narrower bands of 'interprismatic material'. It must be noted that in preparing histological material, the enamel will be sectioned with varying degrees of obliquity, producing a wide variety of prism appearances and crystal orientations.

210 Enamel prisms cut transversely to show variations in crystal orientation. Note the differences in orientation between the head (**A**) and tail (**B**) regions of the prisms. (TEM; × 7,000)

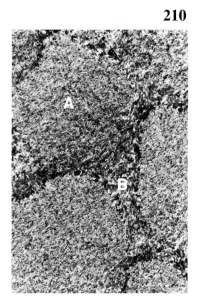

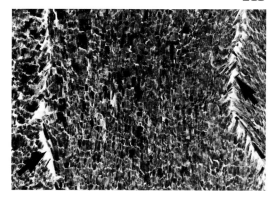

211 Enamel prisms cut longitudinally to show variations in crystal orientation. Note the sudden change in orientation at the prism boundaries (*arrowed*). Although the gaps between the prisms are partly artifactual, there is the suggestion here of large pores which, because of their slit-like appearance, can be described as 'laminar pores'. (TEM; × 13,500)

Although most accounts of enamel highlight the interlocking, keyhole shape of the prism (**202**), alternative arrangements are possible. For example, one can fit a description of round prisms surrounded by interprismatic material. A closer examination, however, reveals that the interprismatic material at one level is the tail section of the keyhole-shaped prism from above (see **209**, surface **C**).

212

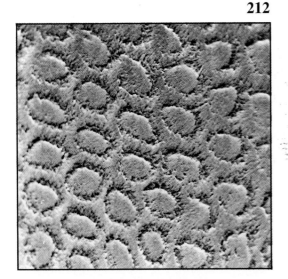

213

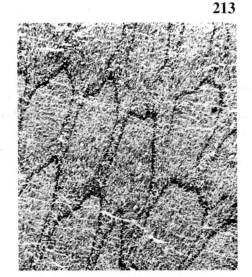

214

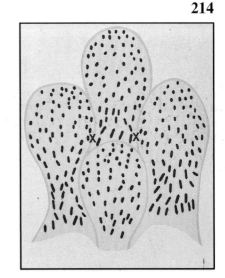

212 Circular prisms with interprismatic material. In some areas, prisms can appear circular with material surrounding them. This surrounding (or interprismatic) material was once thought to form an organic 'sheath' around the prisms. It is now clear, however, that the interprismatic region is also crystalline but gives a different optical effect because the crystals deviate by 40–60° from those in the prism. What is 'interprismatic' is in fact often the tail of one prism adjacent to the head of another. (× 4,300)

213 Transverse section through the enamel showing keyhole appearance of prisms. This ultrathin section of enamel is comparable with the arrangement drawn in surface A of **209**. The prism boundaries have been preferentially stained to show that the boundary of the keyhole-shape is incomplete (TEM with silver staining; × 2,000)

214 Diagram summarising the relationship between various parts of the enamel prism. Note that at **X**, where the end of the tail of one prism is close to the early part of the tail of the adjacent prism, there is little if any divergence in crystal orientation and thus the boundary of the keyhole shape is incomplete.

It is important to realise that the terms employed to describe the shape of the prism lack precision and consequently analogies should not be pursued too far. The 'keyhole' and 'prismatic/interprismatic' descriptors merely provide alternative approaches to what is essentially the same arrangement (with some local variations), which appears differently in different preparations and at different orientations.

215 The appearance of enamel in decalcified sections — enamel prisms cut transversely. The organic content of mature enamel is low. Nevertheless, controlled (and probably incomplete) decalcification will allow retention of some organic material for subsequent staining. Note that the keyhole pattern of the prisms can still be clearly seen. Although it is now known that the prism lacks an organic sheath, there may be a higher level of organic material and water at the prism boundary because of the large pores produced by the abutment of crystals at this junction. This, and the apparently lower solubility of the matrix at the prism boundary, explains the deeper staining of the boundaries. (Note the pattern 2 enamel in the top left corner of the micrograph). (Light blue; × 600)

215

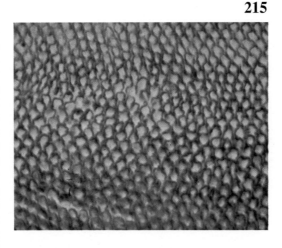

216

216 The appearance of enamel in decalcified sections — enamel prisms cut longitudinally. In this preparation, prism boundaries and cross-striations (see **218**) can be discerned. The prisms, however, are not as well-defined as in fully-calcified ground sections since the reflective and refractive crystals predominantly responsible for the prismatic pattern have been removed. (Procyon red; × 300)

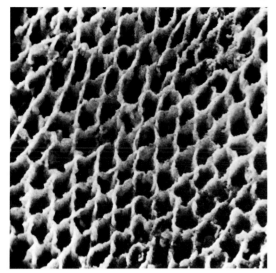 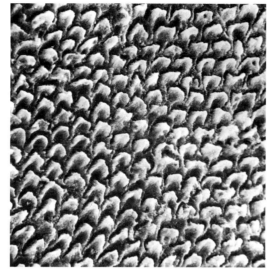 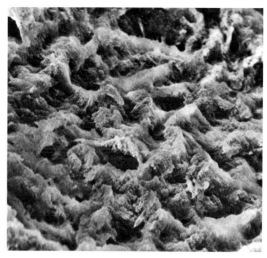

217 The reactions of enamel to demineralising agents has relevance to our understanding of the process of dental caries and of the application of bonding materials. In addition, the differing reactions of the prism core and prism boundary to different demineralising agents is evidence favouring the view that these two regions have dissimilar physical and/or chemical properties. Dilute acids preferentially etch the prism core. Chelating agents preferentially etch the prism boundary. Using strong acids, however, a variety of demineralising patterns can be produced on the same tooth surface. The following three scanning electron micrographs are taken from enamel treated with 30% w/w phosphoric acid for 60 seconds. Three etching patterns can be produced. Pattern 1 (**217a**) shows preferential etching of the prism core. Pattern 2 (**217b**) shows preferential etching of the prism boundary and Pattern 3 (**217c**) shows an even etch which bears no relationship to enamel morphology. The absence of a common etching pattern in strong acids may indicate regional variations in prism structure and properties (**217a**, SEM; × 1,000; **217b**, SEM; × 1,000; **217c**, SEM; × 1,000)

Incremented lines and Hunter–Schreger bands

Two types of incremental lines are found in enamel as a result of the phasic nature of the development of the tissue: cross-striations and striae of Retzius. The cross-striations are 'short-period' markers seen on each individual prism. The striae of Retzius are 'long-period' markers which run obliquely across the whole tissue.

218

219

218 Cross-striations viewed within a ground, longitudinal section of enamel. In transmitted, reflected or polarised light, or by dark-field or phase-contrast illumination (as illustrated here), cross-striations may be seen traversing the prisms at right angles to their long axes. These small lines probably represent daily increments of growth during enamel formation (thereby being related to the circadian cycle). In the enamel of deciduous teeth, the interval between cross-striation is approximately 5µm. In the permanent teeth, however, the interval varies from 2.5-7µm, the lower values being found near the enamel–dentine junction and the surface enamel. (Phase-contrast microscopy; × 350)

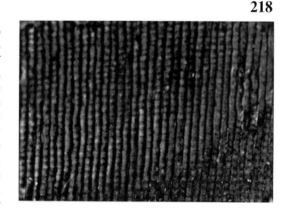

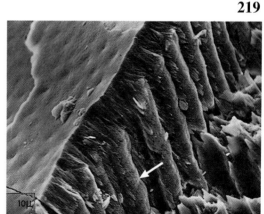

219 Cross-striations seen with the scanning electron microscope. Cross-striations have not been seen with transmission electron microscopy. With scanning electron microscopy, however, fractured enamel prisms show variations in width at regular intervals, with the constrictions (*arrowed*) corresponding to the cross-striations discerned with light microscopy. Cross-striations may relate to a difference in chemical composition of the inorganic phase of enamel formation during the circadian cycle. (SEM; × 400)

Although cross-striations stain intensely with organic dyes in partially demineralised sections (see **216**), no variation in composition has been established. Indeed the very existence of cross-striations has recently been challenged, the appearance being regarded as an artifact due to sectioning across well-aligned groups of prisms. However, this interpretation cannot account for the presence of cross-striations in carefully prepared thin sections, nor for the interrelationship with enamel striae.

220a

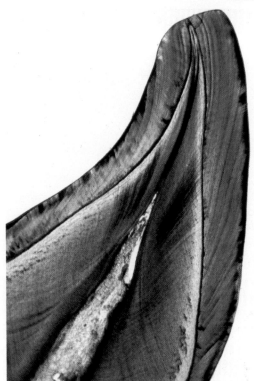

220a The striae of Retzius. In ground sections of enamel viewed in transmitted light, a series of irregularly spaced, brown lines called the striae of Retzius may be seen running obliquely across the tissue and across the prism directions from the enamel–dentine junction. The striae over incisal edges and cusps do not reach the tooth surface (unless there is attrition). However, those on lateral surfaces usually do reach the surface to form perikymata (see **223**). (Ground, longitudinal section through a tooth; × 15)

220b

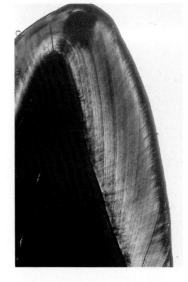

220b Striae of Retzius passing over cusp without reaching the enamel surface. (Ground section; × 20)

221

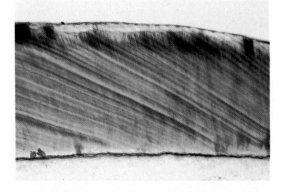

222

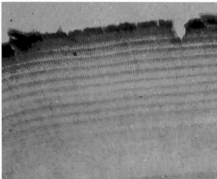

221 Striae of Retzius at higher power. The striae are 20–80μm apart and may vary from 4–15μm in width. They are incremental lines marking the position of the developing enamel at approximately weekly intervals. Indeed, there are about seven cross-striations between consecutive striae (see also page 317).

The pattern of the striae varies from individual to individual, but is similar in different teeth from the same individual. This suggests that a systemic factor is responsible for their development. The enamel of deciduous teeth has fewer striae than for permanent teeth, deciduous enamel forming more rapidly. (Ground longitudinal section of enamel; × 40)

222 Striae of Retzius seen in decalcified enamel from a tooth sectioned perpendicular to its long axis. In transverse sections the striae of Retzius appear as concentric rings, much like the growth rings in a tree. (Demineralised section; light green; × 150)

223a

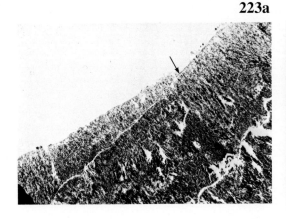

223b

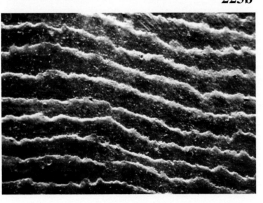

223 Surface terminations of the striae in transmission (223a) and scanning (223b) electron micrographs. The tooth surface shows a series of concentric grooves called perikymata. When the striae reach the surface in areas without wear, they end at the concavities of the perikymata. In **223a**, two striae may be distinguished, one terminating at a perikyma (*arrowed*). This corresponds to the base of the grooves in the scanning electron micrograph (**223b**). (**223a**, TEM, × 1,000; **223b**, SEM, × 200)

224 Prisms and cross-striations showing the 'picket-fence' appearance of a putative stria. In some ground sections viewed at moderately high magnification, step-like lines may be seen crossing the prisms, which might correspond to the striae of Retzius. These lines present a picket-fence appearance and suggest that the striae might be formed along the cross-striations and prism junctions. At high magnifications, however, it is difficult to see equivalent structures to the striae. (Ground, longitudinal section of enamel; × 1,000)

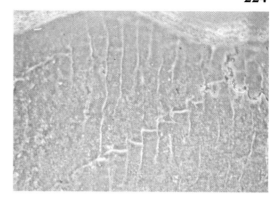

225 Diagrams illustrating the nature and development of the striae of Retzius. It is believed that each stria represents the former outline of the developing front of the enamel. This front, being related to the morphology of the Tomes' processes of the ameloblasts, is sometimes described as having a 'picket-fence' appearance (see also **224**). **225a** suggests that each 'slot' of the picket-fence is related to two structural elements — cross-striations (red) and prism boundaries (blue). However, it is quite rare to obtain the grid-like intersections of cross-striations and prism junctions.

The mechanism responsible for the development of striae is a subject of controversial debate. The rate of enamel formation and the contribution from the various surfaces of the Tomes' process varies on a diurnal basis, resulting in the cross-striations (see **218**). Occasionally, due to some unknown systemic factor, the daily variation in enamel deposition is exaggerated and a greater change in prism dimension results to form a stria. There may also be a variation in composition, but most likely (although not

225a

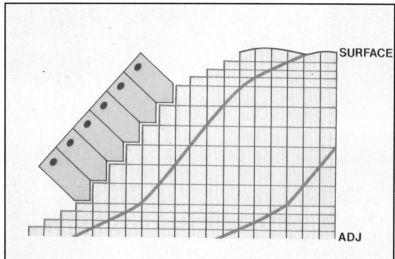

225b

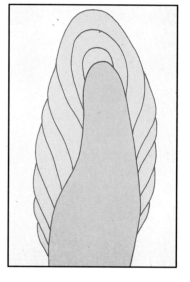

exclusively) a change in crystal orientation with an increase in porosity and organic content.

Virtually all textbook descriptions of the striae emphasise their S-shaped appearance. As daily increments of enamel formation are smaller at the beginning and at the end of amelogenesis, the cross-striations are closer together near the enamel–dentine junction and in surface enamel, and thus the striae develop as S-shaped lines. However, these shapes are not easy to see in histological preparations.

225b shows the pattern of striae in terms of the whole crown. Over unworn cusps and incisal tips, the striae are located completely within the tissue. More laterally, they usually reach the surface in the concavities of the perikymata (see **223**).

In regions where enamel is particularly thin and amelogenesis is slow (e.g. cervical enamel), adjacent striae are close together. In surface enamel which is aprismatic, the striae are incomplete and do not reach the tooth surface.

226

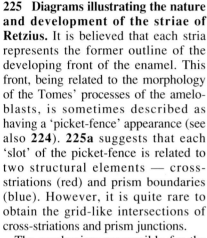

226 Neonatal line (A) in enamel. The striae of Retzius are less pronounced, and may even be absent from, enamel formed prenatally. The disturbance of birth results in the formation of a particularly exaggerated stria, the neonatal line. Since these lines are seen in all enamel forming at the time of birth, they are found in all the deciduous teeth and in the larger cusps of the permanent first molars. (Ground section; × 6)

227 Prism direction at the neonatal line as seen in a ground section of enamel, acid etched, and examined in the scanning electron microscope. At a location consistent with the neonatal line (**A**), the enamel prisms appear to change both their thickness and their direction. (SEM; × 400)

227

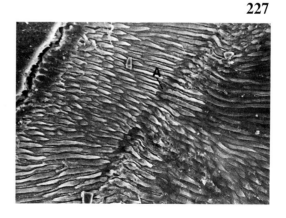

Many textbooks report that the prisms in enamel pass perpendicularly from the enamel–dentine junction to the surface. It seems, however, that the prisms are inclined to both the enamel–dentine junction and to the tooth surface at less than 90° (except for the enamel close to the cervical margin). Indeed, the prisms meet the surface at an angle of approximately 60°.

Furthermore, the prisms do not follow a straight course from the enamel–dentine junction to the surface, their direction reflecting the movements of the ameloblasts during enamel formation (see page 261). The changing direction and arrangement of prisms is responsible for the appearance of histological features of enamel known as Hunter–Schreger bands and gnarled enamel.

228a

228b

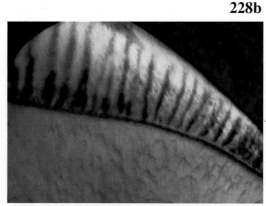

228 Hunter–Schreger bands are seen when enamel is viewed in either reflected light (**228a**) or polarised light (**228b**). They appear as broad (approximately 50μm wide), alternating dark and light bands and are found in the inner 25–50% of the enamel. The bands are the result of variations in the course of adjacent groups of prisms. (Ground, longitudinal sections of enamel; **228a**; × 12; **228b**; × 25)

229

230

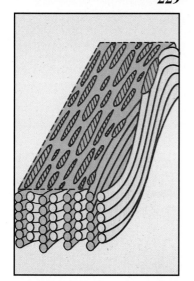

229 Diagram showing direction of prisms and resultant cut surface with alternately reflecting bands. The enamel prism does not follow a straight line but takes a sinusoidal course, making four or five curves before straightening in the peripheral one-third of the tissue. Collectively, the prisms are aligned in horizontal rows or sheets, adjacent rows above and below taking different directions as they leave the enamel-dentine junction. When viewed in longitudinal section, the different prism sheets are cut at different obliquities. If then viewed in reflected light, alternate sheets of prisms will reflect the light in alternately different directions. Some will reflect it to the eyepiece and appear white. Others will reflect it away and appear dark. By changing the direction of the light, the pattern can be reversed. The bands are seen in polarised light because the different sheets exhibit different crystal orientations. The bands are not seen in surface enamel, as here the prisms become aligned in parallel.

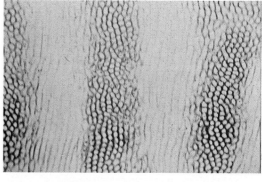

230 Changing prism directions seen in a ground, longitudinal section of enamel. In thin ground sections, when prism junctions can be clearly seen, areas showing sheets of prisms with very different orientations are discernible. The underlying mechanisms during development which allow ameloblasts in different layers to slide past each other are not known.

Functionally, changes in prism directions between different layers may increase the strength of the tissue, making it less prone to fracture and more resistant to wear. (Ground, longitudinal section of enamel; × 300)

231

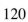

231 Gnarled enamel. In cuspal and incisal enamel, regions may be found which show marked 'decussation' of prisms. Here, there is the suggestion of spiral changes of prism direction to give the appearance known as gnarled enamel. However, gnarled enamel is only seen where (as illustrated here) the section does not pass through the cusp. In other sections, instead of a gnarled appearance it is possible to align the plane of section and the prism directions to show Hunter–Shreger bands. (Ground, longitudinal section through cuspal enamel; × 25)

The enamel–dentine junction

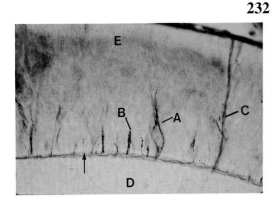

232

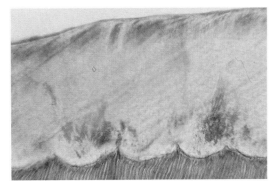

233

233 The scalloped appearance of the enamel–dentine junction. In two dimensions, the junction appears as a series of shell-shaped arches, commonly described as scallops. The arrangement is such that the concavities of the scallops project into the dentine. The scalloped appearance is especially prominent beneath the cusps of the tooth. At the lateral surfaces of the crown, however, the enamel–dentine junction may appear quite smooth. (Ground section of enamel; × 60)

232 The enamel–dentine junction (*arrowed*) and associated structures. A, enamel tuft; **B**, enamel spindle; **C**, enamel lamella; **D**, dentine; **E**, enamel. (Ground, transverse section through enamel; × 60)

234

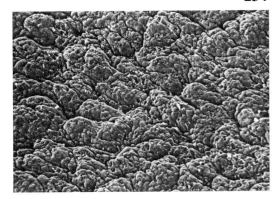

234 The enamel surface of the enamel–dentine junction. If a tooth is fractured in order to separate the enamel and the dentine, the split often occurs in the inner enamel and not at the enamel–dentine junction. If teeth are dehydrated, however, the differing water content of the two tissues causes differential shrinkage and weakens the junction such that fracture of a dried tooth follows the enamel–dentine junction. The interface that is thus revealed by examining the enamel surface is complex in three dimensions, with undulations which fit into depressions of the dentine. It is thought that this arrangement, by enabling a close interlocking of the two tissues, prevents the tissues shearing apart during mastication. (Fractured and dehydrated specimen of enamel viewed by SEM; × 250)

235

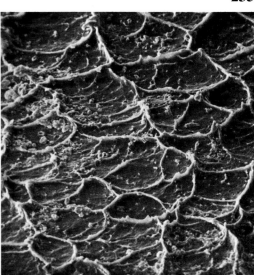

235 Dentine surface of the enamel–dentine junction. The enamel has been removed from this specimen by demineralisation. The wave-like scallops can be seen together with numerous minor irregularities which contribute to the complexity of the interdigitation. (Decalcified surface of enamel–dentine junction viewed by SEM; × 400)

236

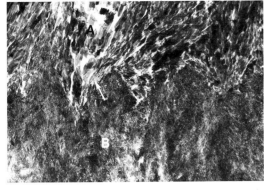

236 Enamel and dentine crystals at the enamel–dentine junction (*arrowed*). The change from small apatite crystals in dentine (**B**) to the larger enamel crystals (**A**) is clear in this specimen. However, there may be a transition zone where crystals are intermediate in size. The intimacy, almost blending, of the tissues contributes to the strength of the enamel–dentine junction. Note that, on the enamel side of the enamel–dentine junction, the relative uniformity of crystal orientation may result in a thin layer of prismless enamel. (TEM of enamel and dentine; × 18,000)

237 Enamel tufts. In ground sections, structures with the superficial appearance of tufts of grass are found in the inner one-third of the enamel, with their bases at the enamel–dentine junction. These structures appear to travel in the same direction as the prisms and can, by altering the plane of focus, be seen in thick sections to be undulating with the sheets of prisms. Tufts are hypomineralised and are therefore evident in demineralised sections of enamel. They recur at about 100μm intervals along the enamel–dentine junction. Each tuft is several prisms wide. It has been suggested that tufts are incompletely mineralised prisms with rather more organic matrix than elsewhere and with the interprismatic material exaggerated. Because of the vertical orientation of these 'faults', they are best seen in transverse sections of the tooth. (Ground transverse section of enamel; × 200)

237

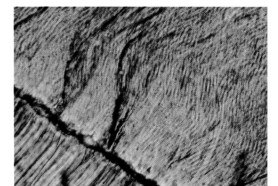

238 Enamel lamellae (A) are hypomineralised sheets which usually run through the full thickness of the enamel. Occasionally, however, they are restricted to the periphery. Like the tufts, they are best seen in transverse sections of the tooth. The lamellae are narrower and longer than tufts and do not extend far in the third dimension. They arise either because groups of prisms fail to complete mineralisation, or because cracks appear in enamel (during development or even after eruption) in which organic material accumulates to divert light in ground sections and to absorb stain in decalcified sections. Lamellae are less common than tufts and are solitary or irregularly arranged. (Decalcified transverse section of enamel; × 150)

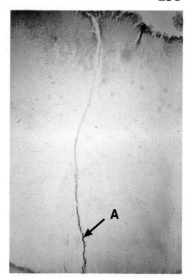

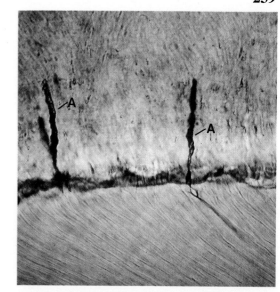

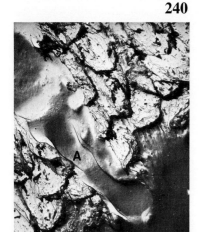

240

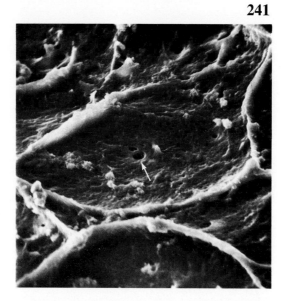

241

239 Enamel spindles (A) are cylindrical, club-shaped structures which extend from the dentine surface 10–40μm into the enamel. They are particularly common beneath cusps and incisal edges. Unlike tufts, spindles are not aligned with the enamel prisms and they are best seen in longitudinal sections of the tooth. Some of the spindles appear to be continuous with dentinal tubules and consequently it is thought that they are formed by odontoblastic processes that insinuated between ameloblasts in the early stages of enamel formation. (Ground, longitudinal section at the enamel–dentine junction; × 250)

240 A dentinal tubule extending across the enamel–dentine junction. The structure labelled **A** is the extension of a dentinal tubule across the scalloped junctional area. It would appear as a 'spindle' in ground section. (Metal replica from fractured tooth surface viewed by TEM; × 2,500)

241 Tubule termination on the dentine surface of the enamel–dentine junction. The small, pore-like structure (*arrowed*) in the centre of a scallop of the enamel–dentine junction has the dimensions of a dentinal tubule and may therefore be a spindle. It is unlikely that the dentinal tubules that enter enamel contain vital cell processes (e.g. odontoblast processes; see pages 134–136). (SEM; × 1,600)

The surface features of enamel

The surface of the enamel has received particular attention because of its significance for the initiation of dental caries and for the adhesion of plastic restorative materials.

Both physically and chemically, surface enamel differs markedly from subsurface enamel. Surface enamel is harder, less porous, less soluble and more radio-opaque than subsurface enamel. It is richer in trace elements, especially fluoride. These properties may contribute to the ability of the surface enamel to resist caries, and to the character of the early enamel lesion.

The outermost layer of enamel may be prismless due to the parallel arrangement of the enamel crystal. Striae of Retzius emerge onto the surface, where they are associated with a series of furrows, the perikymata. The following six electron micrographs illustrate the varying appearances of surface enamel.

242 Perikymata on the enamel surface. Newly erupted permanent teeth show a wave-like pattern of concentric surface rings parallel to the cementum–enamel junction. The elevations are known as imbrication lines (of Pickerill) and the furrows between them are the perikymata. In deciduous teeth, perikymata are infrequent. Perikymata are readily removed by attrition or abrasion and are most often found in protected cervical areas. Note the absence of prism-end markings on this specimen. (SEM; × 500)

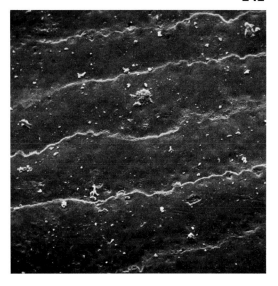

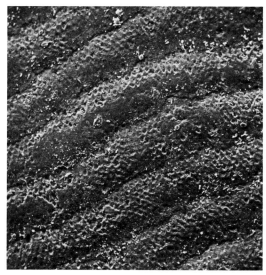

243 Prism-end markings on surface enamel. In some areas, particularly cervically where the reduced enamel epithelium persists for some time after eruption, small pits are seen within the perikymata. These represent the impression of the Tomes' processes of the ameloblasts and are 1–1.5µm in depth. (SEM; × 300)

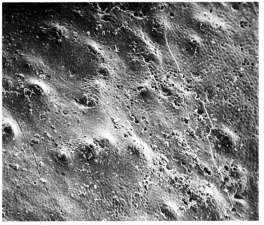

244a

244b

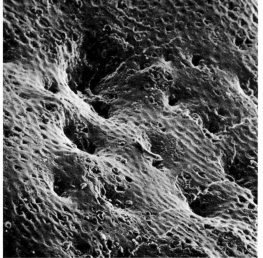

244 Enamel caps (244a) and focal holes (244b). In limited areas of the surface enamel (particularly on the lateral surfaces), small elevations of irregular size and distribution may be seen. The elevations are 10–15µm wide and are known as enamel caps (or surface overlapping projections). It is thought that they may result from enamel being laid down on some non-mineralisable material incorporated into the tissue in the late stages of its development. The focal holes (or isolated deep pits) appear to be formed when the enamel caps are removed by attrition or abrasion. (SEM; **244a**, × 150; **244b**, × 400)

245

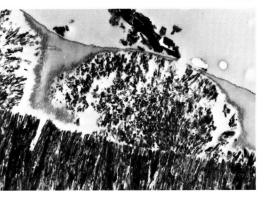

246

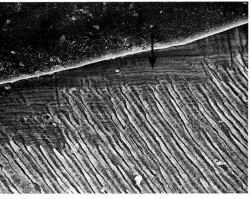

246 Prismless, surface enamel (*arrowed*). The thickness and distribution of prismless enamel differs in deciduous and permanent teeth, in permanent teeth of different types, and also at different sites in the same tooth. Note in the specimen shown the varying thickness of the prismless surface enamel compared with the uniform thickness illustrated in **204**. (SEM; × 200)

245 An enamel broch. These are occasional, large surface elevations (30–50µm in diameter) which occur on the surface of some teeth, particularly premolars. In the broch, the crystals often appear to converge, producing a radial pattern. (TEM; × 10,000)

Comparative anatomy

In addition to the prismatic enamel found in human teeth, three other types of enamel may be found in other animals: enameloid, aprismatic enamel and tubular enamel.

Enameloid

Enameloid is the tissue which covers the dentine of the teeth of fish (with the exception of the coelacanth) and larval amphibians. The tissue differs from other enamels in that, being derived mesodermally and not ectodermally, it should be regarded as a hypercalcified layer of specialised dentine. Indeed, the matrix of developing enameloid is collagenous.

247

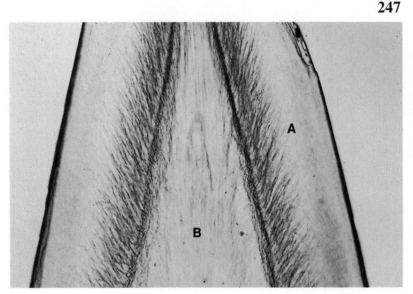

248

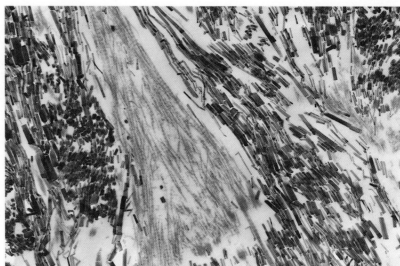

247 Enameloid from the tooth of a piranha (*Serrasalmus rhombeus*). A, enameloid; B, inner core of dentine. Enameloid appears as a relatively structureless, non-prismatic layer. Within the inner enameloid, numerous dark lines may be seen which are continuations of the dentinal tubules. Some fish (for example, the sheeps-head fish, *Sargus ovis*) also have tubules running from the surface of the tooth into the enameloid for varying distances. There may be differences in crystal orientation between the outer and inner zones of the enameloid (a feature which may help counteract the stresses and strains set up within the tissue during feeding). (Ground, longitudinal section; × 120)

248 Mineralising enameloid in the tooth of a dogfish (*Seyliorhinus canicula*). Fluorapatite crystals are being formed within the collagenous matrix of enameloid. The characteristic banding of the collagen can be seen. This collagen is secreted by mesenchymal odontoblast cells. Other matrix components may be secreted by the ectodermal cells of the enamel organ. During maturation of enameloid, the labile collagen fibres disappear, the tooth germ perhaps assisting in its final removal. Chemical analysis of mature enameloid shows that its protein content is similar to ectodermally-derived mammalian enamel. (TEM; × 15,000)

Aprismatic enamel

The teeth of lobe-finned fish (the coelacanth, *Latimeria chalumrae*), of reptiles (excepting the spiny-tailed lizard, *Uromastyx hardwicki*, uniquely possessing a thin layer of prismatic enamel) and of adult amphibians have outer coverings of thin, ectodermally-derived, aprismatic enamel.

Aprismatic enamel results from the parallel arrangement of all the crystals at right angles to the enamel surface, there being no sudden changes in crystal orientation. Developmentally, the parallel arrangement of the crystals is thought to be associated with flattened secretory ends of the ameloblasts (i.e. the absence of Tomes' processes; see pages 260–261).

249

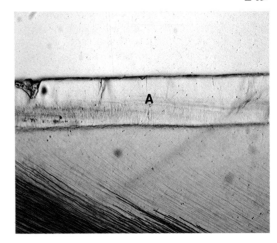

249 Aprismatic enamel (A) from the tooth of a crocodile (*Crocodilus niloticus*). Some incremental lines may be seen running parallel with the enamel surface. (Ground, longitudinal section; × 130)

Tubular enamel

Tubular enamel is a specialised form of prismatic enamel found in most marsupials (excepting the rodent-like teeth of the wombat *Phascolomis*) and in many placental mammals (including the hyrax and certain insectivores and lemurs).

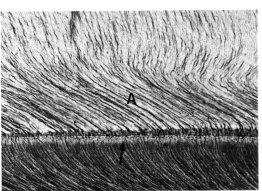

250

250 Tubular enamel (A) of a kangaroo (*Macropus rufus*). As the name suggests, tubular enamel is characterised by the presence of tubules running through the inner portion of prismatic enamel. The tubules may be located both intraprismatically and interprismatically and appear to be continuous with the underlying dentinal tubules. The enamel–dentine junction is arrowed. It has been suggested that, during development, the enamel tubules contain cell processes which are extensions of the ameloblasts. Alternatively, there have been attempts to homologise the enamel tubule with the enamel spindle (see **239**). According to this theory, the enamel tubules are thought to develop around odontoblast processes. (Ground, longitudinal section; × 100)

251

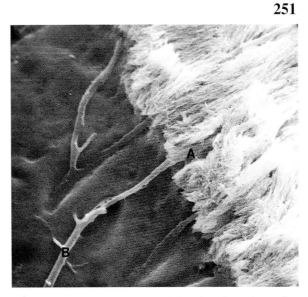

251 Tubules at the enamel-dentine junction of a marsupial tooth (*Trichosurus vulpecula*). Enamel tubules (**A**) and dentine tubules (**B**) have been filled with methylmethacrylate and the mineralised tissues etched away to leave casts. (SEM; × 4,000)

125

Investing organic layers on enamel surfaces

Throughout its life the crown of a tooth is covered by an organic integument. Before the tooth erupts into the oral cavity the crown is covered by the overlying oral mucosa, the coronal part of the dental follicle, and the vestiges of the enamel organ (plus its associated primary enamel cuticle). For information concerning the origins of the dental organ and the dental follicle during early tooth development, see pages 248–252. After emerging into the mouth, parts of the integument of enamel organ origin are lost by degeneration of its epithelial component, and by attrition or abrasion of the underlying cuticular component. In the region of the gingival crevice or sulcus, the primary (or pre-eruptive) enamel cuticle acquires additional matter from the lining epithelium and, coronal to the gingival margin, from saliva. The salivary layer is known as the acquired pellicle. Oral bacteria adhere initially to the enamel cuticle, and later to the acquired pellicle, to form the dental plaque.

Pre-eruptive investing layers

252

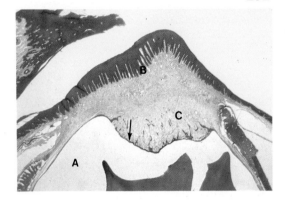

252 The soft tissues covering an erupting tooth comprise oral epithelium (**B**) and the subjacent connective tissue of the dental follicle (**C**). Lining the enamel space (**A**) is an epithelial layer which is the remains of the enamel organ — the reduced enamel epithelium (*arrowed*). (Demineralised, longitudinal section of an erupting tooth *in situ*, H & E; × 10)

253

253 High-power view of the tissue adjacent to the enamel surface. Immediately adjacent to the enamel space (**A**) is the reduced enamel epithelium (**B**). The appearance of this epithelium varies from a thin, flattened layer of cells to a more organised layer of recognisable cuboidal or columnar reduced ameloblasts, deep to which are several more cell layers. In this section, the reduced enamel epithelium appears flattened. Superficial to the reduced enamel epithelium is the fibrous connective tissue of the dental follicle (**C**), and superficial to this is the oral submucosa (**D**). (Demineralised section, H & E; × 160)

254

254 The reduced enamel epithelium in an occlusal fissure. The enamel organ associated with an occlusal fissure appears to be the last to change to a reduced enamel epithelium. In this section, the peripheral cells of the reduced enamel epithelium adjacent to the enamel space (**A**) are still columnar. Note the vascularity of the tissue in this region. (Demineralised section, Mallory's trichome; × 80)

255

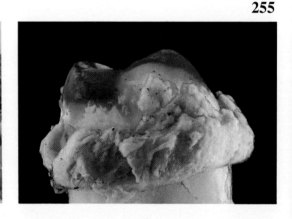

255 Macroscopic appearance of the pre-eruptive investing layers. This unerupted permanent third molar has been stained to show the remains of the dental follicle (yellow) and the vestigial enamel organ (blue). Note that part of the follicle has been lost during the surgical removal of the tooth and that the underlying vestigial enamel organ covers the entire crown. (Alcian blue after fixation in Bouin's solution; × 4)

Investing layers associated with the crowns of erupted teeth

256 Approximal view of an erupted premolar showing the zones of its organic integument. The integument (sometimes referred to as Nasmyth's membrane) covers the entire crown surface. Two zones are stained. The dark blue layer (**A**) is the plaque. The light blue layer (**C**) is the attachment or junctional epithelium which in life links the tooth to the gingiva coronal to the periodontal ligament (see pages 208–210). The unstained zone between them (**B**) comprises the primary (or pre-eruptive) enamel cuticle. Note that the plaque corresponds to a position above the crest of the gingival margin and around the contact point (*arrowed*) where adjacent teeth meet, and that the cuticle lies in the region of the gingival crevice. Apical to the junctional epithelium, the enamel was covered *in vivo* by loosely adherent reduced enamel epithelial cells lost during extraction. Coronal to the plaque, the crown is covered by the primary enamel cuticle together with an organic element of salivary origin (the acquired pellicle). (Alcian blue–Aldehyde fuchsin; × 4)

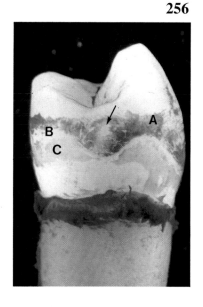

256

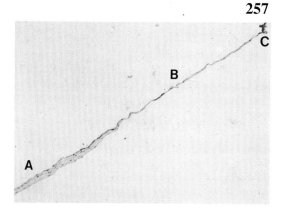

257

257 Organic enamel integument. Using careful demineralising techniques it is possible to lift off the organic integument; consequently the plaque, primary enamel cuticle and junctional epithelium appear as a single continuous entity. **A**, epithelium; **B**, primary enamel cuticle; **C**, plaque. (Ollett's modification of Twort; × 100)

258 Higher magnification of part of the integument after removal from enamel. 258a, superficial surface; **258b**, enamel-related surface; **D**, plaque; **C**, primary (pre-eruptive) enamel cuticle; **E**, junctional epithelium. Note that the surface of the integument adjacent to the enamel shows bands of prism-end markings deep to the plaque (see zone **D**). This indicates the persistence of the pre-eruptively formed primary enamel cuticle on the erupted enamel surface. (**258a**, Toluidine blue and erythrosin, × 20; **258b**, Alcian blue and erythrosin; × 20)

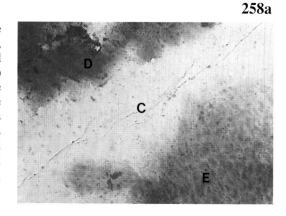

258a

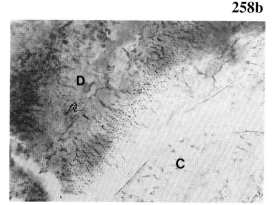

258b

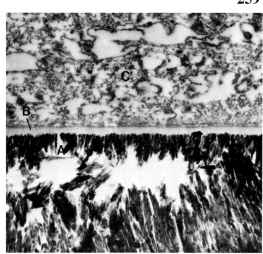

259

259 The enamel integument at the level of the junctional epithelium. This micrograph is taken from a region at the coronal limit of the gingival crevice. The enamel surface (**A**) is covered by the primary enamel cuticle (**B**) and the remaining vestige of an attachment or junctional epithelial cell (**C**). The junctional epithelium is described further on pages 208–210. (TEM; × 13,000)

260 The enamel integument immediately coronal to the junctional epithelium showing the primary enamel cuticle (*arrowed*) on the enamel surface. This section is in the region of the gingival crevice coronal to that illustrated in **259** and therefore lacks a junctional epithelial cell. Note that the cuticle usually has an electron-dense outer border. (TEM; × 10,000)

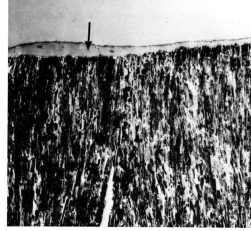

260

261 The primary enamel cuticle and the enamel matrix. The primary enamel cuticle (**A**) is in intimate contact with the underlying organic enamel matrix (**B**). Note the lathe-like spaces occupied *in vivo* by enamel crystals. While generally approximately 30nm thick, the cuticle acquires accretions (**C**) in the region of the gingival crevice. These derive from crevicular epithelium and from plasma, and may increase the cuticle to a thickness of up to about 5μm. (Demineralised section, TEM; × 30,000)

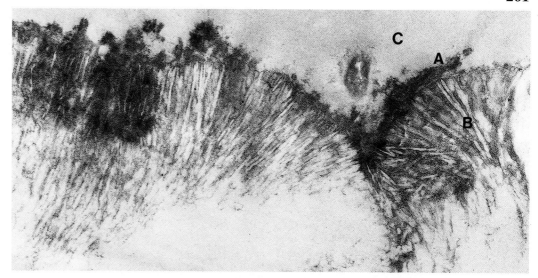

262 Localised thickening of the primary enamel cuticle (*arrowed*) may also occur on its deep aspect, where enamel maturation is incomplete because of the presence at this site of a stria of Retzius (**A**) reaching the surface. (TEM; × 5,100)

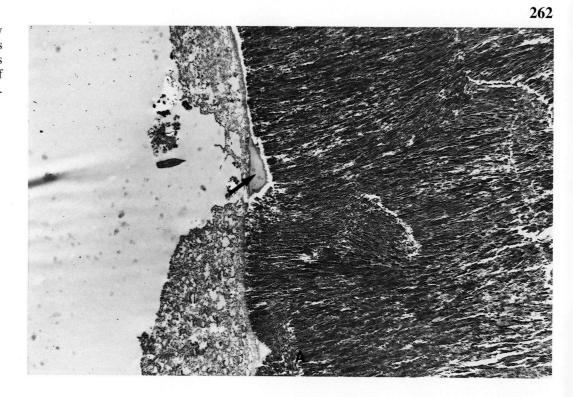

263 Composition of the primary enamel cuticle. The primary enamel cuticle is thought to be composed of protein. Its accretions are mainly proteoglycan or glycoprotein elements from the contiguous soft tissues. Plasma contributions include immunoglobulins, in this case IgG (*arrowed*), which form part of the host defence system against plaque. (TEM with antibody to human IgG; peroxidase method for localisation of IgG; × 34,500)

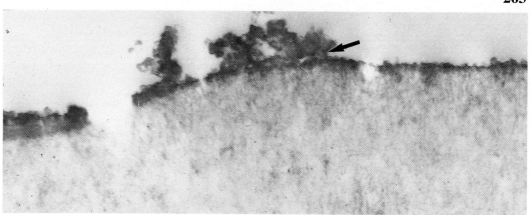

264 The enamel integument coronal to the gingival margin showing bacterial colonisation, forming dental plaque, on the primary enamel cuticle (*arrowed*). **R**, stria of Retzius. (TEM; × 20,000)

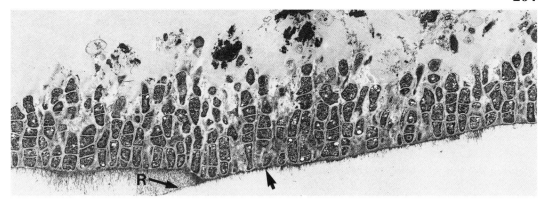

265 The enamel integument above the gingival crest showing bacterial colonisation forming dental plaque. Where the primary enamel cuticle is exposed to the oral environment, it is usually coated with acquired pellicle. This micrograph shows early approximal surface plaque on a clear layer (**A**), which is probably combined primary enamel cuticle and pellicle. Excessive plaque (**P**) accumulation is associated with the causation of both dental caries and chronic inflammatory periodontal disease. (TEM; × 1,500)

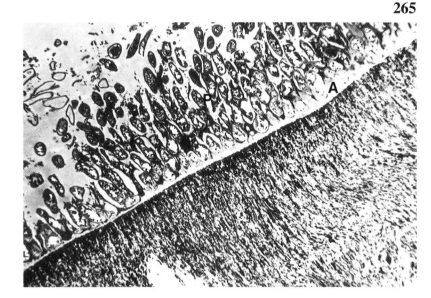

266

266 Enamel surface showing a deposit of dental plaque. In health, the firm apposition of the gingiva to the tooth limits the plaque to the gingival margin. Even slight inflammation allows relaxation of the gingiva, and ingress of bacteria, as shown here. **A**, boundary of dental plaque (SEM; × 1,500)

Where the enamel surface is exposed to wear, either by attrition or abrasion, the vestigial enamel organ is worn away, but the enamel rapidly acquires a layer of acquired pellicle. Indeed, this pellicle always forms a protective coat following any subsequent wear.

Dental calculus is calcified plaque and/or pellicle. It represents an excessive accumulation of salivary mineral and protein, materials which normally serve to mature the surface enamel, and to harden any enamel dentine or cementum surface exposed to wear or demineralisation. The mineral salts within plaque include amorphous calcium phosphate, crystalline octacalcium phosphate and hydroxyapatite.

Dentine

267 The distribution of dentine. Dentine (A) forms the bulk of the tooth, providing the tooth with the shape and rigidity necessary for functioning effectively during mastication. Along the crown, the dentine is covered by enamel; along the root, by cementum. It encloses the dental pulp, with which it shares a common origin from the dental papilla (see **622**). Indeed, the dentine and pulp can be considered as a single developmental and functional unit, often described as the pulpo-dentinal complex. The dentine forms an interdigitating, scalloped junction with the enamel (see **233**), but has a more indistinct junction with the cementum (see **293** and **294**). (Ground, longitudinal section through an incisor tooth; × 4)

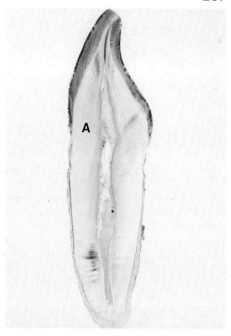

Physical properties of dentine. Dentine is pale yellow in colour. Because the enamel is semi-translucent, dentine gives the crown of the tooth its colour. It is harder than bone and cementum but softer and less brittle than enamel. Dentine has greater compressive and tensile strengths than enamel. Because it is traversed by tubules, the dentine is readily permeable. Regional variations in tubule size and density are reflected in differences in permeability. The specific gravity of dentine is approximately 2.1g/ml.

Chemical composition of dentine. Dentine is composed by weight of approximately 70% inorganic material, 20% organic material and 10% water. By volume, the same components comprise 47%, 32% and 21% respectively. Thus, the non-mineral component is much higher than in enamel. The principal inorganic component is hydroxyapatite (present as plate-like crystallites smaller than those of enamel; see **205**). Trace elements such as fluoride and carbonate are present in the crystallites. The main organic component is Type I collagen (comprising 90% of the matrix), with proteoglycans between the fibres. Other non-collagenous proteins in calcified dentine include phosphoproteins, γ-carboxyglutamate-containing proteins, acidic glycoproteins and plasma proteins. With the exception of plasma proteins, these are absent from the uncalcified predentine on the pulpal surface. Lipids comprise approximately 1.7% of the dentinal organic matrix.

268 The dentinal tubules seen in a longitudinal ground section through dentine. Dentine is permeated by tubules which run from the pulpal surface towards the enamel–dentine and cementum–dentine junctions. *In vivo*, the tubules may contain cellular processes, which are derived from cells lining the pulpo-dentinal junction (the odontoblasts). The tubules taper from about 4µm in diameter at their pulpal ends to 1µm or less peripherally. As the surface area of the dentine is much smaller internally than externally, the tubules are more widely separated at their peripheries. Approximately 80% of the total volume of the dentine near the pulp is composed of tubules, while near the enamel–dentine junction the tubules comprise only about 4% of the tissue by volume. The tubules follow a curved, sigmoid course — the primary curvatures. The convexity of the primary curvatures nearest the pulp chamber faces rootward. In the root and beneath the cusps, the primary curvatures are less pronounced, the tubules running a straighter course. (Ground, longitudinal section; × 25)

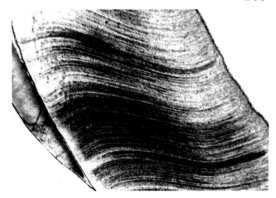

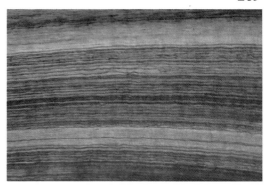

269 Dentinal tubules and secondary curvatures. In addition to the primary curvatures, the tubules also show smaller changes in direction every few micrometres — the secondary curvatures. Where these secondary curvatures coincide in direction, they produce the appearance of a line crossing the dentine — a contour line of Owen (see **297**). (Ground, longitudinal section; × 320)

270 The walls of the dentinal tubules vary according to location, and therefore according to the stage of development of the tissue. In predentine, the wall of a tubule consists of collagen fibres embedded in organic matrix with a thin, amorphous layer on the pulpal surface. In calcified dentine, an apparently proteinaceous membrane (the lamina limitans) overlies the mineralised collagen. In older regions, where peritubular dentine has formed, a similar film overlies the amorphous mineral. In this specimen of fractured dentine, the surface layers have been removed by acid etching. The tubules to the left have been exposed longitudinally and those to the right transversely. (SEM; × 1,750)

270

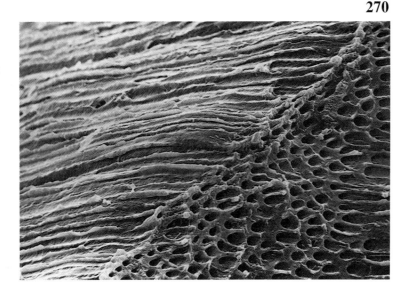

271

271 Branching of the dentinal tubules near the enamel–dentine junction (*arrowed*). The dentinal tubules are not single discrete tubes running through the dentine, but give off narrow branches along their course. Branching is particularly marked near the enamel–dentine junction. In the root, the dentinal tubules not only branch at their ends but also form loops which are thought to be responsible for the appearance of the granular layer (of Tomes, see page 140). (Ground, longitudinal section; Picrothionin; × 320)

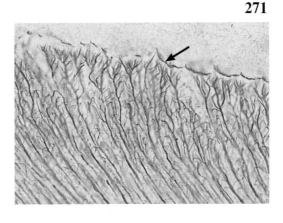

272 Transverse ground section showing dentinal tubules. In ground sections, the dentinal tubules (**A**) appear as circular regions. The concentration of tubules varies from 15,000/mm² in outer dentine to 65,000/mm² in inner dentine. Between the tubules lies the bulk of the dentine, referred to as intertubular dentine (**B**). When first formed the lumen of the tubule is approximately 4μm in diameter, but it is reduced by the deposition on its wall of peritubular dentine (**C**). Because of its position, a more correct term for this layer might be intratubular dentine. In the section shown, the large amount of peritubular dentine deposited in the tubules has reduced the lumen to a very small diameter. The mounting medium used has not penetrated the tubules and, because of the air and debris trapped within them, the tubules appear as black dots. (Partially demineralised and stained with eosin; × 1,500)

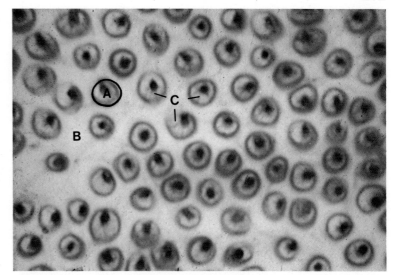

273 Transverse decalcified section of dentinal tubules. Compared with ground sections, two basic differences are seen in a decalcified transverse section through the tubules. An odontoblast process may be seen within the lumen of the tubule, and the peritubular dentine is lost so that the lumen of the tubule appears larger. (Harris' haematoxylin; × 1,000)

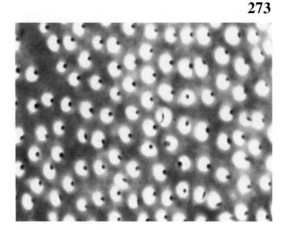

The contents of dentinal tubules

274 Peritubular dentine (A) can be distinguished from intertubular dentine (B) as a zone of increased electron density lining the internal surface of the dentinal tubule. Peritubular dentine is more highly mineralised than intertubular dentine. Unlike intertubular dentine, the matrix of peritubular dentine is not collagenous, though its precise composition has yet to be determined. In demineralised sections at the electron microscope level, the matrix appears as an amorphous material. The mineral component of peritubular dentine is calcium phosphate, but not in the form of hydroxyapatite crystallites. Although commonly considered amorphous, it has been reported as crystalline octocalcium phosphate. Some crystallites have a hexagonal shape and appear as compact platelets slightly smaller than (but similar to) those of intertubular dentine. Other crystalline species may also be present. Although the bulk of peritubular dentine is hypercalcified relative to the intertubular dentine, hypocalcified areas bound its inner and outer surfaces. Peritubular dentine is formed at about the same time as (or soon after) intertubular dentine. By the time primary dentine formation is complete, all peripheral tubules have a lining of peritubular dentine that extends from the enamel–dentine junction to within 100–150μm of the predentine. Eventually, the tubules become occluded, being most evident beneath attrition, though it can occur in unerupted teeth. Total occlusion may involve not only gradual accretion of peritubular dentine but precipitation of other material in the core of the tubule. Little is known about this material but it does differ from what has been termed peritubular dentine. In tubules exposed by attrition, some occluding components may be derived from saliva. (TEM; × 6,000)

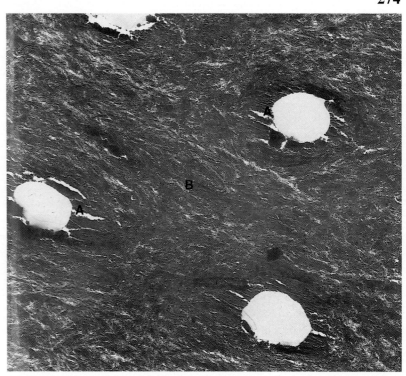

275–277 The relationship between peritubular dentine formation and tubule diameter at various levels within the dentine.

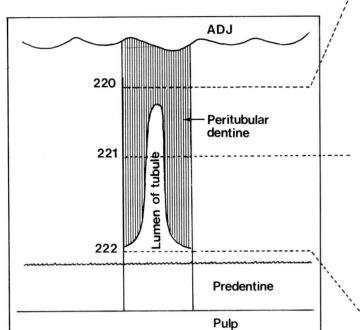

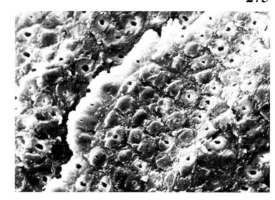

275 Near the enamel–dentine junction the tubule may be filled or nearly filled with peritubular dentine. (SEM; × 1,200)

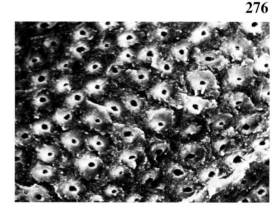

276

276 Towards the middle of the dentine a distinctive zone of peritubular dentine is seen. The thickness of the peritubular zone and consequently the degree of tubular occlusion varies considerably. (SEM; × 1,200)

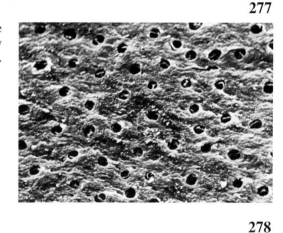

277

It has been suggested that variations with age in the reactions of the pulp to a noxious stimulus through the dentine may be related, at least in part, to variations in the amounts of peritubular dentine formed. Thus, in the young tooth where the tubules are relatively open, the passage of a stimulus through the dentine may be more rapid than in an older tooth where the tubules may be occluded with peritubular dentine.

277 Near the pulp where the tubule is newly formed, there may be little or no peritubular dentine. (SEM; × 540)

278

278 Translucent dentine. Associated with physiological aging, especially in root dentine, the dentinal tubules become completely occluded by mineral in a process similar to that of peritubular dentine formation (**274**) The contents of the tubules acquire the same refractive index as the intertubular dentine. When a ground section of a root is placed in water (as illustrated here), with a refractive index different from that of dentine, affected regions of dentine appear translucent (not being filled with water). Tubules become infilled at the root apex adjacent to cementum and extend cervically and towards the root canal with age The amount of translucent dentine increases linearly with age and is not affected by function or external irritation. In cross-section of the root, translucent zones have a butterfly shape, being wider at the mesial and distal margins. (Ground section ; × 5)

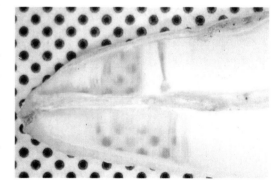

279 Each dentinal tubule is occupied by a protoplasmic extension of the odontoblast cell of the pulp (see 317) — the odontoblast process. When examined with the electron microscope, most of the dentinal tubules do not contain a cell process at the periphery (i.e. towards the enamel–dentine junction). This appearance may be due to the difficulty of preserving cell structures in such a remote location in mineralised tissue. However, even if the odontoblast processes are limited to the inner dentine, they are extremely long compared to the size of the cell body.

The odontoblast process is bounded by a cell membrane. In calcified dentine, the process contains microtubules, microfilaments and vesicles responsible for the transport and discharge of materials into the peri-odontoblastic space (see below). Nearer its base in the predentine, the odontoblast process contains more vesicles, the occasional mitochondrion, and strands of endoplasmic reticulum.

Where the tubule is occupied by an odontoblast process, there is often a space of variable size between the process and the tubule wall (the peri-odontoblastic space), which is presumably filled with tissue fluid.

In addition to the odontoblast processes, some dentinal tubules contain the terminals of sensory, non-myelinated axons, particularly in the regions beneath the cusps.

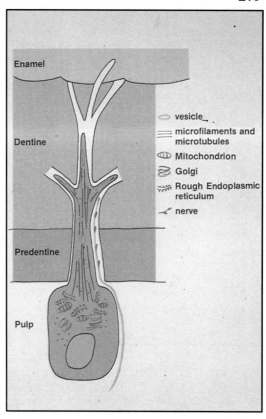

280 The odontoblast process in transverse section. Many of the elements included in the preceding diagram are found in this process, sectioned here in the unmineralised predentine, including microtubules, microfilaments, vesicles and mitochondria. (TEM; × 80,000)

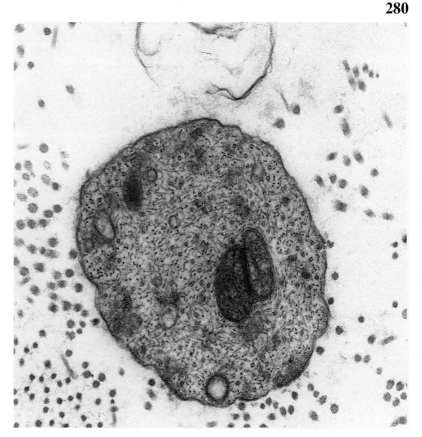

281 Dentinal tubules in peripheral dentine. With currently available fixation techniques, it is not possible to produce convincing images of cell processes in peripheral dentine. The images seen vary somewhat, but a common one is shown in this micrograph which shows amorphous, non-cellular material in the tubules. (TEM; × 8,000)

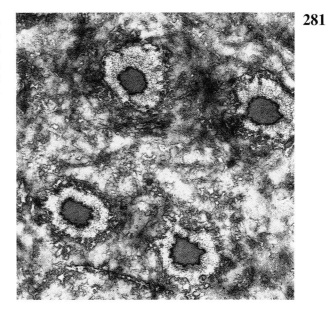

282 Dentinal tubules in intermediate dentine. In the inner third of calcified dentine, a variety of intratubular appearances are seen. Some tubules clearly contain cell processes, others are apparently empty and others contain non-cellular material. (TEM; × 3,000)

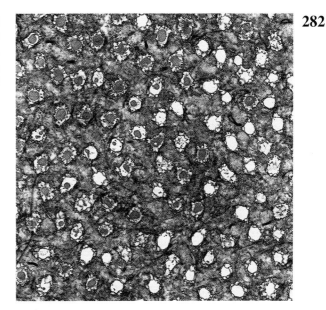

283 Dentinal tubules in inner calcified dentine. All tubules in inner dentine are occupied by odontoblast processes. In this example, from cuspal dentine, most of the tubules also contain sensory nerve terminals. (TEM; × 10,000)

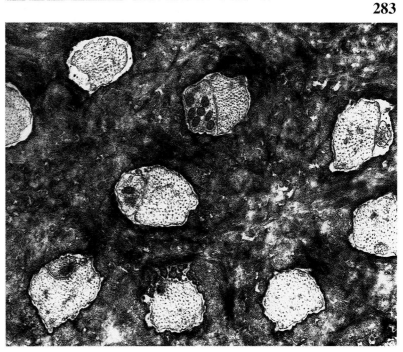

284 Intratubular structures in peripheral dentine. Different histological techniques can produce different interpretations of structure. Scanning electron micrographs of peripheral dentine (i.e. towards the enamel–dentine junction) reveal structures in the tubules which may be cell processes. This micrograph shows a branching tubular structure (*arrowed*) near the enamel–dentine junction of human dentine which has been decalcified and treated with collagenase. However, it is difficult to establish by this technique whether there are cellular structures within the tubules or merely organic sheaths (the lamina limitans) lining the tubules. (SEM; × 3,000)

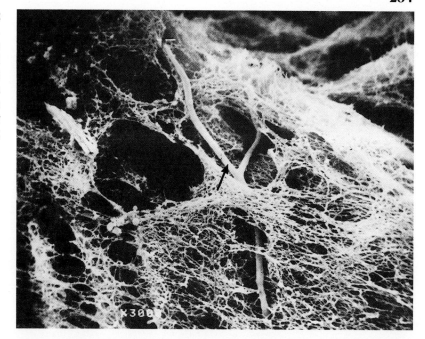

285 Components of the cytoskeleton in peripheral dentine. Techniques which recognise individual proteins may be used to detect the presence of intracellular material in peripheral dentinal tubules. Antibodies to vimentin, tubulin and actin (components of the intracellular tubule–filament system) react with tubule contents and can be revealed by fluorescent microscopy. In this micrograph the fluorescence in the tubules of a human molar is caused by labelled antibodies to the cytoskeleton protein tubulin. This method suggests that at least some peripheral tubules contain these substances. (Ultraviolet fluorescence after labelling with anti-tubulin antibodies and fluorescein-labelled goat anti-rabbit serum; × 4,200)

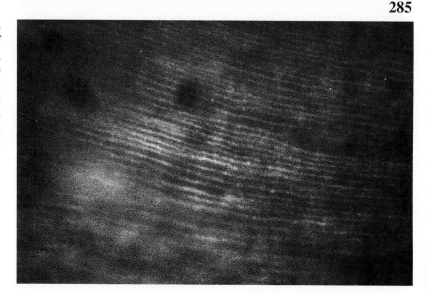

The present evidence concerning the controversy regarding the extent of the odontoblast processes in the dentinal tubules suggests that the processes occupy the tubules in their entirety only during the early stages of development. In the adult tissue, however, the extent of the odontoblast processes probably varies considerably, but in some sites may extend into the peripheral dentine.

286 The odontoblast process in the maturing tooth. This diagram describes three possible fates for the odontoblastic process. For all three situations (**A**, **B** and **C**), the process occupies the full length of the tubule during the early stages of development (**i**). In **A**, it remains along the full length of the tubule, throughout both intertubular dentine formation (**ii**) and peritubular dentine formation (**iii**). For **B**, the odontoblast process reaches a predetermined, finite length and retreats bodily (peritubular dentine forming within the dentinal tubule after the process has retreated). For **C**, the odontoblast process shortens at its distal end, becoming incorporated into the matrix of the peritubular dentine.

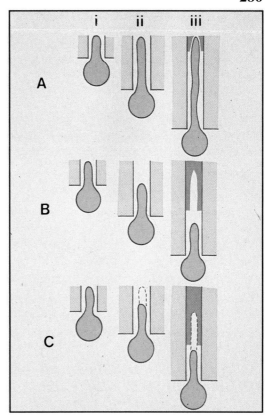

287 The pulp–predentine junction. The odontoblasts (**A**) form a continuous layer on the pulpal surface of the predentine (**B**). When techniques are employed that cause minimal tissue shrinkage, no space is seen between the odontoblast layer and the predentine. Note also that, in the predentine, the odontoblast processes (**C**) completely fill the dentinal tubules with no evidence of peri-odontoblastic spaces. (TEM of a surface replica obtained by freeze–fracture and coating the fractured surface with heavy metal by evaporation. The surface coating is then separated; × 2,000)

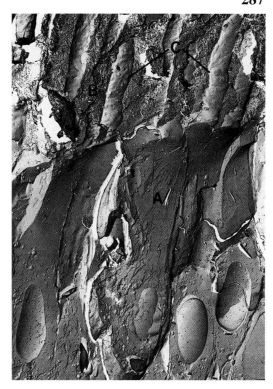

288 Sensory nerves terminating in the dentinal tubules may contribute to the sensitivity of the tissue. These terminals are limited mainly to the dentine of the crown beneath the cusps and are sparse in cervical and root dentine. This micrograph shows a single tubule containing both an odontoblastic process (**B**) and a sensory nerve terminal (**A**).

The axon in an innervated tubule is narrower than the odontoblast process. It contains microtubules, a few microfilaments and often mitochondria. Vesicles are rare in the nerve terminals or in the odontoblast process adjacent to them. There are no structurally specialised contacts between the axon and process to suggest synaptic linkage. It is probable that the process supports the axon metabolically (much as would a Schwann cell). (TEM; × 70,000)

The sensory nature of intratubular axons can be demonstrated by tracer techniques. Radioactive amino acids (e.g. tritium-labelled proline) injected into the trigeminal ganglion are converted into proteins and transported down the axons to the peripheral terminations. These terminals can be detected by coating labelled sections with photographic emulsion. After lengthy exposures, the radioactivity converts silver halides in the emulsion to silver grains that may be seen in the microscope after photographic development.

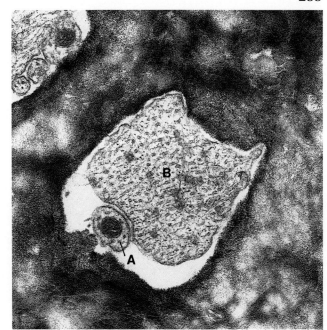

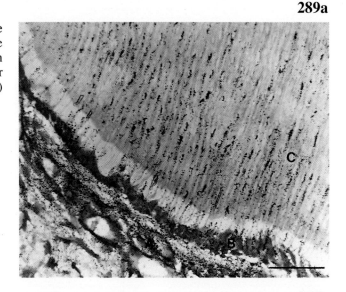

289a Light microscope autoradiograph showing the position of nerve endings in rat dentine. The presence of radioactively labelled nerve endings is demonstrated by the black silver grains developed in photographic emulsion painted over the section. Silver grains occur over the sub-odontoblastic plexus (of Raschkow) (**A**), the odontoblast layer (**B**) and over the dentinal tubules in the inner circumpulpal dentine (**C**). (× 730)

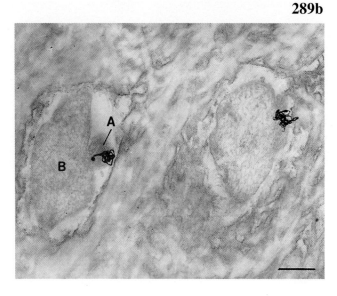

289b Labelled nerve (A) adjacent to an odontoblast process (B) in coronal rat dentine. Developed silver grains can be detected over the nerve-like processes which accompany odontoblast processes in the dentinal tubules. This evidence confirms that these structures are afferent axons, whose cell bodies lie in the trigeminal ganglion. Almost all the radioactivity remains within the nerve terminals for at least 7 days after injection and does not transfer to other cells in significant amounts. (TEM autoradiograph; × 20,000)

Sensory mechanisms in dentine

290 Sensory mechanisms in dentine. The functional significance of the dentinal innervation is not clear. One of the most important clinical features of dentine relates to its sensitivity. Three main hypotheses have been put forward to account for its sensitivity, implicating (i) nerves in dentine; (ii) the odontoblast processes; and (iii) fluid movements in the dentinal tubules. Arguments against the view that pain is due to direct stimulation of nerves in the dentine relate to their relative scarcity and to the fact that they appear to be absent in the outer parts of dentine. In addition, the application of local anaesthetics to the surface of dentine does not abolish the sensitivity. Referring to the second hypothesis, there is no physiological evidence to date which indicates that the odontoblast process is analogous to a nerve fibre and can similarly conduct impulses pulpwards. Furthermore, the process may not extend to the enamel–dental junction (see pages 135 and 136), while the application of substances designed to prevent transmission of such impulses is without effect. The most plausible hypothesis to explain the transmission of sensory stimuli suggests that all effective stimuli applied to dentine cause fluid movement through the tubules, and that this movement is sufficient to depolarise nerve endings in the inner parts of tubules, at the pulp–predentine junction and in the sub-odontoblastic neural plexus (**A**). Some stimuli, such as heat, osmotic pressure and drying, would tend to cause fluid movement outwards (**B**), while others such as cold would cause movement inwards (**C**). Movement in either direction would mechanically distort the terminals. These stimuli have been shown to cause such fluid movement *in vitro*. Chemicals (in strong solution) and thermal stimuli induce a response much more quickly than can be explained by conduction or diffusion. This, too, is consistent with the hydrodynamic hypothesis. In animal experiments, however, the response of intradental nerves to chemical stimuli is often slow and may be more readily explained by diffusion. It may be that both 'direct' and 'hydrodynamic' mechanisms operate, but that the hydrodynamic force predominates whenever there is pulpal inflammation and a lowering in threshold of intrapulpal nerves to the small mechanical forces generated by fluid flow.

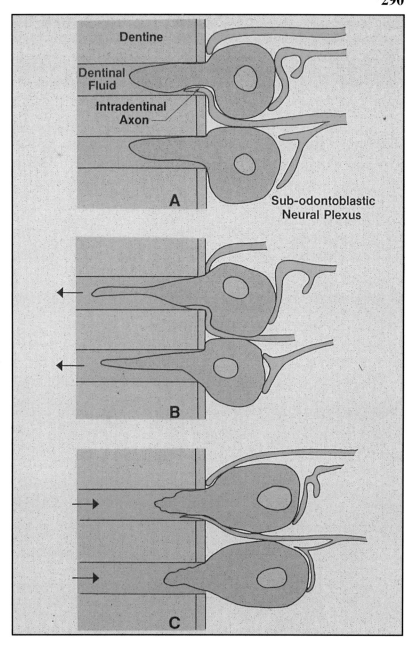

Regional differentiation of dentine

291 Regional differentiation of dentine. Dentine is not a uniform tissue but differs from region to region. The bulk of the dentine, termed circumpulpal dentine (**A**), differs in terms of structure and composition from the outer dentine lining the enamel–dentine junction, mantle dentine (**B**). In the root, the mantle dentine becomes continuous with a hyaline layer (**C**) which lies above a granular layer (**D**). The term primary dentine is used to describe the first-formed dentine which produces the typical form of the tooth. Secondary dentine is deposited during the later functional life of the tooth inside the primary dentine. Secondary dentine may be subdivided into regular (**E**) and irregular (**F**) varieties, depending upon its structure (see pages 143 and 144). The innermost, uncalcified layer of dentine lining the pulp is termed the predentine (**G**). **H**, enamel; **I**, cementum.

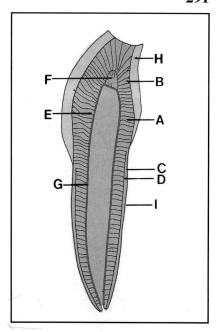

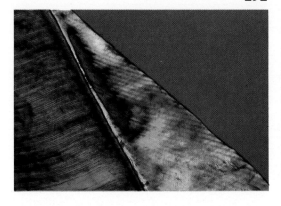

292 Enamel–dentine junction in the cervical region, shown in polarised light. Mantle dentine appears as the orange layer immediately beneath the enamel–dentine junction. The use of polarised light allows a visible distinction to be made between the mantle dentine and the circumpulpal dentine, which here appears blue. The mantle dentine is a thin layer approximately 20μm wide; it is the first dentine formed. The main distinguishing feature of the mantle dentine is the orientation of a large proportion of its collagen fibres perpendicular to the enamel–dentine junction. The fibres of the circumpulpal dentine are mainly parallel to the enamel–dentine junction. Such differences in orientation account for the different appearances in polarised light. Mantle dentine also differs from circumpulpal dentine in being hypomineralised. The dentinal tubules in mantle dentine branch more profusely than those in circumpulpal dentine. (Ground, longitudinal section; × 50)

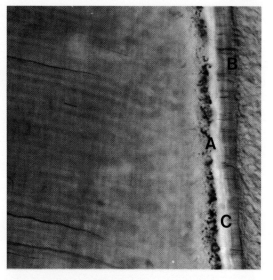

293 Root dentine showing the granular and hyaline layers. The granular layer (**A**) is seen as a thin, dark, granular region just beneath the cementum (**B**), lying along the whole length of the root. It is hypomineralised compared with the circumpulpal dentine. Its appearance has been related to the presence of minute interglobular areas produced as the result of incomplete mineralisation, or alternatively to the scattering of light from air trapped in dilatations or loops of the terminal parts of the dentinal tubules. This layer is not seen in demineralised sections.

Immediately superficial to the granular layer is the clear and relatively structureless hyaline layer (**C**) which is approximately 15μm wide. The hyaline layer may be difficult to distinguish from the adjoining layer of acellular cementum. (Ground section; × 160)

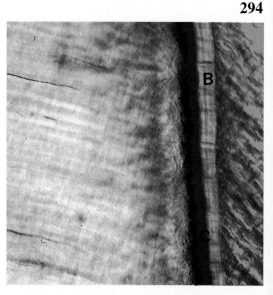

294 The granular and hyaline layers in polarised light. The ground section illustrated in **293** is here viewed through polarised light with a quartz-sensitive tint. The appearance of the granular layer (**A**) is similar to that seen in ordinary transmitted light. However, the hyaline layer (**C**) is sharply demarcated from the overlying acellular cementum. Its purple colour indicates a lack of birefringence due to the mixed orientation of its fibres. **B**, cementum. (Ground section; × 160)

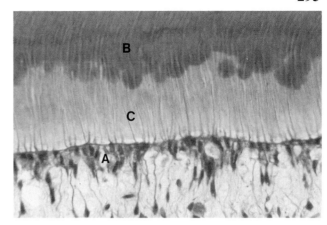

295 The predentine. Between the odontoblast layer (**A**) and the darker staining circumpulpal dentine (**B**) lies a pale zone, the predentine (**C**). The width of predentine varies from 10 to 40μm. The border between the circumpulpal dentine and predentine is the mineralising front, predentine being unmineralised. The predentine layer is always present; it is not merely a feature of the tissue during the early stages of development. Its thickness varies according to the rate of dentine formation, being thicker in young teeth where dentine forms rapidly. Even in decalcified sections (as illustrated here), a difference in staining properties can clearly be seen between dentine and predentine. This occurs because, at the time of mineralisation, there is a modification of the composition of the organic matrix. It has been suggested that the principal role of the odontoblast process in predentine is to secrete material, whereas in calcified dentine it is to modify and resorb some components. (Decalcified section of pulp and inner regions of dentine, H & E; × 500)

Structural lines in dentine

A number of lines have been described running roughly at right angles to the dentinal tubules. However, controversy exists concerning the seemingly irreconcilable differences between the descriptions and explanations of these structures by different authorities. The following description of structural lines in dentine is essentially a compromise. Two basic types of line can be distinguished, those related to the curvatures of the dentinal tubules — Schreger and Owen's lines — and those related to disturbances in dentinogenesis or the rhythmic deposition of dentine — mineralising lines and von Ebner lines.

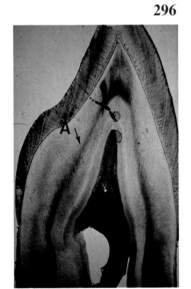

296 A Schreger line (A) results from the congruence of the primary curvatures of the dentinal tubules, and is related to the crowding of the odontoblasts which takes place as the size of the developing front is reduced during dentine deposition. In ground, transverse section, two Schreger lines may be seen as concentric rings. (Ground, longitudinal section through dentine; × 5)

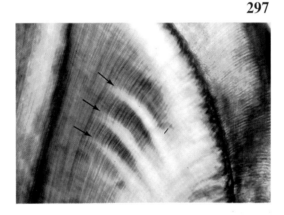

297 The contour lines of Owen (*arrowed*). Where the secondary curvatures of the dentinal tubules become coincident, the optical effect so produced gives rise to a contour line of Owen. In primary dentine, Owen's lines are rare. The most consistent Owen's line is seen at the junction of the primary and regular secondary dentine (see **305**). (Ground, longitudinal section; polarised light; × 120)

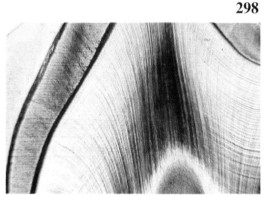

298 Von Ebner's lines run at right angles to the dentinal tubules and are approximately 20μm apart. Dentine matrix is laid down at a rate of 4μm per day. With each increment, the orientation of the deposited collagen fibres changes slightly. More severe changes in orientation occur approximately every five days, accounting for the presence of the von Ebner's lines. (Ground, longitudinal section through dentine; × 12)

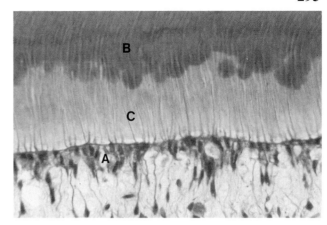

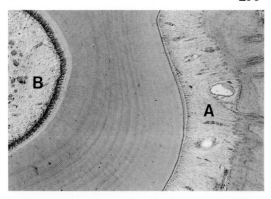

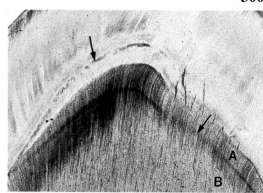

299 Mineralising lines are incremental lines due to variations in mineralisation. They may be seen microradiographically in ground sections, and in demineralised sections with certain stains. Mineralisation follows a 12-hour rhythm, but sometimes activity is more exaggerated and results in lines visible microscopically. The concomitant changes in matrix composition allow these lines to be seen in decalcified material. Such lines are not as regularly spaced as von Ebner lines. Because the mineralising lines take on the shape of the mineralising front at different stages of dentinogenesis, they often have a more jagged appearance than the von Ebner lines. Since the mineralising front is not necessarily parallel to the inner surface of the predentine, mineralising lines often lie at an angle to the von Ebner lines. **A**, periodontal ligament; **B**, pulp. (Decalcified, transverse section of root dentine, H & E; × 80)

300 Neonatal lines (*arrowed*) in dentine and enamel. In the deciduous teeth and the first permanent molar, an accentuated incremental line is seen separating the pre- (**A**) and postnatally formed dentine (**B**). In the specimen shown, the neonatal lines are unusually clear and pigmented, having come from the tooth of a patient who had suffered from icterus neonatorum (a disorder associated with disconjugation of bile pigment). (Ground, longitudinal section; × 25)

Interglobular dentine

301 Interglobular dentine (*arrowed*). A considerable proportion of the mineral in dentine is laid down in the form of globules, the calcospherites (see page 268). Where the calcospherites do not completely fuse, hypocalcified areas between the globules occur and these may persist in mature dentine (particularly in the coronal, circumpulpal dentine close to the enamel–dentine junction) as interglobular areas. The irregular interglobular spaces appear dark in ground sections viewed by transmitted light (as illustrated here) because of internal reflection of the light. Note that dentinal tubules are not interrupted by the interglobular areas but pass through them (although peritubular dentine is absent). **A**, enamel. (Ground, longitudinal section; van Gieson; × 300)

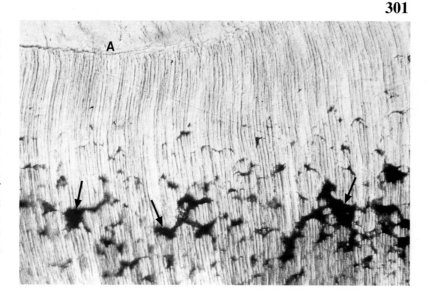

Secondary dentine and other post-eruptive features

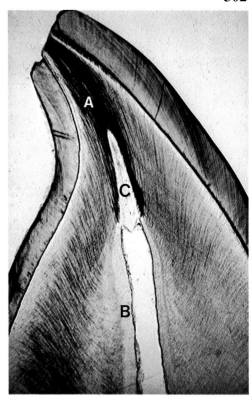

Post-eruptive changes in the structure of dentine may be related to age changes or to reactions to noxious or pathological stimuli. With age, dentine formation continues slowly, and the term regular secondary dentine is used to describe this tissue. Since regular secondary dentine is laid down at the pulpal end of the primary dentine, the pulp cavity decreases in size with age. Peritubular dentine generally increases with age and may completely obliterate the tubule. In response to noxious stimuli, the odontoblasts may 'evacuate' the tubules, giving rise to the so-called dead tract, and/or seal off the tubules at their pulpal ends with irregular secondary dentine, or form sclerotic dentine.

302 A dead tract (A), regular secondary dentine (B) and irregular secondary dentine (C). This is a longitudinal ground section through dentine. The dead tract shown has been produced in response to attrition. Its dark appearance is said to be related to the retention of air in the 'emptied' tubules which have not been penetrated by the mounting medium. Areas simulating dead tracts can be produced during the preparation of a ground section. A 'true' dead tract may be recognised by areas of sclerotic dentine bounding the tract laterally and pulpally. Occasionally, dead tracts are found in the dentine of unerupted teeth, possibly associated with atrophic degeneration of the odontoblast process due to excessive crowding during development. (Ground, longitudinal section; × 15)

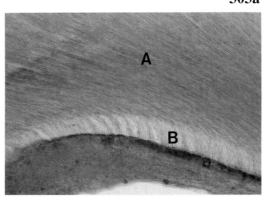

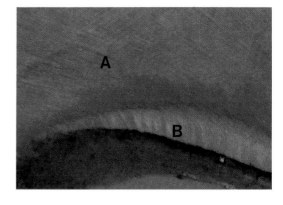

303a Primary dentine (A) and regular secondary dentine (B). Regular secondary dentine may not be easily distinguished from primary dentine. There are usually fewer tubules in secondary dentine. There is often a sudden change in tubule direction from that taken by the tubules of primary dentine, thus forming a pronounced contour line. Peritubular dentine is poorly developed in secondary dentine. (Ground, longitudinal section; × 80)

303b The same specimen as 303a. The colour differences illustrate the change in direction of the matrix and tubules from primary to secondary dentine. (Ground longitudinal section viewed in polarised light with a quartz sensitive tint; × 80)

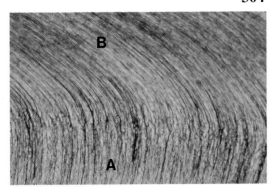

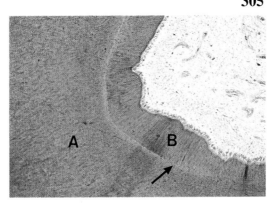

304 Dentinal tubules in regular secondary dentine. In this ground section, individual tubules can clearly be seen to continue across the junction between the regular secondary dentine (A) and the primary dentine (B). (Ground section; × 125)

305 The contour line of Owen (*arrowed*) separating the primary (A) and secondary (B) dentine. (Decalcified section of dentine, Silver stain; × 32)

306 Primary dentine (A) and irregular secondary dentine (B). This is a section of dentine in the floor of the pulp chamber. Where dentine is subjected to acute damage (e.g. dental caries), some of the underlying odontoblasts die, while others lay down a form of repair tissue called irregular secondary dentine. Where there are tubules in this secondary dentine, they are few in number and irregularly arranged.

Note that regular secondary dentine is deposited in larger amounts on the floor of the pulp chamber than on the roof of the chamber, suggesting that it is mainly an age change rather than a response to attrition or irritation. Irregular secondary dentine is often known as irritation or response dentine in recognition of the common cause of its formation. (Ground, longitudinal section through dentine; × 20)

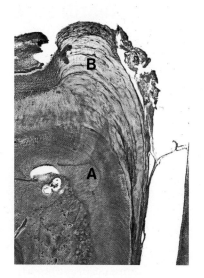

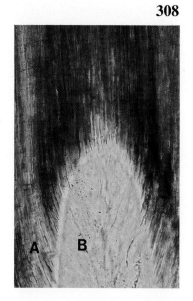

308 Dentinal tubules in primary (A) and irregular secondary dentine (B). Irregular secondary dentine (sometimes referred to as tertiary dentine) has many fewer tubules than primary dentine and only a small proportion of tubules are continuous across the two tissues. (Ground section; × 50)

307 Irregular secondary dentine (A) filling a pulp horn. (Decalcified, longitudinal section of dentine, H & E; × 50)

309a Sclerotic dentine. This is produced by a chronic stimulus (such as dental caries) and may be found bordering a dead tract (**302**). In areas of sclerotic dentine, the tubules are occluded by mineral which has a fine texture like that of peritubular dentine. In primary dentine affected by caries, the mineral usually appears to be apatite, but plate-like crystals of octocalcium phosphate have also been encountered. The infilling of tubules is thought to be controlled by odontoblasts, but the precise details are not known. (Ground, longitudinal section; × 20)

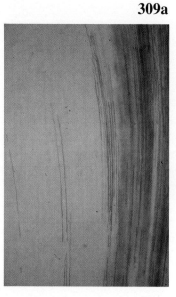

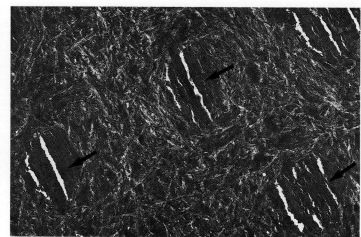

309b High-power view of sclerotic dentine showing transversely sectioned tubules filled in with mineral (*arrowed*). (TEM; × 7,000)

Comparative anatomy

Two basic types of dentine may be recognised in living vertebrates; orthodentine and vasodentine. Orthodentine is characterised by the presence of tubules within the tissue, while in the main, vasodentine is devoid of tubules, having vascular channels within it.

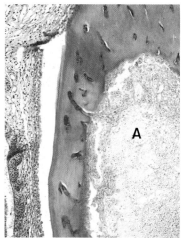

310 Vasodentine in a hake tooth (*Merluccius merluccius*). In the forming of dentine in some fish, blood capillaries become entrapped. Tubules may be scarce or absent within the vasodentine. The significance of the capillaries within the vasodentine is not known. **A**, pulp. (Decalcified, longitudinal section, H & E; × 90)

Unlike human orthodentine, which is arranged around a single pulp chamber, the orthodentine of crossopterygian fishes, many fossil amphibians (especially the so-called 'labyrinth-odonts') and a few lizards is arranged as a series of complicated folds of the pulp. Such dentine is referred to as plicidentine.

311 Plicidentine at the base of a tooth of a monitor lizard (*Veranus sp.*). Note the folds of dentine, each with a central core of pulp tissue. (Ground, transverse section; × 8)

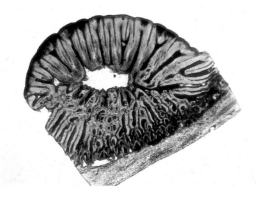

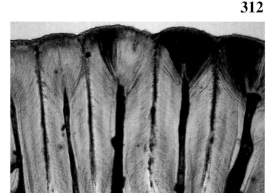

312 High-power view of plicidentine of a monitor lizard (*Veranus sp.*) showing the tubular nature of the dentine. (Ground section; × 30)

In some fish there is no clearly defined pulp cavity. Instead, the pulp cavity becomes divided by dentinal trabeculae. Because this tissue has a resemblance to bone, it has been termed osteodentine.

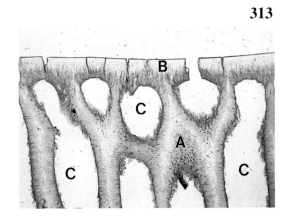

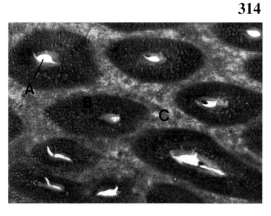

313 Tooth of an eagle ray (*Myliobatis aquilla*) showing osteodentine. The osteodentine (**A**) shown here is regularly arranged in the form of parallel trabeculae. **B**, covering enameloid; **C**, pulp spaces. (Ground, longitudinal section; Basic fuchsin; × 80)

314 Cross-section through osteodentine in a tooth of an eagle ray (*Myliobatis aquilla*). In cross-section, the osteodentine is seen to be traversed by vascular pulp canals (**A**) which are surrounded by concentric laminae of dentine termed denteons (**B**). Unlike bone, however, these laminae do not contain cells but house the processes of odontoblasts whose cell bodies line the vascular spaces. Between the denteons lies calcified interstitial tissue (**C**) which is generally devoid of cells. (Decalcified section; Mallory; × 65)

Dental pulp

The dental pulp is the loose connective tissue which occupies the pulp chamber in the centre of the tooth. It is the mature form of the dental papilla. The morphology of the chamber varies from tooth to tooth and has been described on pages 42 and 43. In the crowns of molar teeth the pulp extends under the cusps into pulp horns (or cornua). It is present in each root canal of multirooted teeth. At the apical constriction of the root canal the pulp becomes continuous with the periodontal ligament. Smaller accessory canals pass laterally through the root dentine to reach the periodontal ligament. Dentine is the calcified tissue of the pulp as cementum is the calcified tissue of the periodontal ligament; the cement–dentine junction at the apical constriction marks the boundary between the two.

315

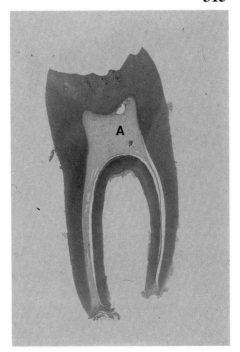

315 Decalcified section through a whole tooth to display the dental pulp (A). The dental pulp has many features in common with other soft connective tissue, consisting of cells (principally fibroblasts) embedded in an extracellular matrix of fibres (mainly collagen) and ground substance. The tissue has an extensive nerve and vascular supply. By weight, the pulp is 75% water and 25% organic material. The dental pulp is surrounded and supported by dentine, providing an inflexible shell that gives the pulp tissue many of its characteristic properties (e.g. its high tissue fluid pressures). The pulp and its precursor (the dental papilla, see **622**) are responsible for the formation of the dentine. After the relatively rapid formation of primary dentine, secondary dentine is formed slowly throughout life, and more rapidly in response to stimuli such as caries or attrition which threaten the integrity of the pulp. The bulk of the pulp provides nutritive support for this major synthetic role focused in the odontoblast layer at the periphery of the tissue. Although there is no turnover of dentine to compare with the remodelling of bone, the odontoblasts of the pulp extend cell processes into the dentine to allow some modifications of the tissue. The dental pulp acts as a sensory organ, but usually only when dentine is exposed. (Decalcified, longitudinal section through a tooth; H & E; × 3)

316

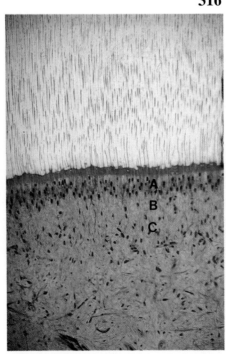

316 Regions of the dental pulp. The major functions of the pulp are fulfilled by a layer of dentine-forming cells (the odontoblasts) located at the periphery of the tissue. The odontoblasts (**A**) form a clearly defined layer in contact with the dentine. This layer is thicker in the crown than in the root of the tooth. Beneath the odontoblast layer, there is often (but not always) an apparently cell-free zone (of Weil) (**B**) which contains a plexus of nerves and capillaries. Deep to this is a region of increased cell density (the cell-rich zone). The cell-rich zone (**C**) gradually blends with the central bulk of the pulp which, apart from containing nerves and vessels, is a sparse mixture of cells and fibres. The cell-free zone is usually absent in radicular pulp. The appearance of the cell-free zone is less apparent in material prepared for electron microscopy (which shrinks much less than tissue prepared for light microscopy), and it may therefore be exaggerated by (if not created by) the method of processing. Even if it is a real feature, 'cell-free' is a misnomer as many cell processes cross the region, and it contains nerves and blood vessels. It would therefore be more accurate to describe it as a nucleus-free zone. (Decalcified section of the pulp and dentine; H & E; × 200)

Cells of the dental pulp

The pulp contains one cell type, the odontoblast, which is characteristic to this tissue as well as other cell types common to all soft connective tissues. Numerically, the predominant cell is the fibroblast. Occasional defence cells are found, even in normal pulps. The remaining cell types are those associated with the neurovascular supply.

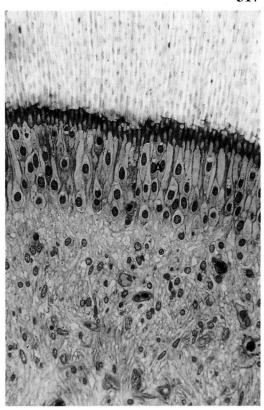

317 The odontoblast layer (A). The odontoblasts are columnar cells that form a clearly defined layer adjacent to the dentine. Their appearance varies according to the rate of dentinogenesis. In general, odontoblast nuclei are placed basally in the cell but lie at different levels within the layer, giving a false appearance of stratification (pseudostratification). This arrangement is probably the result of crowding (as dentine formation continually decreases the pulpal surface area). It is much less evident in radicular pulp, where dentine formation is less extensive. (Decalcified section at the pulp–dentine junction, Toluidine blue; × 650)

318 The odontoblast. Once primary dentine has been formed, odontoblasts continue to produce dentine at a very slow rate throughout the life of the tooth. The ultrastructure of the odontoblast reflects this reduced level of activity in that the organelles responsible for protein synthesis (Golgi apparatus, rough endoplasmic reticulum and mitochondria) are still present in the supranuclear region but in relatively small amounts. One large process extends into the dentine but several smaller processes link odontoblasts to adjacent odontoblasts and to pulpal fibroblasts.

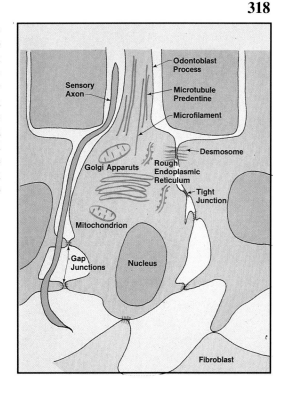

319 Ultrastructure of the odontoblast. Not all features of an odontoblast can be seen in a single section. Several of the elements described in **318** are seen in this electronmicrograph (**N**, nucleus; **R**, rough endoplasmic reticulum; **M**, mitochondrion). The odontoblast produces the precursors of Type I collagen and the glycoproteins that form the dentine. These are packaged within the Golgi apparatus into vesicles for transport along the odontoblast process. For more detail on the odontoblast, see **611**. (TEM; ×9,300)

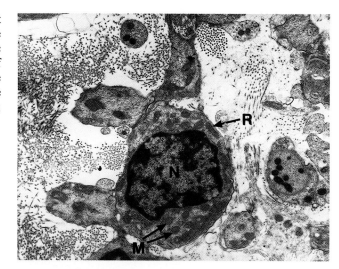

320 Junctions between odontoblasts. Odontoblasts are linked to each other by a variety of cell contacts. Occasionally, junctional complexes containing a desmosome and a tight junction are seen linking cells near to the pulp–predentine border. However, these are unusual. Single desmosome-like junctions and tight junctions may be seen, but the commonest form of linkage is the gap junction.

The different junctions may play different roles. Desmosomal junctions are mainly involved in maintaining the mechanical integrity of the layer. Tight junctions and desmosomes can control the permeability of the layer. Gap junctions, while probably contributing some mechanical adhesion, are more significantly involved in cell-to-cell communication, allowing the passage of some small-molecular-weight elements. Gap junctions were first described in situations where they acted as electronic synapses in excitable tissues and it has been suggested that the odontoblast is linked to nerves by these junctions. While there is no doubt that unsheathed axons pass through the odontoblast layer, there is no convincing evidence that they are linked directly to the odontoblasts. There are also numerous gap junctions between odontoblasts and the underlying fibroblasts.

The overall effect of these junctional arrangements is to maintain the integrity of the odontoblast layer, limiting its permeability (possibly with directional differences) and coordinating the activity of adjacent cells. **G**, gap junction, and **D**, desmosome, between two odontoblasts (**OD**). (TEM; ×45,000)

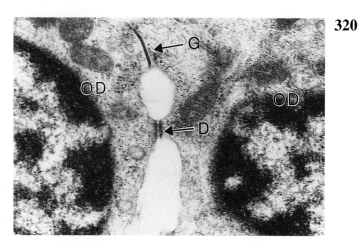

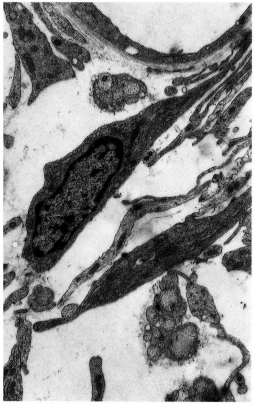

321 The pulpal fibroblast. Most of the cells in the dental pulp have the appearance of the ubiquitous fibroblast. In its quiescent state, it is essentially ovoid in shape (with processes extending to connect with other cells), and it has relatively little cytoplasm around the nucleus. Consequently there are few organelles and it is probably more accurate to describe the pulpal fibroblast as a fibrocyte. When activated, pulpal fibroblasts become markedly basophilic, their cytoplasm enlarges and there is a significant increase in organelles associated with protein synthesis. They then secrete the precursors of both pulpal collagen and ground substance.

In the sub-odontoblastic region, there are cells which seem to retain much of their embryonic potential and can, when stimulated, differentiate into odontoblasts and produce dentine. At rest, these mesenchymal-type cells are indistinguishable from fibroblasts. (TEM; ×20,000)

The principal defence cell in the pulp is the histiocyte or fixed macrophage. It is similar in appearance to the fibroblast and it is difficult to distinguish between them. A more granular cytoplasm and smaller nucleus are the only distinguishing features of the histiocyte at the light microscope level. Its ultrastructural appearance is shown in **405**. In inflammation, histiocytes become free macrophages. Occasional lymphocytes are seen in normal pulps but are common in chronic inflammation. Polymorphonuclear leukocytes are only found during inflammation.

Fibres and ground substance of the dental pulp

Collagen is the predominant protein in the dental pulp (comprising 34% of the total in human pulp). Of this collagen, 60% is present as Type I collagen, the remainder as Type III. Collagen forms 3–5% of the wet weight of human pulp, a low proportion in comparison with other soft connective tissues. There are some regional variations in distribution, the concentration being lowest in the coronal pulp. Fibronectin is also found in the dental pulp. It is an extracellular glycoprotein present in many connective tissues and basement membranes. It acts as a mediator of cell adhesion, linking cells to each other and to extracellular components. The fibronectin is distributed in a reticular pattern throughout the pulp (with increased levels in blood vessel walls). It is sometimes seen as small (10nm) non-striated filaments between the larger collagen fibres. The matrix of pulp therefore differs from dentine by the presence of significant amounts of Type III collagen and fibronectin.

It has been suggested that a small number of oxytalan fibres occur in the pulp. However, it is unlikely that they are present as they are commonly regarded as being related to elastic fibres, which are absent from the matrix of the pulp.

The major component of the ground substance is proteoglycan. These large macromolecules consist of a protein core with side chains of glycosaminoglycans (GAG) and oligosaccharides. All normally occurring connective tissue GAG (chondroitin-4-sulphate, chondroitin-6-sulphate, dermatan sulphate, heparan sulphate, hyaluronan and keratan sulphate) can be demonstrated in the pulp. In mature pulps, in which primary dentinogenesis is complete, hyaluronan (60%), dermatan sulphate (28%) and chondroitin sulphate (12%) predominate. The proteoglycans are large molecules and occupy a considerable proportion of the volume of the tissue. Many of the physical properties of the tissue (e.g. resilience and permeability) are a function of these constituents. Non-collageneous proteins other than proteoglycans have not been described in the pulp.

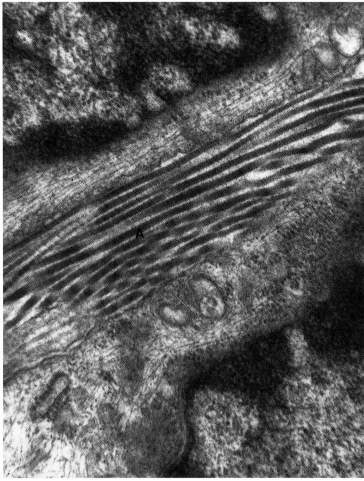

322 Collagen fibrils in the pulp (A). Type I collagen occurs as randomly arranged fibrils 100nm in diameter, with the characteristic 64nm primary periodic banding. These fibrils vary in density and distribution in the pulp, but increase with age. Type III collagen is present as fine, branched filaments 15nm in diameter, or as dark material adherent to fibroblasts. Both types of collagen are produced by pulpal fibroblasts. Reticular fibres, traditionally described on the basis of their argyrophilia (silver staining), are common in young pulps. The ultrastructural and biochemical correlates to the reticular fibres seen in the light microscope have not been determined. One suggestion is that they are due to carbohydrate elements of the ground substance. (TEM; × 134,000)

Blood supply of the dental pulp

The vascular supply to the pulp enters via the apical foramina of the roots. There are often several foramina entering each root canal, forming an apical delta. The largest vessels to enter are arterioles (maximally 150μm in diameter) but these soon branch into smaller vessels. The arterioles ascend towards the crown, giving off many side branches *en route*. The arterioles terminate in a rich sub-odontoblastic capillary plexus. The capillaries drain into venules which run more centrally in the pulp and drain through the apical foramen. The veins lack valves and reduce in number as the root apex is reached.

323

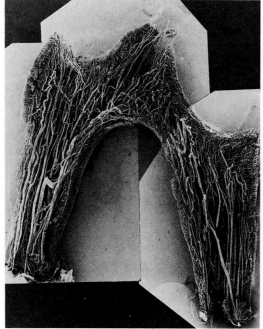

324

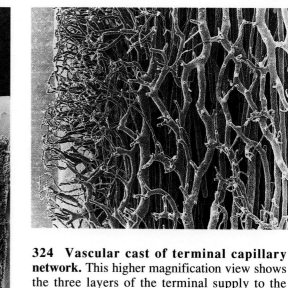

323 Vascular cast of mandibular molar of a dog. This three-dimensional representation of the pulpal vasculature is made by perfusing plastic resin through the carotid arteries and then dissolving away both hard and soft tissues. In this preparation, the terminal capillary network on the exposed surface of the pulp has also been removed. Arterioles run coronally along the sides of the root canal; the venules drain in the centre of the canal. Larger vessels run relatively straight routes to the cornua. Side branches subdivide to form a terminal capillary network beneath the dentine. (SEM; × 8)

324 Vascular cast of terminal capillary network. This higher magnification view shows the three layers of the terminal supply to the odontoblast layer. The flat-ended loops of capillaries are most superficial; beneath these lie the capillary network and beneath this the venular network. Underneath these layers are arterioles running straight to the coronal area. (SEM; × 11)

325a

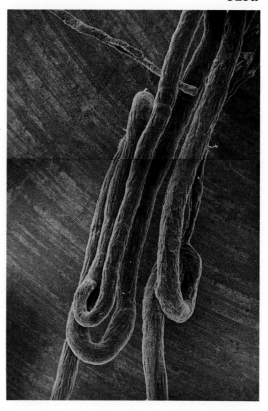

325b

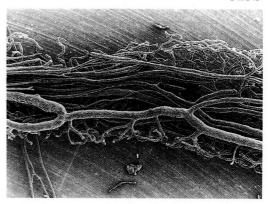

325 Arteriolar loops and venous–venous anastomoses. Two characteristics of the pulpal microvasculature are shown: a U-turn loop on one of the main arterioles (**325a**), a venous–venous anastomosis (**325b**). These arrangements probably play a role in the regulation of blood flow within the pulp, not only altering its level, but also its regional distribution during dentinogenesis and its response to inflammatory insults. (SEM; **325a**, × 150; **325b**, × 160)

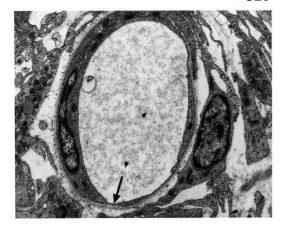

326 Fenestrated capillary in the sub-odontoblastic region. Approximately 4–5% of the pulpal capillaries shows fenestrations (*arrowed*). These are particularly pronounced between and beneath the odontoblasts. The fenestrations appear as circular openings in the endothelial cell. (TEM; freeze-fracture; × 12,600)

327 Ultrastructure of a fenestrated capillary in the pulp. Fenestrated capillaries have a thick endothelium (60–100nm). The fenestrations themselves are 60–80nm in diameter. The basal lamina is continuous over the pores. Fenestrated capillaries are more permeable than continuous capillaries, and probably play a role in the rapid supply of substrate to synthesising cells. (TEM; × 31,500)

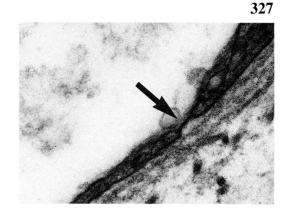

Pulpal lymphatics are difficult to demonstrate convincingly. Lymphatic capillaries are 'leaky' blind-ended vessels and lack blood cells within them. Elements fitting these criteria can indeed be found in the pulp. Evidence for the existence of lymphatic vessels in the pulp also come from studies using particulate tracer materials and lymphography; particulate tracer material placed into the pulp eventually appears within the regional lymph nodes and retrograde lymphography deposits material into pulpal vessels.

Innervation of the dental pulp

The dental pulp has a rich innervation. The nerve fibres enter the pulp via the apical foraminae and lateral canals. The number of nerves entering varies with tooth type and the stage of development. It has been estimated that a fully developed human premolar has approximately 2500 axons at its root apex.

328 Neurovascular bundle in the radicular pulp. Both myelinated (dark green) and non-myelinated (light green) nerves enter the dental pulp. The non-myelinated nerves constitute 70–80% of the total, and are categorised as 'C' fibres (including pain fibres and vasomotor fibres). 90% of the myelinated axons are narrow and would be categorised into the Aδ size range. They are thought to be devoted exclusively to pain transmission. There is some evidence that narrowing of the parent axons occurs to some extent outside the pulp and that a higher proportion of the fibres may belong within the Aβ size range. Within the root canal and pulp chamber, the nerve fibres generally accompany blood vessels (although some axons can be found some distance from the blood vessels). As the nerves travel up the root canal and pulp chamber, they branch considerably such that the number of axons at the mid-coronal level can be more than four times as numerous as those in the apical pulp. Only a small proportion of the nerve fibres (probably 10% or less) end in the radicular pulp, the rest continue to the coronal pulp.

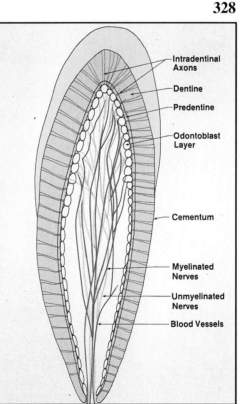

329 Sympathetic fibres in the dental pulp. A small proportion of the non-myelinated axons entering the apical pulp are sympathetic in origin, although it is difficult to estimate their numbers accurately. In this preparation, the section has been treated with glyoxylic acid, which combines with the catecholamines to form a material that fluoresces in ultraviolet light. (Sucrose phosphate glyoxylic acid fluorescence; × 100)

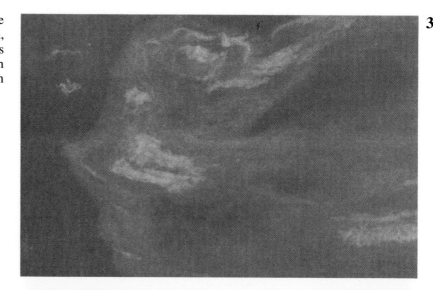

330 Sympathetic axons containing dense-cored vesicles. Sympathetic axons contain catecholamine transmitters. If an animal is injected with a false neurotransmitter (such as 6-hydroxydopamine), this will be taken up (but not released) and will be easier to find microscopically. This electron micrograph shows some axons containing such dense-cored vesicles (*arrowed*). They are contained in the same Schwann cell pocket as some unlabelled axons which may be sensory. Simultaneous activation of sensory and sympathetic fibres amplifies the activity in sensory nerves. This close approximation of sensory and sympathetic axons may explain this interaction.

The pulpal sympathetics are principally concerned with controlling the calibre of arterioles, although roles in sensory activities and in the control of dentinogenesis have also been suggested. While the pulpal sympathetic fibres are known to be noradrenergic, they also contain vasoactive intestinal polypeptide. A parasympathetic supply to the pulp has been suggested but has never been convincingly demonstrated. (TEM; × 31,000)

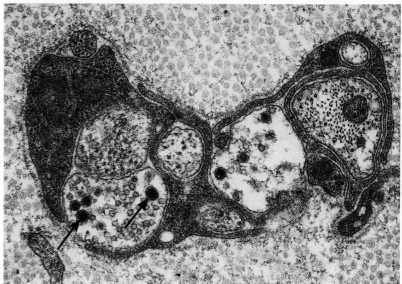

Understanding the role of the pulpo–dentinal innervation is complicated by the discovery of several peptides in pulpal axons, including substance P, calcitonin-gene-related peptide (CGRP), vasoactive intestinal peptide (VIP), encephalins and neuropeptide Y. Some occur in combination, e.g. substance P and CGRP. The precise role of these peptides is unknown. Furthermore, it is not clear why so many different peptides should be present. Although some peptides may be involved in the sensory transduction process, there is as yet no direct evidence for this. Many of these peptides have profound effects on local blood flow and may be released physiologically by axon reflexes. Some of the peptidergic axons proliferate in response to damage and consequently their major function may be to respond to insults.

331

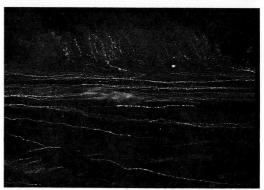

331 Substance P-containing sensory axons in the dental pulp. Substance P is a vasoactive agent which, when released, causes a transient increase in pulpal blood flow, followed by a much longer period of impaired microcirculation. It is probably a component of neurogenic inflammation. Substance P has a similar effect on the sensitivity of sensory nerves — a transient increase followed by a prolonged reduced responsiveness. In this preparation, the section has been treated with a labelled antibody to substance P. The substance P-containing fibres appear to be non-myelinated, sensory C fibres. (× 300)

152

332 Calcitonin-gene-related peptide in pulpal axons. These midline sections of rat maxillary first molars show nerve fibres that are immunoreceptive for CGRP, four days after drilling a cervical cavity (**a**) or in the contralateral normal tooth (**b**). The boundary between coronal and radicular dentine is indicated by a broken line in the control; the estimated equivalent site in the injured tooth is shown by dots. Normally, there are very few CGRP nerve branches in the cervical pulp. After injury, many CGRP nerve fibres are found in the cervical odontoblast layer and subjacent pulp (*between arrowheads*). Electron microscopy confirms that those fibres have sprouted into the area in response to injury (Taylor *et al.*, *Brain Research*, **461**(1988) 371–378). (Decalcified sections; × 650)

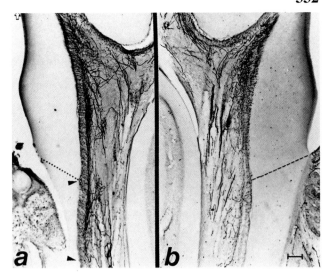

333 Terminal branching of sensory fibres in the dental pulp. As the nerve fibres pass into the coronal pulp, they branch repeatedly and the branches pass towards the periphery. This preparation is a very thick (60μm) section stained with silver, allowing the stained nerve fibres to be followed over a considerable distance. The branches pass towards the periphery, subdivide and intertwine beneath the odontoblasts and form the sub-odontoblastic plexus (of Raschkow). Some axons will pass between the odontoblasts and end on the surface of the predentine. Others will continue and enter dentinal tubules and travel up to 200μm alongside the odontoblastic process. (Linder's silver stain; × 140)

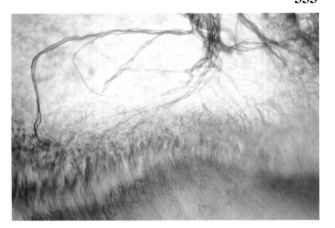

334 The sub-odontoblastic plexus of Raschkow. The terminal and subterminal branches of intrapulpal nerves form a plexus in the cell-free zone beneath the odontoblasts. This plexus is not evident until after the tooth has erupted. The fibres are non-myelinated and as far as is known, entirely sensory. Branches from the plexus pass into the odontoblast layer. Some go on to form the marginal plexus between the odontoblast layer and the predentine; others continue into the dentine to accompany odontoblast processes in the dentinal tubules. The sub-odontoblastic plexus may be one site of sensory activation in the pulp–dentine complex. The nerve fibres in this area have several characteristics that would make this likely. As shown in this micrograph, many of the axons are incompletely ensheathed (**A**). When traced in serial section, some axons leave the protection of the Schwann cell completely and terminate in the extracellular space. Such axons would be very susceptible to changes in the local environment. The axons branch profusely, providing a broad surface area for activation. Within the Schwann cell there are often many axons in a single pocket and the spread of signals from axon to axon is possible. (TEM; × 40,000)

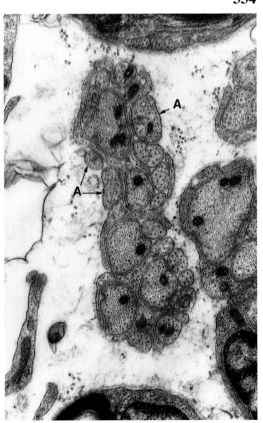

335 The marginal, predentinal plexus (of Bradlaw). In the crown of the tooth, some unsheathed axons (*arrowed*) are located between the odontoblast layer and the predentine. It is perhaps a little overstated to call it a plexus as most of the axons seen here are in transit to the dentinal tubules. Some axons may end here and these (plus those continuing on into the dentine) may be activated at this point (particularly by stimuli, applied to the dentine, that cause fluid movement through the dentinal tubules). (TEM; × 85,000)

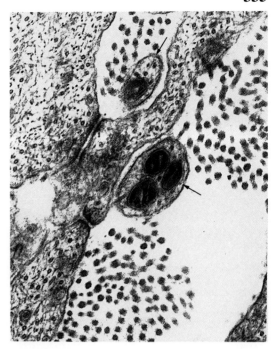

Age changes in the dental pulp

The change from the developmental tissue (the dental papilla) to the mature tissue (the dental pulp) is gradual and a matter of degree rather than a dramatic transformation. During the developmental stages the synthetic activity of the odontoblasts and fibroblasts is high and the cells are large with prominent organelles associated with protein synthesis. With maturity the activity subsides to a low but constant level, but the tissue remains ready to accelerate should this be demanded by some outside stimulus. Similarly the differences between the mature pulp and the aged pulp are slight. There have been relatively few quantitative studies on ageing pulps. Consequently the qualitative impression of declining cellularity and increasing fibrosity has not been confirmed. Older odontoblasts tend to be cuboidal rather than columnar and the odontoblast layer becomes narrower. The vasculature and nerve supply of the dental pulp is said to diminish with age.

336 Pulp stones. Calcification is the most obvious feature associated with the ageing pulp. While it can occur occasionally in young pulps, over 90% of old human teeth show some degree of pulpal calcification. The calcification can take various forms. First, it can be diffuse, beginning around the neurovascular bundles. Second, and more commonly, discrete pulp stones may appear. These may be either true denticles (consisting of tubular dentine surrounded by an odontoblast layer) or false denticles (consisting of concentric layers of calcified material with no odontoblast layer). False denticles occur more frequently than true denticles. Although initially lying free within the pulp (free pulp stones), they may become enclosed by secondary dentine formation (attached pulp stones). They are not associated with any symptoms. **A**, dentine. (Decalcified sections; H & E; **336a**, × 20; **336b**; × 60)

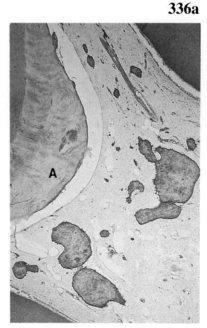
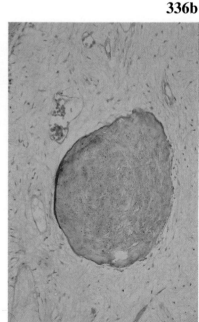

154

Cementum

337 The distribution of cementum (A). Cementum is the thin layer of calcified tissue covering the dentine of the root. It is one of the four tissues that support the tooth in the jaw (the periodontium), the others being the alveolar bone, the periodontal ligament and the gingivae. While restricted to the root in man, cementum is present on the crowns of some mammals as an adaptation to an herbivorous diet. Cementum varies in thickness at different levels of the root. It is thickest at the root apex and in the interradicular areas of multi-rooted teeth, and thinnest cervically. The thickness cervically is 10–50μm, and apically, 50–200μm (although it may exceed 600μm). Cementum is contiguous with the periodontal ligament on its outer surface and is firmly adherent to dentine on its deep surface. Its prime function is to give attachment to collagen fibres of the periodontal ligament. As cementum is slowly formed throughout life (with its surface being covered by a layer of uncalcified matrix or precementum), this allows for continual reattachment of the periodontal ligament fibres. Some regard cementum as a calcified component of the ligament. Developmentally, cementum is derived from the investing layer of the dental follicle (see **577**). Like dentine, it is deposited throughout life and there is always a thin layer of uncalcified matrix on its surface. While similar in chemical composition and physical properties to bone, cementum is avascular and has no innervation. It is also less readily resorbed, a feature that is very important for permitting orthodontic tooth movement. The reason for this feature is unknown but it may be related to: differences in physicochemical or biological properties between bone and cementum; the properties of the precementum; the increased density of Sharpey's fibres (particularly in acellular cementum); the proximity of epithelial cell rests to the root surface (see page 178); and/or the position of blood vessels nearer to the alveolar bone. (Ground, longitudinal section of a tooth; × 4)

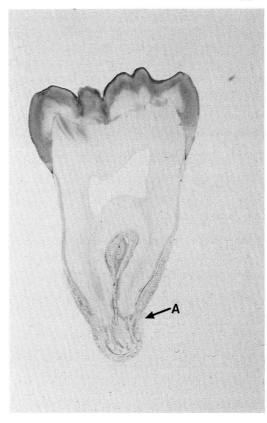

Physical properties of cementum. Cementum is pale yellow with a dull surface. It is softer than dentine. Permeability varies with age and the type of cementum, the cellular variety being more permeable. In general, cementum is more permeable than dentine. Like the other dental tissues, permeability decreases with age. The relative softness of cementum, combined with its thinness cervically, means that it is readily removed by abrasion when gingival recession exposes the root surface to the oral environment. Loss of cementum will expose dentine.

Chemical properties of cementum. On a wet weight basis, cementum contains 65% inorganic material, 23% organic material and 12% water. By volume, the inorganic material comprises approximately 45%, organic material 33%, and water 22%. The degree of mineralisation varies in different parts of the tissue. Some acellular zones may be more highly calcified than dentine. The principal inorganic component is hydroxyapatite, although other forms of calcium are present at higher levels than in enamel and dentine. The hydroxyapatite crystals are thin and plate-like and similar to those in bone. They are on average 55nm wide and 8nm thick. Their length varies, but values derived from sections cut with a diamond knife are underestimates due to shattering of the crystals along their length. As with enamel, the concentration of trace elements tends to be higher at the external surface. This, for example, is true of fluoride levels which are also higher in acellular than in cellular cementum. The organic matrix is primarily collagen. The collagen is virtually all Type I.

338 The cement–enamel junction. In any single section of a tooth, three arrangements of the junction between cementum and enamel may be seen. Pattern 1, where the cementum overlaps the enamel for a short distance, is the predominant arrangement in 60% of sections. Pattern 2, where the cementum and enamel meet at a butt joint, occurs in 30% of sections. Pattern 3, where the cementum and enamel fail to meet and the dentine between them is exposed, occurs in 10% of sections. Although one of these patterns may predominate in an individual tooth, all three patterns may be present.

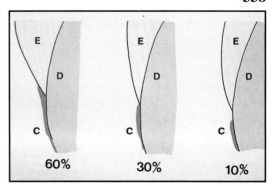

339 Scanning electron micrograph of the cement-enamel junction. In this example, the cementum (**A**) overlaps the enamel (**B**). (SEM; × 250)

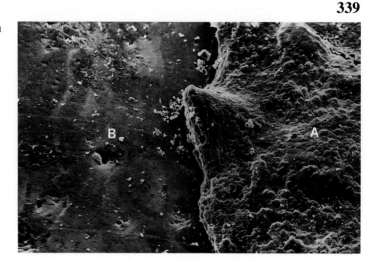

Classification of cementum

The various types of cementum encountered may be classified in two different ways. One classification is based upon the presence or absence of cells, the other upon the nature and origin of the organic matrix.

Classification of cementum based on the presence or absence of cells

340 Cellular and acellular cementum. Cellular cementum, as its name indicates, contains cells (cementocytes); acellular cementum does not. In the most common arrangement, acellular cementum(**A**) covers the root adjacent to the dentine, whereas cellular cementum (**B**) is found mainly in the apical area and overlying the acellular cementum. Deviations from this arrangement are common and sometimes several layers of each variant alternate. Being formed first, the acellular cementum is sometimes termed primary cementum and the subsequently formed cellular variety, secondary cementum. Cellular cementum is especially common in interradicular areas.

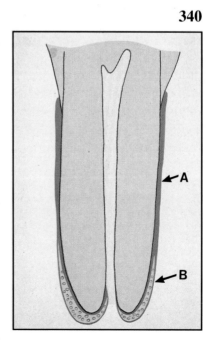

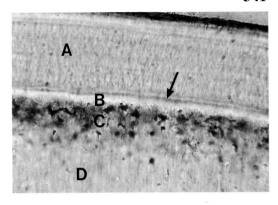

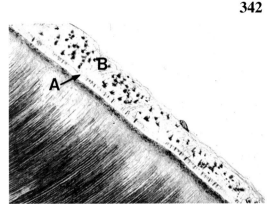

341

342

343

342 Cellular cementum (B) overlying acellular cementum (A). This is the usual arrangement at regions of the root where cellular cementum is present. Note the greater thickness of the cellular layer. Many of the structural differences between cellular and acellular cementum are thought to be related to the faster rate of matrix formation for cellular cementum. Indeed, the essential difference is that, as cellular cementum develops, the formative cells (the cementoblasts, see page 278) become embedded in the tissue as cementocytes. The different rates of cementum formation is also reflected in the wider precementum layer and the more widely spaced incremental lines in cellular cementum (see **348**). (Ground section; × 50)

341 Acellular cementum (A). In this section at the cervical region of the root, no cellular cementum overlies the acellular cementum. The acellular cementum appears relatively structureless. In the outer region of the radicular dentine (**D**), the granular layer (of Tomes, **C**) can be seen and outside this the hyaline layer (of Hopewell-Smith, **B**). These layers are also described on page 140. The dark line between the hyaline layer and the acellular cementum (*arrowed*) may be related to the afibrillar cementum patchily present at this position. (Ground section; × 200)

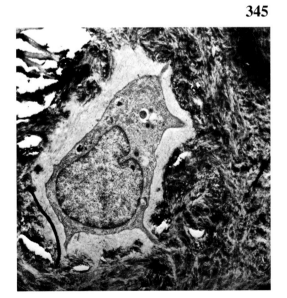

344

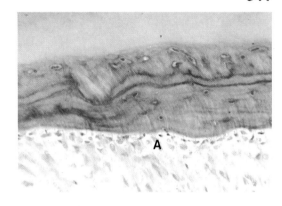

343 Lacunae and canaliculi in cellular cementum. The spaces that the cementocytes occupy in the tissue are called lacunae, and the channels that their processes extend along are the canaliculi. Adjacent canaliculi are often connected, and the processes within them exhibit gap junctions. In ground sections, the cellular contents are lost; air and debris filling the voids give the dark appearance. In thicker layers of cellular cementum *in vivo*, it is highly probable that many of the lacunae do not contain vital cells. Compared with osteocytes in bone, cementocytes are more wide-

ly dispersed and more randomly arranged. In addition, their canaliculi are preferentially orientated towards the periodontal ligament, their chief source of nutrition. Unlike bone, of course, the cementocytes are not arranged circumferentially around blood vessels in the form of osteons (Haversian systems).

In this high-power view of a section of cellular cementum, the preferential orientation of the lacunae indicates that the external surface is above and to the left. (Ground section; × 500)

344 Lacunae containing cementocytes seen in decalcified section. In decalcified sections, the cellular contents of the lacunae are retained, albeit in a shrunken condition. A layer of active cementoblasts responsible for secreting the cementum matrix is seen on the periodontal ligament surface (**A**). The pale zone (3–5μm in width) between the cementoblast layer and the cementum is unmineralised matrix (precementum). (Decalcified section; H & E; × 200)

345

345 A cementocyte within a lacuna. Although derived from active cementoblasts, once they become embedded within the cementum matrix, cementocytes become relatively inactive cells. This is reflected in their ultrastructural appearance. Their cytoplasmic/nuclear ratio is low and they have sparse, if any, representation of the organelles responsible for energy production and synthesis. Some unmineralised matrix may be seen in the perilacunar space. The cementocyte processes here appear short, but this is because they extend out of the plane of the section. The processes can extend for distances several times longer than the diameter of the cell body. (TEM; × 4,500)

Although the most usual relationship between acellular and cellular cementum is for the cellular variety to overlie the acellular, other arrangements are common.

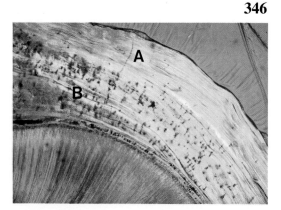
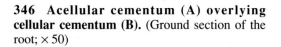

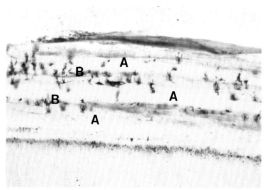

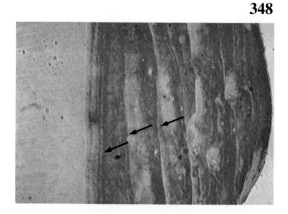

346 Acellular cementum (A) overlying cellular cementum (B). (Ground section of the root; × 50)

347 Alternating acellular (A) and cellular cementum (B). In some areas, the two variants of cementum alternate irregularly, probably representing variations in the rate of deposition. (Ground section; × 60)

348 Incremental lines of Salter (*arrowed*) in cellular and acellular cementum. Cementum is deposited in an irregular rhythm, resulting in unevenly spaced incremental lines. Unlike enamel and dentine, the precise periodicity between the incremental lines is unknown, although there have been unsuccessful attempts to relate it to an annual cycle. In acellular cementum, incremental lines tend to be close together, thin and even. In the more rapidly formed cellular cementum, the lines are further apart, thicker, and more irregular. The appearance of incremental lines in cementum is mainly due to differences in the degree of mineralisation, but these must also reflect differences in composition of the underlying matrix since, as shown here, the lines are readily visible in decalcified sections. (Decalcified section; Mallory; × 50)

Table 15: Summary of differences between acellular and cellular cementum.

Acellular	Cellular
No cells	Lacunaeand canaliculi containing cementocytes and their processes
Border with dentine not clearly demarcated	Border with dentine clearly demarcated
Rate of development relatively slow	Rate of development relatively fast
Incremental lines relatively close together	Incremental lines relatively wide apart
Precementum layer narrow	Precementum layer wide

Classification of cementum based on the nature and origin of the organic matrix

Cementum derives its organic matrix from two sources: from the inserting Sharpey's fibres of the periodontal ligament, and from the cementoblasts. When derived from the periodontal ligament, the fibres are referred to as the extrinsic fibres. These Sharpey's fibres continue into the cementum in the same direction as the principal fibres of the ligament (i.e. perpendicular or oblique to the root surface; see page 167). When derived from the cementoblasts, the fibres are referred to as intrinsic fibres. These run parallel to the root surface, and approximately at right angles to the extrinsic fibres. It is therefore possible to classify cementum according to the nature and origin of the fibrous matrix.

Extrinsic fibre cementum. For this type of cementum, all the collagen is derived as Sharpey's fibres from the periodontal ligament (the ground substance itself may be produced by the cementoblasts). This type of cementum corresponds with primary acellular cementum. It is therefore formed slowly and the root surface is smooth. The fibres are well mineralised.

Mixed fibre cementum. For this type of cementum, the collagen fibres of the organic matrix are derived from both extrinsic fibres (from the periodontal ligament) and intrinsic fibres (from cementoblasts). The extrinsic and intrinsic fibres can be readily distinguished. First, the intrinsic fibres run between the extrinsic fibres with a different orientation. Indeed, the greater the number of intrinsic fibres in mixed fibre cementum, the greater the separation of the extrinsic fibres. Second, the fibre bundles are of different sizes. The extrinsic fibres are ovoid or round bundles about 5–7μm in diameter; the intrinsic fibres are 1–2μm in diameter.

If the formation rate is slow, the mixed fibre cementum may be acellular and well mineralised. If the formation rate is fast, mixed fibre cementum may be cellular and the fibres less well mineralised (especially their cores).

Intrinsic fibre cementum. This type of cementum is comprised only of intrinsic fibres running parallel to the root surface. The absence of Sharpey's fibres means intrinsic fibre cementum has no role in tooth attachment. It may be found in patches in the apical region. It may be a temporary phase, with extrinsic fibres subsequently gaining a reattachment, or it may represent a permanent region without attaching fibres.

349

350

349 Mixed fibre cementum. In this region the mineralised intrinsic fibres (**A**) are present in relatively small amounts such that the mineralised extrinsic fibres (**B**) are close together. (SEM; anorganic preparation; × 3,000)

350 Intrinsic fibre cementum at root apex. Note the absence of Sharpey's fibres and the parallel distribution of the bundles of mineralised intrinsic fibres. (SEM; anorganic preparation; × 150)

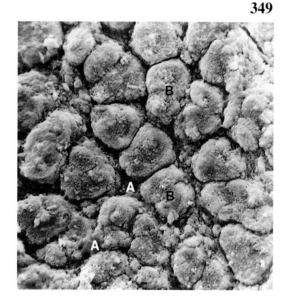

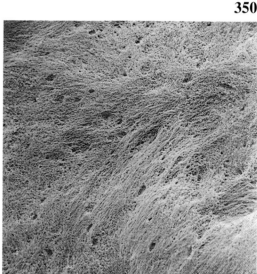

The extrinsic, mixed and intrinsic fibre cementum types all contain collagen fibres. However, there is a further type of cementum which contains no collagen fibres. This afibrillar cementum is sparsely distributed and consists of a well mineralised ground substance which may be of epithelial origin. Afibrillar cementum is a thin, acellular layer (difficult to identify at the light microscope level), which covers cervical enamel or intervenes between fibrillar cementum and dentine.

351

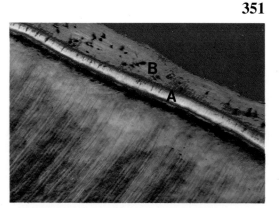

352

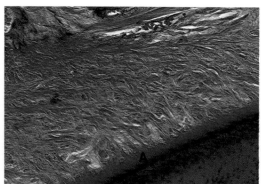

353

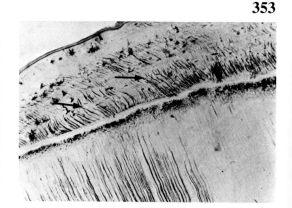

351 Fibre orientation in acellular and cellular cementum. The root surface is seen in polarised light, the different colours reflecting different orientations of the collagen fibres. The acellular cementum (**A**) contains primarily extrinsic fibres arranged perpendicular to the root surface. The overlying cellular cementum (**B**) contains extrinsic fibres as well as many intrinsic fibres running parallel to the root surface. Thus, there is a colour difference between the two layers. (Ground, longitudinal section, polarised light; × 50)

352 Attachment of the periodontal ligament fibres to cementum. The fibres of the periodontal ligament are seen to run into the organic matrix of precementum (**A**) which is secreted by cementoblasts. Subsequent mineralisation of precementum will incorporate the extrinsic fibres as Sharpey's fibres into cementum. (Decalcified section; Masson's blue trichrome; × 200)

353 Extrinsic fibres in ground sections. The extrinsic fibres are grouped into relatively large bundles and may not be completely calcified within cementum. This is especially the case in the more rapidly formed cellular cementum. The unmineralised organic matrix (e.g. the core of the fibre bundle) may be lost during preparation of a ground section and replaced with air or debris. This results in the total internal reflection of transmitted light, giving the appearance of thin black lines (*arrowed*). (Ground section; × 100)

354a

354 Insertion of Sharpey's fibres into cementum. 354a, ground section: the inserting collagen fibres darken as they enter the cementum due to their partial mineralisation. 354b, decalcified section: the grouping into a bundle and cross banding are apparent. **C**, cementum; **D**, periodontal ligament. (TEM; **354a**, × 8,000; **354b**, × 15,000)

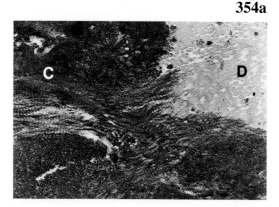

354b

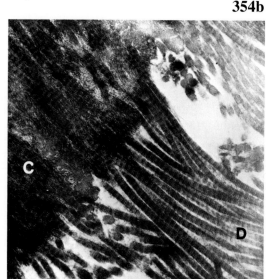

160

The ultrastructural appearance of cementum

This varies with the level of the tissue examined.

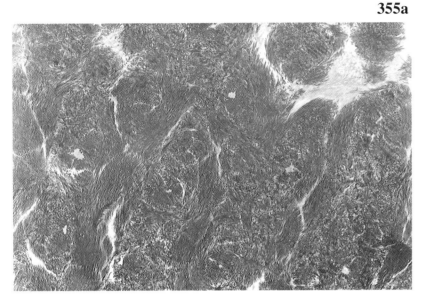

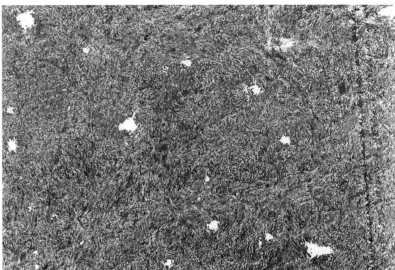

355a Cementum near the periodontal surface. Cementum at the surface region is not homogeneous, due to ongoing calcification and the presence of Sharpey's fibres. The calcification of precementum is probably initiated in the early phases by the presence of the underlying root dentine mineral, and continues on and around the collagen fibres (both those formed by the cementoblasts and those included as attachment fibres from the periodontal ligament). The outer part of the cementum, where Sharpey's fibres predominate, may be considered as calcified periodontal ligament. Unlike dentine, no calcospherites are present within precementum. (TEM; × 2,500)

355b Cementum near the cement–dentine junction. At deeper levels, acellular cementum resembles peripheral dentine. Indeed, a demarcation is often difficult to see. The small channels seen at this level may be canaliculi derived from more superficial cementocytes, but some may be the terminals of dentinal tubules which traverse the border between the two tissues. (TEM; × 2,500)

356 Intermediate cementum near the cement–dentine junction. Intermediate cementum (**A**) is that tissue close to the dentine surface which is characterised by wide, irregular branching spaces. Intermediate cementum is most commonly found in the apical region of cheek teeth. The spaces in intermediate cementum may interconnect with dentinal tubules. The nature and origin of the spaces is controversial. One suggestion is that they may be related to entrapped epithelial cells. Indeed, cell remnants containing tonofilaments characteristic of epithelial cells have been described in this region. Alternatively, they may be enlarged terminals of dentinal tubules. **B**, granular layer. (Ground section; × 250)

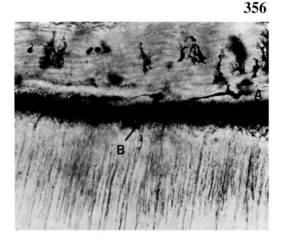

Resorption and repair of cementum

Although cementum is less susceptible to resorption than bone under the same pressures (e.g. with orthodontic loading), most roots of permanent teeth still show small, localised areas of resorption. The cause of this is not known, but may be associated with microtrauma. The resorption is carried out by multinuclear odontoclasts (see page 283) and may continue into the root dentine.

357

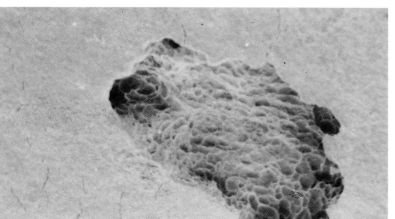

357 Surface of root showing localised area of resorption of cementum. (SEM; × 300)

358

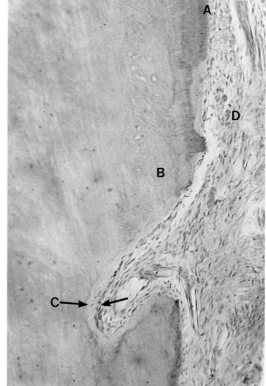

358 Repair of cementum following a localised region of root resorption. In this section, odontoclasts have resorbed through the thin layer of acellular cementum (**A**) and penetrated into the root dentine (**B**). Repair is occurring and a layer of formative cells (cementoblasts, *arrowed*) have deposited a thin layer of matrix (precementum) in the deficiency. An irregular and dark staining reversal line (**C**) separates the repair tissue from the underlying dental tissues. **D**, periodontal ligament. (Decalcified section of a root; H & E; × 90)

Resorption deficiencies may be filled by deposition of mineralised tissue. Indeed, a line known as a reversal line may be seen separating the repair tissue from the normal underlying dental tissues.

The repair tissue resembles cellular cementum. The formative cells have a similar ultrastructure to cementoblasts. Lines resembling incremental lines may be seen and there is a zone of uncalcified repair tissue homologous to precementum. However, differences can be noted between the repair tissue and cementum. First, the width of the uncalcified zone of reparative cementum (15µm) is greater than that for precementum (4µm). Second, its degree of mineralisation is less (as judged by electron density). Third, its crystals are smaller. Fourth, calcific globules are present, suggesting that mineralisation is not proceeding evenly.

These differences may be related to the speed of formation of the repair tissue. Where this is very slow, the repair tissue cannot be distinguished histologically or in its mineralisation pattern from primary cementum. However, where the repair tissue is formed rapidly (as in resorbing deciduous teeth), it closely resembles woven bone.

Root fractures may, on some occasions, repair by the formation of a cemental callus. Unlike the callus that forms around fractured bone, the cemental callus does not remodel to the original dimensions of the tooth.

Other features and clinical considerations are cementicles, hypercementosis, and the appearance of the apical constriction of the root.

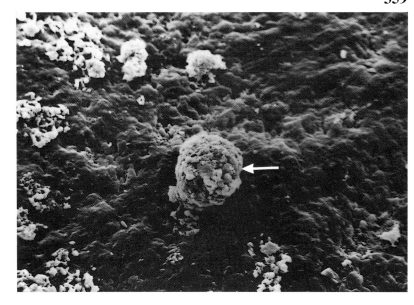

359 Cementicles are small, globular masses of cementum found in approximately 35% of human roots. They are not always attached to the cementum surface but may be located free in the periodontal ligament. Cementicles may result from microtrauma, when extra stress on the Sharpey's fibres causes a tear in the cementum. This micrograph shows a cementicle (*arrowed*) attached to the root surface. Cementicles are more common in the apical and middle third of the root and in root furcation areas. (SEM; × 1,000)

Cementum continues to be deposited slowly throughout life. The thickness of cementum increases about threefold between the ages of 16 and 70, although whether this proceeds in a linear manner is not known. It may be formed at the root apex in much greater amounts as a result of compensatory tooth eruption in response to attrition (wear) at the occlusal surface. Where there has been a history of chronic periapical inflammation, cementum formation may be substantial, giving rise to local hypercementosis. Hypercementosis affecting all the teeth may be associated with Paget's disease. It may cause problems during tooth extraction.

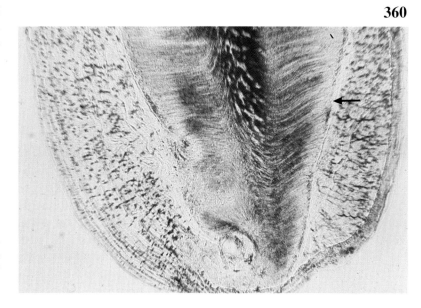

360 Hypercementosis as shown by increased thickness of cellular cementum (arrow shows cement–dentine junction). (Ground section near the root apex; × 30)

Where the root canal exits the apex of the tooth, cementum is deposited not only over the apex but also for a short distance (usually 0.5–1.5mm) from the anatomical apex. This results in a narrowing of the canal at this point, the apical constriction. This represents the junction of the pulp and periodontal tissue (although there is no visible demarcation in the soft tissue). In clinical procedures of root canal therapy which call for the removal of a diseased or decayed pulp, this is the point to which the cleansing should be extended.

Periodontal ligament

The periodontal ligament is the dense fibrous connective tissue which occupies the periodontal space between the root of the tooth and the alveolus. It is derived from the dental follicle (see **577**). Above the alveolar crest, the ligament is continuous with the connective tissues of the gingiva; at the apical foramen, it is continuous with the dental pulp. The continuity with the gingiva is important when considering the development of periodontitis from gingivitis. The continuity with the pulp explains why inflammation from this dental tissue (often related to dental caries) spreads to involve the periodontal ligament and the other apical supporting tissues.

361 The relationship of the periodontal ligament and the periodontal space (*arrow*) to the other tissues of the periodontium. **A**, alveolar bone; **B**, gingiva; **C**, root of tooth lined by cementum. Although the average width of the periodontal space is said to be 0.2mm, there is considerable variation both between teeth and within an individual tooth. The space has been described as hour-glass in shape, being narrowest in the mid-root region, near the fulcrum about which the tooth moves when an orthodontic load (tipping load) is applied to the crown. The width of the periodontal space also varies according to the functional state of the periodontal tissues. The space is reduced in non-functional and unerupted teeth and is increased in teeth subjected to heavy occlusal stress. With age, the periodontal space narrows slightly. The periodontal spaces of the permanent teeth are said to be narrower than those of the deciduous teeth. (Decalcified, longitudinal section of a tooth *in situ*; H & E; × 4)

361

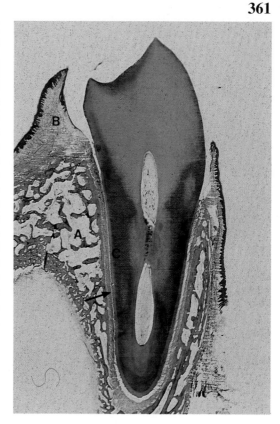

A considerable amount of research has been conducted in recent times into the structure, function and composition of the periodontal ligament. This has occurred not only because the tissue is associated with important dental functions (in particular the mechanisms of tooth support and tooth eruption; see pages 185–187 and 284–287 respectively) but also for clinical reasons. As mentioned above, the tissue is involved with inflammatory periodontal disease (a common cause of tooth loss). With the application of orthodontic loads, the periodontal tissues must adjust to permit tooth movements. Despite the amount of research undertaken, many of the important features of the periodontal ligament remain poorly understood and consequently there is much controversy. We are only now beginning to understand the extent of specialisation of the tissue (see page 184), but we still do not know why the tissue remains a soft connective tissue and does not completely calcify, even though it is enclosed by bone externally and cementum internally.

The periodontal ligament has the following functions:

1. It is the tissue of attachment between the tooth and alveolar bone. It is thus responsible for resisting displacing forces (the tooth support mechanism) and it protects the dental tissues from damage caused by excessive occlusal loads (especially at the root apex).
2. It is responsible for the mechanisms whereby a tooth attains, and then maintains, its functional position. This includes the mechanisms of tooth eruption, tooth support (particularly the recovery response after loading), and drift.
3. Its cells form, maintain and repair alveolar bone and cementum.
4. Its mechanoreceptors are involved in the neurological control of mastication (see page 101 for reflex jaw activities).

164

The periodontal ligament has been likened to a fibrous joint (a gomphosis) and to periosteum. As will become apparent, however, such comparisons are not accurate (either from a structural or functional point of view).

In common with other dense fibrous connective tissues, the periodontal ligament consists of a stroma of fibres and ground substance containing cells, blood vessels and nerves.

Fibres of the periodontal ligament

The connective tissue fibres are mainly collagenous (comprising well over 90% of the periodontal ligament fibres), but there may also be small amounts of oxytalan and reticulin fibres and, in some species, elastin fibres.

Collagen of the periodontal ligament

The periodontal collagen is mostly Type I collagen. This variety of collagen is the major protein component of most connective tissues (including bone and skin) and contains two identical α_1 chains and a chemically different α_2 chain. It is low in hydroxylysine and glycosylated hydroxylsine. Unusually, however, the periodontal ligament is relatively rich in Type III collagen (about 20%). This variety consists of three identical α_1 III chains. It is high in hydroxyproline, low in hydroxylysine, and contains cysteine. The function of Type III collagen is unknown.

Much of the collagen is gathered together to form bundles which are approximately 5μm in diameter. These bundles are termed the principal fibres of the periodontal ligament. The principal fibres appear to be more numerous (but smaller) at their attachments to cementum than at the alveolar bone (see **379**).

362

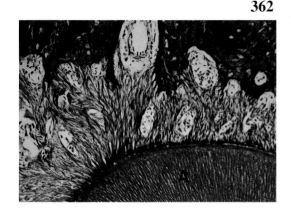

363

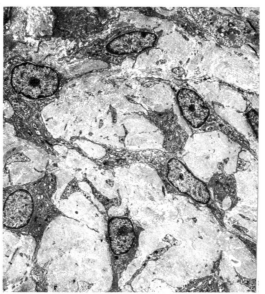

364

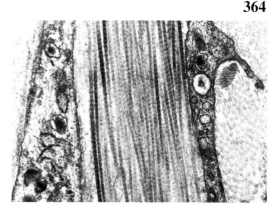

362 Principal collagen fibres passing across the periodontal space from the root (**A**) to the alveolar bone (**B**). Note also the vascular nature of the periodontal ligament. (Decalcified, transverse section through the periodontal ligament; Gomori's silver stain; × 250)

364 High-power view of a fibroblast process enveloping a principal fibre. Note the individual collagen fibrils within the principal bundle sectioned longitudinally. (TEM; × 10,000)

363 The close association between the principal fibres and the fibroblasts of the periodontal ligament. The fibroblasts are responsible for the synthesis and degradation of collagen. Cellular processes surround or envelop the fibre bundles; indeed, processes from adjacent cells are joined by intercellular contacts (see **395**) to form a cellular network. Many of the isolated islands of cytoplasm present in this section are cell processes from fibroblasts whose cell bodies are beyond the plane of section. (TEM; × 3,000)

Collagen fibrils are the banded subunits of the collagen fibre. They are formed by the packing together of individual tropocollagen molecules. The diameters of the collagen fibrils reflect the mechanical demands put upon the connective tissue.

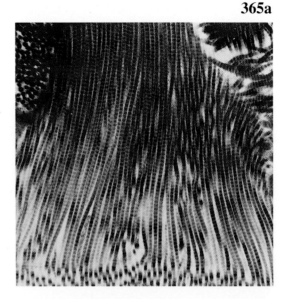

365 High-power view of collagen fibrils within a principal fibre of the periodontal ligament. 365a, fibrils sectioned longitudinally; **365b**, fibrils sectioned transversely. The fibrils in longitudinal section display the banding characteristic of collagen. The fibrils in transverse section appear to be small and of uniform diameter. (TEM; **365a**, x 16,000; **365b**, × 100,000)

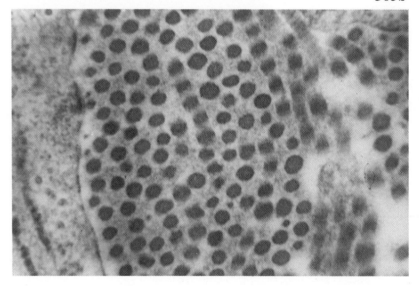

366 Histogram showing the range of collagen fibril diameters in the periodontal ligament. The histogram shows that there is a sharply unimodal distribution of collagen fibrils in the periodontal ligament (range ~20–70nm) with a mode of approximately 42nm. This confirms that the periodontal fibrils are small and of essentially uniform diameter. The pattern of distribution is reminiscent of collagen in connective tissues placed under compression and differs markedly from the bimodal distribution with large fibrils usually associated with tissues under tension (e.g. tendon). Recent research indicates that the distribution for periodontal collagen alters neither with changes in periodontal function nor with age. Indeed, the lack of change with age differs from many other fibrous connective tissues.

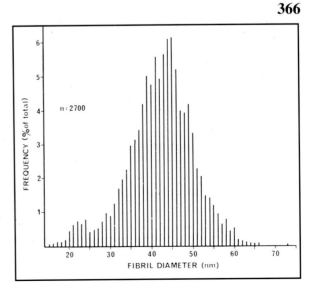

166

367 The orientation of the principal fibres of the periodontal ligament seen in longitudinal section of a multirooted tooth. The principal collagen fibres show different orientations in different regions of the periodontal ligament. They comprise: **1**, dento-alveolar crest fibres; **2**, horizontal fibres; **3**, oblique fibres; **4**, apical fibres; **5**, interradicular fibres.

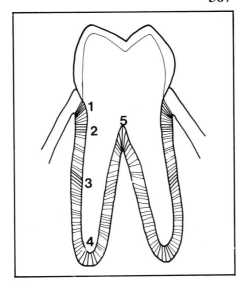

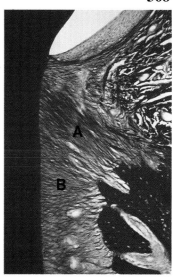

368 The dento-alveolar crest fibres (A) and the horizontal fibres (B) of the periodontal ligament. (Decalcified, longitudinal section through the ligament in the region of the alveolar crest; van Gieson; × 80)

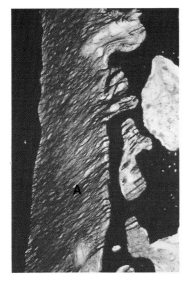

369 The oblique fibres (A) of the periodontal ligament. (Decalcified, longitudinal section; van Gieson; × 80)

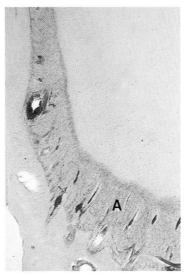

370 The apical fibres (A) of the periodontal ligament. (Decalcified, longitudinal section through the ligament in the region of the root apex; H & E; × 30)

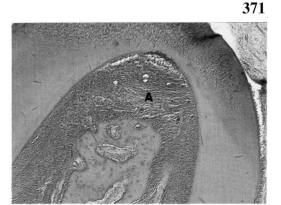

371 Interradicular fibres (A) of the periodontal ligament. (Decalcified, longitudinal section of the ligament in the region of a root bifurcation; orange green and light green; × 40)

It has been usual to ascribe specific functions to each of the groups of principal fibres. For example, it has been suggested that the orientation of the oblique fibres shows that they form a suspensory ligament which translates pressure on the tooth into tensional forces on the alveolar wall. However, no physio-logical evidence exists to support such a concept (see pages 185–187) and many of the structural features of the periodontal ligament (e.g. the collagen fibril diameters) suggest compression (see pages 166 and 187).

Controversy exists concerning the extent of individual principal fibres across the width of the periodontal ligament. One view holds that there are distinct tooth-related and bone-related fibres, and that these intercalate near the middle of the ligament at an intermediate plexus. However, recent evidence suggests that the fibres cross the entire width of the periodontal space but branch *en route* and join neighbouring fibres to form a complex three-dimensional network.

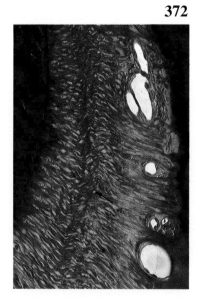

372 Longitudinal section through the periodontal ligament producing an appearance of an intermediate plexus (*arrowed*). While remodelling of fibres in the intermediate plexus provides a convenient model to explain how such axial tooth movements as eruption may be sustained, the plexus is usually only seen in longitudinal sections of continuously growing incisors (of rodents and lagomorphs). It is not seen in cross-sections of the tissue. Thus, the plexus is an artifact which is probably related to the fact that the collagen fibres in the periodontal ligaments of continuously growing incisors are arranged mainly in the form of sheets rather than bundles. (Decalcified, longitudinal section; Alcian blue; × 200)

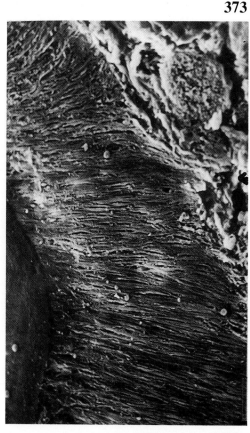

373 Continuity of the principal fibres across the periodontal space. This is a periodontal ligament cut transversely. No intermediate plexus can be seen, the fibres branching and joining with each other. (SEM; × 500)

Despite the lack of histological evidence for an intermediate fibre plexus, it has been proposed that there is a 'zone-of-shear' — a site of remodelling in the periodontal ligament which allows a tooth to move during eruption. The location of this zone is in dispute. Some believe that it lies near the centre of the periodontal ligament, the avascular, tooth-related part of the ligament moving with the erupting tooth. Using tritium-labelled proline, it is claimed that there is a zone in the mid-region of the periodontal ligament where there is greatest uptake of the label. However, other studies have been unable to support this, demonstrating uniform uptake of various labels over the whole width of the ligament. In contrast, by counting the number of intracellular collagen profiles in the periodontal fibroblasts (see page 175) which indicate degenerating collagen, there is said to be greater remodelling in the centre of the tissue. Nevertheless, the physiological significance of a central location for the zone of shear is thrown into doubt by experiments on the resected rodent incisor, which indicate that the zone of shear is close to the root surface.

374 The effects of root resection on the periodontal ligament. Root resection involves the surgical removal of the growing base of the rodent incisor. Because this incisor continues to erupt, it passes up the socket, leaving a space below its base. Accordingly, if the zone of shear occurs centrally within the periodontal ligament, the tooth-related part of the ligament should move with the tooth, leaving behind the bone-related tissue only (i.e. approximately half of the tissue, **B**). In fact, the whole width of the ligament is left behind the erupting tooth (**A**), indicating that the zone of shear is close to the tooth surface. This is further supported by experiments where lathyrogens are administered in the diet. The lathyritic periodontal ligament results from the specific inhibition by the drug of the formation of collagen crosslinks and is characterised by a longitudinal cleft down the ligament adjacent to the tooth surface.

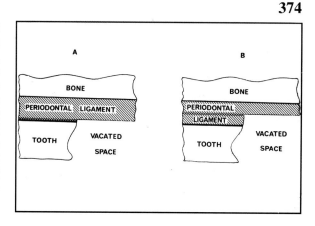

In addition to the principal fibre groups, the periodontal ligament was thought to contain numerous collagen fibres with random orientation, forming an indifferent fibre plexus.

However, this plexus is now known to be produced artifactually as a consequence of tissue preparation.

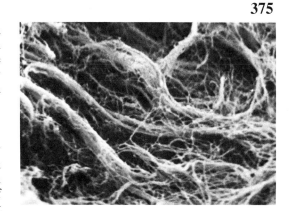
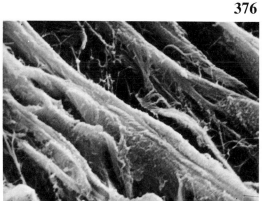

375 Periodontal ligament prepared with a rotating abrasive disc. Specimens prepared in this manner show the periodontal ligament to be mainly composed of a mass of fine, randomly orientated fibres, giving the appearance of an indifferent fibre plexus. (SEM; × 3,500)

376 Periodontal ligament prepared by slicing through a demineralised tooth with a sharp razor blade. Unlike the previous SEM in **375**, the ligament consists almost entirely of branching principal fibres without an indifferent fibre plexus. Thus, the method of specimen preparation is important in determining the appearance of the ligament. (SEM; × 3,500)

The principal fibres of the periodontal ligament do not necessarily run a straight course as they pass from the region of the alveolar bone to the tooth. Indeed, they are said to be wavy, although it is not known whether the waviness is real or represents an artifact due to histological preparation. If real, it could have important implications for the biomechanical properties of the ligament and consequently the mechanism of tooth support (see pages 185–187).

A specific type of waviness seen in collagenous tissues (including the periodontal ligament) is called crimping. Collagen crimps are best seen under the polarising microscope.

377 Crimping of collagen in the periodontal ligament as viewed under polarised light. The fibres are seen to be banded between crossed polars, reflecting an underlying periodicity along the fibre. The period is about 16μm and the angular deflection from the fibre axis is in excess of 20°. It is important to realise that the banding does not rely on seeing shapes (waves in particular), the alternating dark and bright bands being evident in otherwise straight and smooth cylindrical fibres. In functional terms, it has been proposed that the crimp is gradually pulled out when the ligament is subjected to mechanical tension, until the crimp eventually disappears. (Transverse section of the central region of the rabbit incisor periodontal ligament; polarising optical micrograph; × 200)

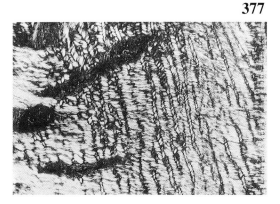

378 Crimping displayed in a single teased-out collagen fibre from the periodontal ligament. Note that the banding relates to the wavy course of the fibrils in the bundle (**378a**, polarising optical micrograph; **378b**, Nomarski differential interference contrast of same field as **378a**; × 200)

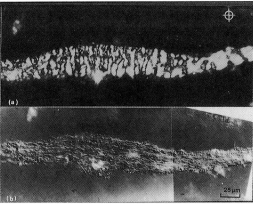

The principal fibres of the periodontal ligament which are embedded in cementum and in the bone lining the tooth socket are termed Sharpey's fibres.

379

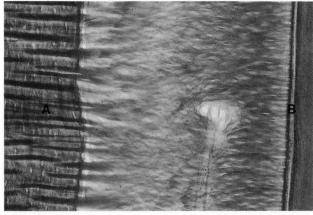

380

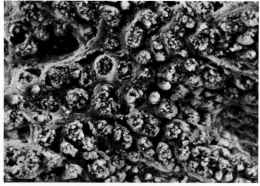

381

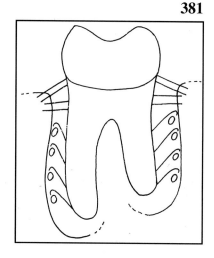

379 The insertion of periodontal fibres into alveolar bone (A) and cementum (B). The horizontal lines in the bone and cementum represent the Sharpey's fibres. Note that the principal fibres are more numerous but smaller at their attachments to cementum than at the alveolar bone. (Decalcified section; van Gieson; × 250)

380 Electron micrograph of Sharpey's fibres in the alveolar bone. The mineralised parts of the fibres appear as projecting stubs covered with mineral clusters. The occurrence of mineralisation at approximately right angles to the long axes of the fibres may indicate that in function the fibres are subjected to tensional forces. (SEM; × 300)

381 The location and distribution of Sharpey's fibres from the periodontal collagen along the tooth socket. This diagram is conjectured from data obtained from a variety of species and suggests that the fibres near the alveolar crest show pronounced Sharpey's fibre insertions. Elsewhere, many of the principal fibres in the periodontal ligament do not insert into bone but perhaps terminate around the blood vessels of the ligament.

Sharpey's fibres are also considered with bone and cementum, on pages 197–198 and 160 respectively.

The rate of turnover of collagen within the periodontal ligament is faster than virtually all other connective tissues. Indeed, the half-life of collagen has been reported as being between 3 and 23 days. The rate appears to vary in different parts of the same tooth, being highest towards the root apex. However, turnover seems to be relatively even across the width of the periodontal ligament, perhaps providing evidence against the existence of separate tooth-related and bone-related parts to the tissue (see page 168). The reason for the high rate of turnover is not known but it is reasonable to suppose that the high rate may relate to the considerable functional demands placed upon the tooth in terms of remodelling as a reaction to occlusal stress and to tooth movements. However, the ligaments of teeth subjected to greatly reduced masticatory loads do not show different rates of turnover from teeth subjected to normal loads. Furthermore, the periodontal ligaments of teeth erupting very rapidly do not have different turnover rates from the ligaments of fully erupted teeth.

Recent studies indicate that measuring rates may not reflect total protein turnover and that there may be several protein pools having different turnover rates, each contributing to a different extent to overall protein turnover in the periodontal ligament. Indeed, control of matrix morphostasis may be more dependent on extracellular processing (e.g. fibrillogenesis, proteolysis) than upon initial rate of protein secretion.

The possible role of the periodontal collagen in tooth support and tooth eruption is considered further on pages 186 and 285 respectively.

Oxytalan fibres of the periodontal ligament

Depending upon species, the periodontal ligament contains either oxytalan fibres or elastin fibres. In man, the periodontal ligament contains oxytalan fibres. In order to demonstrate periodontal oxytalan fibres at the light microscope level, it is necessary to oxidise tissue sections strongly prior to staining with certain elastin stains. Unlike collagen, oxytalan fibres are not susceptible to acid hydrolysis. Although little is known about their composition, their ultrastructural characteristics suggest that they are immature elastin fibres (pre-elastin).

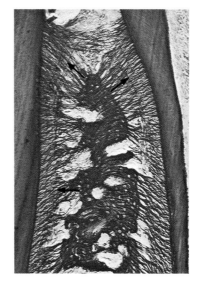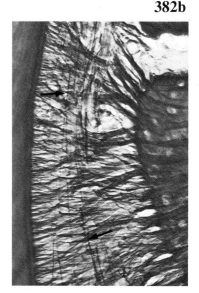

382 The course of oxytalan fibres (*arrowed*). The oxytalan fibres are attached into the cementum of the tooth and course out into the periodontal ligament in various directions, rarely being incorporated into bone. In the cervical region, they follow the course of gingival and transseptal collagen fibres, but within the periodontal ligament proper they tend to be more longitudinally orientated, crossing the oblique fibre bundles more or less perpendicularly. In the outer part of the ligament, the oxytalan fibres are said to often terminate around blood vessels and nerves. The oxytalan fibres vary in size from 0.5µm–2.5µm in diameter (as assessed with the light microscope) and constitute no more than about 3% of the extracellular fibre composition. (Decalcified, longitudinal section through the periodontal ligament; potassium monopersulphate, aldehyde fuchsin counterstained with van Gieson; **382a**, × 40; **382b**, × 120)

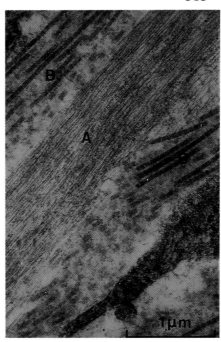

383 An oxytalan fibre. The oxytalan fibre (**A**) can be recognised at the ultrastructural level as a collection of unbanded fibrils arranged parallel to the long axis of the fibre. Each fibril is approximately 15nm in diameter and an interfibrillar amorphous material is present in variable amounts. In cross-section, the oxytalan fibre is oval and its dimensions are smaller than reported using the light microscope. They are thought to resemble pre-elastin in that, unlike mature elastin, the oxytalan fibre does not possess a central amorphous core. **B**, collagen fibres showing their characteristic banding and demonstrating the different size of the fibrils compared with oxytalan. (TEM)

The functions of the oxytalan fibres remain unknown. They are said to be thicker and more numerous in teeth which carry abnormally high loads, including abutment teeth for bridges and teeth being moved for orthodontic reasons. Thus, it appears that oxytalan may have a role in tooth support (perhaps also indicated by the relationship with the periodontal vasculature). However, experimental evidence shows that the oxytalan fibres are unchanged in the periodontal ligaments of teeth with greatly reduced masticatory loading. Elastin fibres are restricted to the walls of the blood vessels, although in some animals (e.g. herbivores) they replace the oxytalan fibres. Reticulin fibres are related to basement membranes within the periodontal ligament (i.e. associated with blood vessels and epithelial cell rests) and are a variety of collagen.

Ground substance of the periodontal ligament

Because of its relative inaccessibility and complex biochemical nature, little detailed information concerning this important component of the periodontal ligament is available. Although we are used to thinking of the ligament as a collagen-rich tissue, in reality it is a tissue rich in ground substance. Indeed, even the collagen fibre bundles are composed of about 60% ground substance by volume.

384

384 Electron micrograph of the extracellular matrix of the periodontal ligament. Note that the matrix is rich in ground substance, even within the collagen fibre bundle. (TEM; × 100,000)

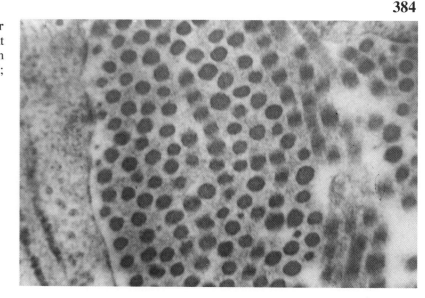

The ground substance of the periodontal ligament consists mainly of hyaluronate glycosaminoglycans, proteoglycans and glycoproteins. The proteoglycans are compounds containing anionic polysaccharides (glycosaminoglycans) covalently attached to a protein core. Two proteoglycans have been isolated in the periodontal ligament: proteodermatan sulphate and a proteoglycan containing chondroitin sulphate/dermatan sulphate hybrids which has been designated PG1. All components of the periodontal ligament ground substance are presumed to be secreted by fibroblasts.

The ground substance is thought to have many important functions (ion and water binding and exchange, control of collagen fibrillogenesis and fibre orientation). Tissue fluid pressure has been found to be high in the periodontal ligament, being about 10mmHg above atmospheric pressure. Indeed, the tissue fluid has been implicated in the tooth support and eruptive mechanisms (see page 287).

The composition of the ground substance in the periodontal ligament varies according to the developmental state of the tissue (**385**) and according to location (**386**).

385

385 Glycosaminoglycans in the periodontal ligament at different stages of development (from bovine incisors). Δ, hyaluronate; ▫, proteodermatan sulphate; ○, PG1 proteoglycan. Group 1 specimens are of dental follicle. Group 2 is the initial stage of formation of the periodontal ligament. Sharpey's fibre attachments were discernible in Group 3. Groups 4 and 5 were for erupting teeth (the typical orientation of collagen fibres being first observed in Group 5). Group 6 specimens were from fully erupted teeth. Note that there is a marked change in the amount of hyaluronate as development proceeds from the dental follicle to the initial periodontal ligament. This is a trend which occurs during embryonic development of other connective tissues. For the proteoglycans, note that the PG1 proteoglycans show a significant increase during eruption. Note HYP = hydroxyproline, enabling determinations of ground substance components relative to collagen content.

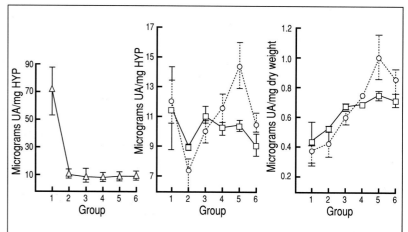

386 Glycosaminoglycans (sulphated GAG) at different sites in the periodontal connective tissues (from sheep incisors).

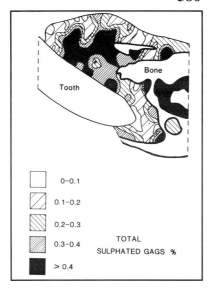

TOTAL SULPHATED GAGS %

0–0.1
0.1–0.2
0.2–0.3
0.3–0.4
> 0.4

Much interest has recently been shown in a complex glycoprotein called fibronectin. This protein is thought to promote attachment of cells to the substratum, especially to collagen fibrils. Furthermore, as cells preferentially adhere to fibronectin, it may be involved in cell migration and orientation. Considering these functions, together with the high rate of turnover in the periodontal ligament, it is not surprising that fibronectin may have considerable biological significance within the ligament. Immunofluorescent techniques at the light microscope level have revealed that fibronectin is uniformly distributed throughout the periodontal ligament in both erupting and fully erupted teeth. Ultrastructural studies have localised the glycoprotein over collagen fibres and at certain sites at the cell–collagen interface. As loss of fibronectin has been observed during the terminal maturation of many connective tissue matrices, its continued presence within the periodontal ligament may be indicative of the ligament retaining 'immature', fetal-like characteristics. Another glycoprotein termed tenascin has recently been identified in the periodontal ligament. Like fibronectin, tenascin is more characteristic of a fetal-like connective tissue than a fully 'mature' connective tissue. Unlike fibronectin, tenascin is not uniformly localised throughout the ligament but is concentrated adjacent to the alveolar bone and the cementum. The role of these glycoproteins in the functions of the periodontal ligament awaits clarification.

Cells of the periodontal ligament

The predominant connective tissue cell within the periodontal ligament is the fibroblast. Cells covering the surface of both cementum and alveolar bone are also considered part of the ligament (i.e. cementoblasts, cementoclasts, osteoblasts and osteoclasts). In addition, the periodontal ligament contains undifferentiated mesenchymal cells, defence cells and epithelial cells (rests of Malassez).

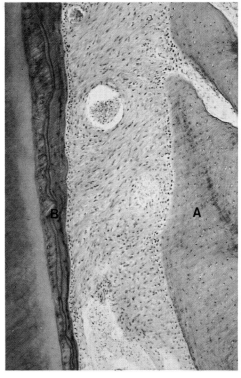

387 The distribution of cells in the periodontal ligament. The type and number of cells varies according to the functional state of the ligament. In addition to the numerous fibroblasts within the ligament, the surfaces of the alveolar bone (**A**) and cementum (**B**) are lined with osteoblasts and cementoblasts, indicating active deposition of bone and cementum in this specimen. (Decalcified, longitudinal section through the periodontal ligament; H & E; × 80)

The fibroblasts in the periodontal ligament seem to have a variety of shapes with many fine cytoplasmic processes, although they are usually described as being fusiform. However, the overall shape can only be determined by consideration of the cell outlines in different planes. When this is done, the periodontal fibroblasts often appear as flattened, disc-shaped cells.

388

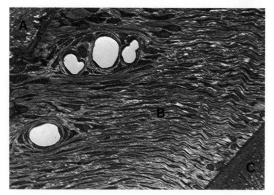

388 A periodontal ligament (B) comprising numerous fibroblasts. A, alveolar bone; **C,** cementum. (Decalcified, longitudinal section through the periodontal ligament; Toluidine blue; × 300)

389

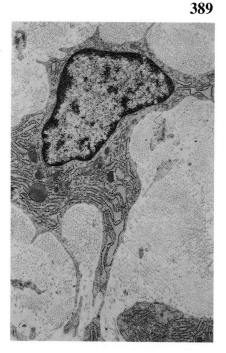

389 Periodontal fibroblasts, being active cells, have low nuclear–cytoplasmic ratios, and each nucleus contains one or more prominent nucleoli. The typical periodontal fibroblast is rich in the intracytoplasmic organelles associated with the synthesis and export of proteins. It therefore shows a well-developed rough endoplasmic reticulum, Golgi apparatus and many mitochondria. (TEM; × 4,000)

Much has been made of the possibility that the periodontal fibroblasts are motile–contractile cells, and that they are thereby capable of generating a force responsible for tooth eruption (see page 286). Much of the evidence for migratory or contractile activities comes from research on the behaviour and appearance of periodontal fibroblasts *in vitro*. *In vitro*, periodontal fibroblasts can organise a fibrous network and can generate significant forces. However, the behaviour and appearance depends upon the method of culture.

390

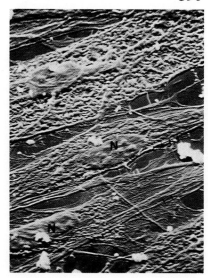

390 The appearance of periodontal fibroblasts cultured on plastic. These cells assume the properties of motile cells. They are thin and highly polarised with respect to both shape and location of organelles. In particular, there are numerous microtubules and microfilaments (as stress fibres) which run along the length of the cell. Cells with these characteristics have not been seen in the periodontal ligament *in vivo*. **N,** nucleus. (SEM; × 1,200)

391 The appearance of periodontal fibroblasts cultured on collagen gels. During contraction of the gel, the periodontal fibroblasts assume the appearance of myofibroblasts (see **658b**). Myofibroblasts are cells which have the properties of both fibroblasts and smooth muscle cells, and are found in contracting wounds. They are characterised ultrastructurally by having polarity of shape, crenulated (folded) nuclei, and numerous microfilaments (as shown here). Adjacent cells contact by means of gap junctions. While periodontal fibroblasts *in vivo* may show occasional gap junctions (see **395**), they show no other features characteristic of myofibroblasts. (TEM; × 30,000)

391

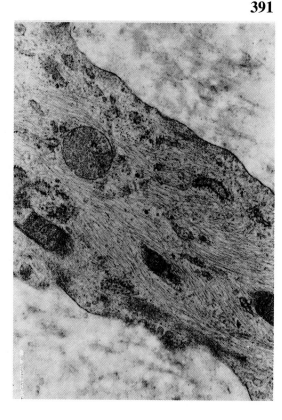

174

Thus, although the evidence from *in vitro* studies suggests that the periodontal fibroblasts have the potential to be migratory and/or contractile cells, under normal functional conditions *in vivo* the cells are primarily involved in protein synthesis and secretion.

In addition to synthesising and secreting proteins, there is now evidence that the cells are responsible for collagen degradation. This contrasts with earlier views that degradation was essentially an extracellular event involving the activity of proteolytic enzymes such as collagenases. The main evidence indicating that the periodontal fibroblasts are also 'fibroclastic' is the presence of organelles termed intracellular collagen profiles.

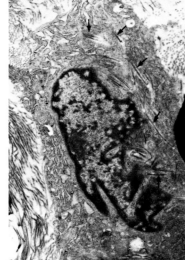

392a

392a **Periodontal fibroblast showing intra-cellular collagen profiles (*arrowed*).** (TEM; × 5,000)

392b **Banded collagen fibrils (*arrowed*) seen within an elongated membrane-bound vacuole.** It is thought that the intracellular collagen vacuoles are associated with the degradation of collagen which has been 'ingested' from the extracellular environment. (TEM; × 25,000)

392b

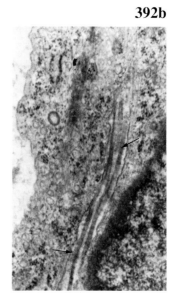

393

393 **The temporal sequence for intracellular digestion of collagen in the periodontal ligament. A,** banded fibril surrounded by an electron-lucent zone. This is the stage when a collagen fibril is first phagocytosed by the fibroblast. **B,** banded fibrils surrounded by an electron-dense zone. At this stage, the phagosome fuses with primary lysosomes to form a phago-lysosome in which there is a gradual increase in electron density of the matrix. **C,** fibrils with indistinct banding surrounded by an electron-dense zone. This, the terminal stage, indicates that enzymatic degeneration of the fibril has proceeded to the point where the fibril loses its characteristic structure. (TEM)

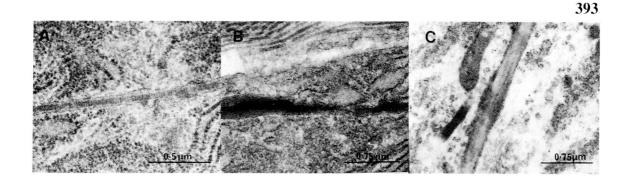

The time taken to degrade collagen intracellularly is not known, although it is suggested to be about 30 minutes (a similar time to that required for synthesis).

It has been argued that the collagen profiles within periodontal fibroblasts are not truly intracellular and that the collagen merely lies in surface invaginations. Accordingly, the degradation would still be an extracellular phenomenon. It has also been suggested that, because the periodontal fibroblasts may be synthesising collagen in excess of requirements, the profiles contain collagen which is being degraded without ever having been secreted extracellularly. Overall, however, the evidence does suggest that the collagen is ingested from the extracellular compartment of the periodontal ligament and that the profiles are intracellular.

Cilia and intercellular contacts are features of the fibroblasts in the periodontal ligament which are not usually seen in the fibroblasts of other fibrous connective tissues.

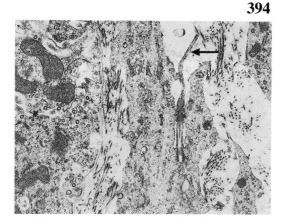

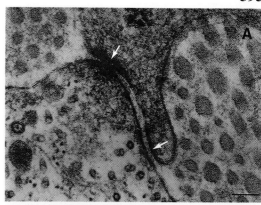

394 A cilium (*arrowed*) lying within an invagination of the cell membrane of a periodontal ligament fibroblast. The cilium differs from those seen in other cell types in that it contains no more than nine tubule doublets (compared to the usual 9 plus 2 configuration). The significance of the cilia in fibroblasts is unknown, although it has been suggested that they may be associated with control of the cell cycle and/or inhibition of centriolar activity. (TEM; × 11,000)

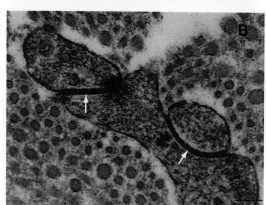

395 Intercellular contacts (*arrowed*) between the fibroblasts of the periodontal ligament. A, simplified desmosome; **B,** gap junction. Intercellular contacts are a feature of fibroblasts in fetal-like connective tissues. The simplified desmosome is the most frequently seen of the contacts. There is little information concerning the functional significance of these organelles in the periodontal fibroblast. (TEM; **A,** × 80,000; **B,** × 80,000)

In addition to the fibroblasts, the connective tissue cells of the periodontal ligament include cementoblasts and cementoclasts and the osteoblasts and osteoclasts. Cementoblasts are the cement-forming cells lining the surface of cementum.

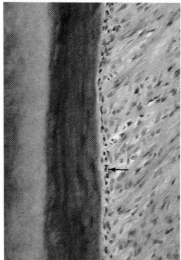

396 A layer of cementoblasts (*arrowed*) lining the cementum. (Decalcified, longitudinal section of periodontal ligament; H & E; × 160)

397 A cementoblast (A) lining cementum. Cementoblasts are not as elongated as periodontal fibroblasts, being squat, cuboidal cells. They are rich in cytoplasm and have large nuclei. Like fibroblasts, they contain all the intracytoplasmic organelles necessary for protein synthesis and secretion. The nucleus of a cementoblast is distinctly vesicular, with one or more nucleoli. The appearance of a cementoblast will depend upon its degree of activity. Cells actively depositing acellular cementum do not have prominent cytoplasmic processes. However, cells depositing cellular cementum exhibit abundant basophilic cytoplasm and cytoplasmic processes, and their nuclei tend to be folded and irregularly shaped. **B,** precementum. (TEM; × 3,700)

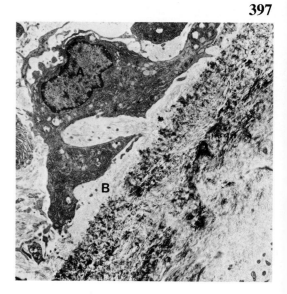

Osteoblasts are the bone-forming cells lining the tooth socket. They closely resemble cementoblasts.

398 A layer of osteoblasts *(arrowed)* **lining the alveolar bone.** This layer is only prominent when there is active bone formation. Each osteoblast appears cuboidal and exhibits a basophilic cytoplasm which is related to the extensive endoplasmic reticulum within the cell. The prominent, round nucleus tends to lie towards the basal end of the cell. A pale, juxtanuclear area indicates the site of the Golgi material. When bone is not forming, its surface is occupied by flattened, inactive bone-lining cells. Note the Sharpey's fibres passing between osteoblasts. (Decalcified, longitudinal section of periodontal ligament, H & E; × 230)

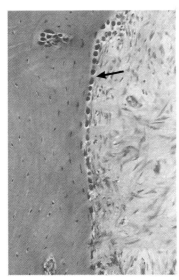

398

399

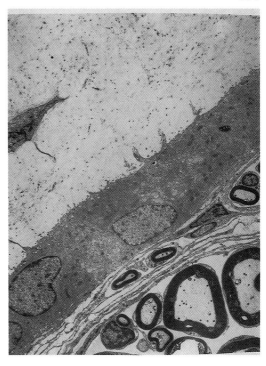

399 Ultrastructural features of the osteoblast. Like the periodontal fibroblasts, active osteoblasts contain an extensive rough endoplasmic reticulum and numerous mitochondria and vesicles. However, their Golgi material appears more localised and extensive. Microfilaments are prominent beneath the cell membrane at the secreting surface. The cells contact one another by means of desmosomes and tight junctions. The cell surface adjacent to bone has many fine cytoplasmic processes, some of which contact underlying osteocytes by tight junctions to form part of a transport system throughout the bone. (TEM; × 6,000)

Osteoclasts and cementoclasts (or odontoclasts) are found in areas where bone and cementum are being resorbed. Recent evidence shows that these cells are actively involved in the resorption process. Osteoclasts and cementoclasts have the same cytoplasmic features. These cells are now known to arise from blood cells of the macrophage type.

400

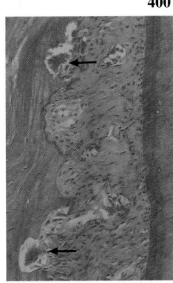

400 Resorbing alveolar bone and the osteoclast. The surface of the alveolar bone shows a number of resorption concavities termed Howship's lacunae in which lie the osteoclasts *(arrowed)*. Osteoclasts show considerable variation in size and shape, ranging from small mononuclear cells to large multinuclear cells. The part of the cell which lies adjacent to bone often has a striated appearance, the so-called brush border. (Decalcified, longitudinal section of the periodontal ligament, H & E; × 130)

401

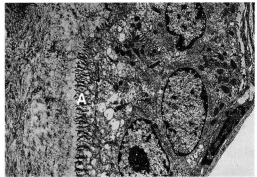

401 Ultrastructural features of a multinucleated osteoclast. The brush border (**A**) comprises many tightly packed microvilli which may be coated with fine, bristle-like structures. At the circumference of the brush border, the plasma membrane tends to become smooth and the cytoplasm beneath it more dense. It has been suggested that this modified annular zone may serve to limit the diffusion of hydrolytic enzymes, thereby creating a microenvironment in which resorption can take place. The osteoclast contains numerous mitochondria distributed throughout the cytoplasm, except for the region immediately beneath the brush border. The rough endoplasmic reticulum is less conspicuous than in osteoblasts, but Golgi material is prominent (especially in juxtanuclear areas). Most of the remaining cytoplasm contains large numbers of vesicles of different sizes and types; some contain acid phosphatase. (TEM; × 3,000)

Aggregations of epithelial cell rests, the rests of Malassez, are a normal feature of the periodontal ligament. They are the remains of the developmental epithelial root sheath of Hertwig (see pages 272–273).

402a

402b

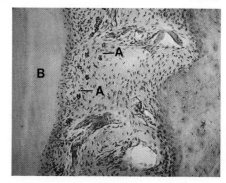
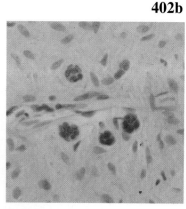

402 The position of the epithelial rests (A), close to the cementum (B). Epithelial rests can be distinguished from adjacent fibroblasts by the close packing of their cuboidal cells and their tendency to stain more deeply. The rests lie about 25μm from the cementum surface. Differences have been observed in the distribution of epithelial cells according to site and age. During the first and second decades they are most prevalent in the apical zone, whereas between the third and seventh decades the majority are located cervically in the gingiva above the alveolar crest. **402b** shows that in cross-section the epithelial cells appear cluster-like, though tangential or serial sections show that they form a network of interconnecting strands parallel to the long axis of the root. (Decalcified section through periodontal ligament, H & E; **402a**, × 240; **402b**, × 250)

403 Ultrastructural appearance of the epithelial cell rests. The cluster arrangement of the cells is reminiscent of a duct-like structure. The cells are separated from the surrounding connective tissue by a basal lamina. The nucleus of each cell is prominent and often shows invaginations. The scanty cytoplasm is characterised by the presence of tonofibrils, some of which insert into the desmosomes that are frequently found between adjacent cells, and into hemidesmosomes between the cells and the basal lamina. Tight junctions are also found between the cells. Mitochondria are distributed throughout the cytoplasm, while the rough endoplasmic reticulum and Golgi material are poorly developed. A primary cilium is often present, although its function is not understood. (TEM; × 4,500)

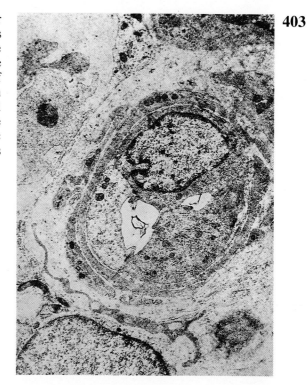

403

404 Tangential section through the epithelial rests, showing a network appearance. (Iron haematoxylin; × 60)

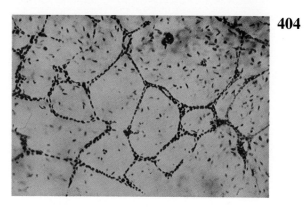

404

Histochemical and electron microscope studies reveal little activity in the epithelial cells. However, they may proliferate to form cysts or tumours if appropriately stimulated (e.g. by chronic inflammation). Following orthodontic movement, there is no regeneration of the epithelial rests, although there is regeneration of connective tissue on the compression side.

Defence cells within the periodontal ligament include macrophages, mast cells, and eosinophils. These are similar to defence cells in other connective tissues.

405 Ultrastructural features of a macrophage. Macrophages are responsible for phagocytosing particulate matter and invading organisms. They also synthesise a range of molecules with important functions such as interferon (the antiviral factor), prostaglandins, and factors that enhance the growth of fibroblasts and endothelial cells. Macrophages are derived from blood monocytes. Their structure depends upon their state of activity. The resting macrophage differs from the fibroblast in that there is a paucity of rough endoplasmic reticulum, there are thin, finger-like projections from the cell surface, and the macrophage has many lysosomes and other membrane-bound vesicles of varying density. When active, macrophages have many mitochondria and vesicles and may possess many branching processes. (TEM; × 6,000)

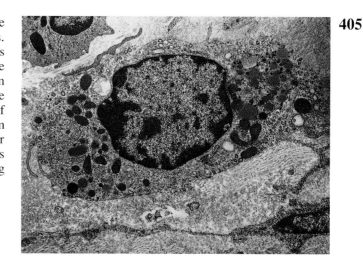
405

406 The ultrastructural appearance of the mast cell. Mast cells are often associated with blood vessels. They show a large number of intracytoplasmic granules (a feature which explains the intense staining reaction with basic analine dyes for light microscopy). The granules are dense, membrane-bound vesicles and are of varying sizes. Other cytoplasmic organelles are relatively sparse. When the cell is stimulated, it degranulates. Numerous functions have been ascribed to the mast cell, including the production of histamine, heparin, and factors associated with anaphylaxis. (TEM; × 5,000)

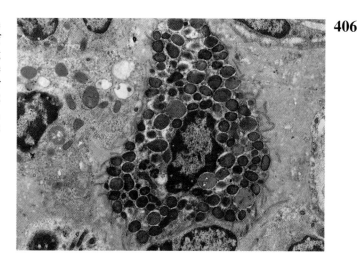
406

407 The ultrastructural features of an eosinophil. These cells are only occasionally seen in the normal periodontal ligament. Note the characteristic granules (peroxisosomes) which possess one or more crystalloid structures. The cells are capable of phagocytosis. (TEM; × 2,500)

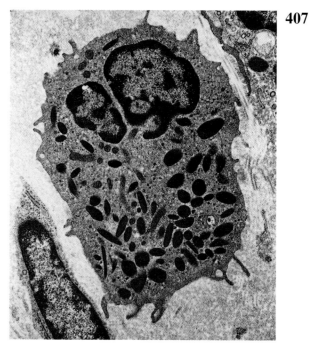
407

Cell kinetics in the periodontal ligament

As osteoblasts and cementoblasts of the periodontal ligament become incorporated into alveolar bone and cellular cementum, replacement cells must be provided within the ligament to permit osteogenesis and cementogenesis to continue. Periodontal fibroblasts are also generated throughout the life of the tissue. It is not known whether periodontal fibroblasts, cementoblasts and osteoblasts all arise from a common precursor or whether each cell type has its own specific precursor cell. Although progenitor cells can be identified by their ability to incorporate tritium-labelled thymidine, little is known about their origin and life-cycle.

Studies have shown that approximately 0.5–3% of cells within the periodontal ligament are initially labelled following injection of tritium-labelled thymidine. Such variation may be related to diurnal periodicity, or to age, or to location within the ligament, as well as to individual variation. As for other tissues, there is a reduction of the labelling index with age.

Dividing cells are located predominantly paravascularly and migrate towards the bone and cementum surfaces. The relatively low labelling index seen in the normal physiological state can be significantly increased by, for example, orthodontic loading and wounding. However, orthodontic pressure and injury may recruit progenitors that are distinctly different cell types (osteoblastic versus fibroblastic).

Blood vessels and nerves of the periodontal ligament

408

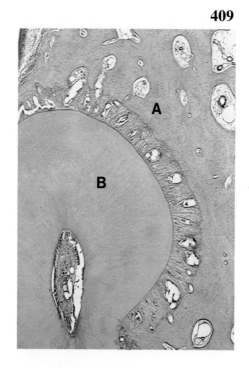

409

410

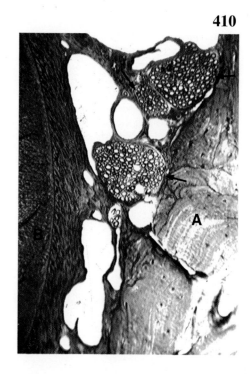

408 The rich blood supply to the periodontal ligament is derived from the appropriate superior and inferior alveolar arteries, though arteries from the gingiva (such as the lingual and palatine arteries) may also be involved. The arteries supplying the periodontal ligament are not primarily derived from those entering the pulp at the apex of the tooth, but from a series of perforating arteries passing through the alveolar bone. The dual source of the main arterial supply allows the periodontal ligament to function following removal of the root apex as a result of various endodontic treatments.

409 The major vessels of the periodontal ligament lie between the principal fibre bundles, close to the wall of the alveolus. They have an average diameter of 20μm. The vessels branch and anastomose to form a capillary plexus around the teeth. **A**, alveolar bone; **B**, dentine. (van Gieson; × 30)

410 Semi-thin section of periodontal ligament in which the blood vessels are seen as large spaces. Nerve bundles are arrowed. **A**, alveolar bone; **B**, dentine. (Toluidine blue; × 100)

180

411 A crevicular plexus of capillary loops (**A**) completely encircles the tooth within the connective tissue beneath the region of the gingival crevice. Each loop consists of one or two thin (8–10μm in diameter) capillary ascending limbs and one or two post-capillary sized venules. The crevicular capillary loops are separated from other more marginally situated loops in the gingival surface (**B**) by a distinct gap (*arrowed*). The crevicular capillary loops arise from a circular plexus (**C**), which is comprised of one to four intercommunicating vessels (6–30μm in diameter) lying at the level of the junctional epithelium. The circular plexus anastomoses with both the gingival and periodontal ligament vessels.

Species differences may occur in the pattern of the vasculature, which may also be affected by inflammation. More complex glomerular-like structures have also been described. The functional significance of the complex vasculature in this region is not fully understood, although it may be related to the provision of a dentogingival seal. It may provide a means for blood flow reversal and rapid redistribution of the blood under varying occlusal loads, and as a reaction to pathological stimuli. (SEM of vascular cast; × 80)

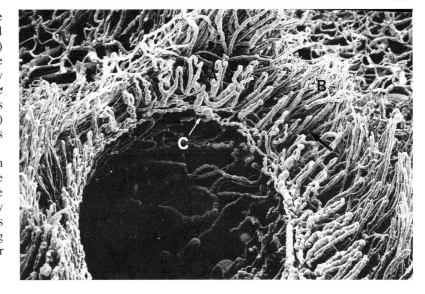

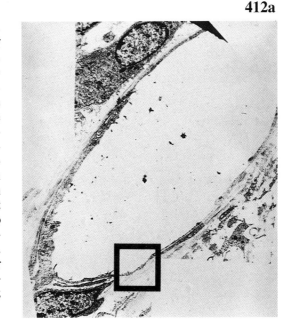

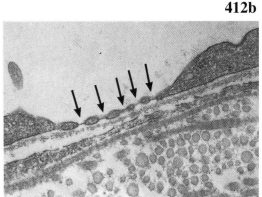

412 Fenestrated capillaries within the periodontal ligament. Note in **412a** the thinning of the endothelium in the boxed area, where fenestrations are present. **412b** is a high power view of the boxed region shown in **412a.** The fenestrations are arrowed. Fibrous connective tissues usually have continuous capillaries. The presence of fenestrated capillaries in large numbers (up to 40×10^6 per mm³ of tissue) is therefore a specialised feature of the periodontal ligament. Fenestrated capillary beds differ from continuous capillary beds in that the diffusion and filtration capacities are greatly increased. It is possible that the fenestrations are related to the high metabolic requirements of the periodontal ligament (viz. high rate of turnover). Experimental evidence suggests that the number of fenestrations also relates to the stage of eruption (see page 287). (TEM; **412a**, × 10,000; **412b**, × 35,000)

The veins within the periodontal ligament do not usually accompany the arteries. Instead, they pass through the alveolar walls into intra-alveolar venous networks. Anastomoses with veins in the gingiva also occur. A dense venous network is particularly prominent around the apex of the alveolus.

The nerve fibres supplying the periodontal ligament are functionally of two types: sensory and autonomic. The sensory fibres are associated with the modalities of pressure and pain. The autonomic fibres are associated mainly with the supply of the periodontal blood vessels. Compared with other dense fibrous connective tissues, the periodontal ligament is well innervated.

The nerve fibres entering the periodontal ligament are derived from two sources. Some nerve bundles enter near the root apex and pass up through the periodontal ligament, others enter the middle and cervical portions of the ligament as finer branches through openings in the alveolar walls.

Periodontal nerve fibres are both myelinated and unmyelinated. The myelinated fibres are on average about 5μm in diameter (although some are as large as 15μm) and are sensory fibres only. The unmyelinated fibres are about 0.5μm in diameter and are both sensory and autonomic.

It has been suggested that about 75% of mechanoreceptors within the periodontal ligament have their cell bodies in the trigeminal ganglion while the remaining 25% of cell bodies lie in the mesencephalic nucleus.

413

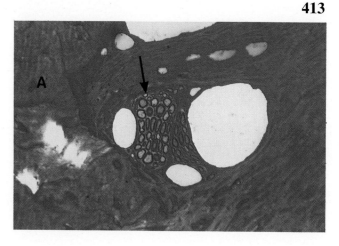

413 The rich nerve supply to the periodontal ligament. Nerve bundles are arrowed. **A**, alveolar bone; (Decalcified, transverse section through a tooth and its periodontal ligament; Toluidine blue; × 150)

At the light microscope level, a plethora of forms which are assumed to represent nerve endings have been described within the periodontal ligament. These forms vary from simple free endings to more elaborate arborising structures, although they still only mediate two sensory modalities — pain or pressure.

Most attention has been paid to the periodontal mechanoreceptors. The discharge of afferent impulses from mechanoreceptors has been recorded from single nerve fibres dissected free from the inferior alveolar nerve in animals. The discharge appears to vary according to the direction and amplitude of the displacing force. Periodontal mechanoreceptors exhibit directional sensitivity in that they respond maximally to a force applied to the crown of the tooth in one particular direction. Their conduction velocities place them within the A_β group of fibres. The response characteristics can vary from slowly adapting through to rapidly adapting fibres.

414

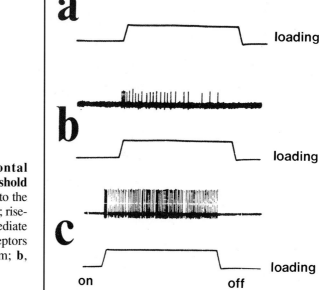

414 The responses of three periodontal ligament mechanoreceptors to suprathreshold ramp–plateau stimuli of 1 newton applied to the crown of the canine tooth (duration 3 seconds; rise-time 50ms). **a**, rapidly adapting; **b**, intermediate adapting; and **c**, slowly adapting. The receptors were located in the same tooth: **a**, 1.5mm; **b**, 3.0mm; and **c**, 5.5mm from the fulcrum.

The question arises as to whether the slowly adapting, intermediate adapting and rapidly adapting mechanoreceptors are truly different types of receptor. Where it has been possible to examine histologically nerve endings which have been physiologically characterised, it seems that the endings of the mechanoreceptors are similar, being unencapsulated Ruffini-like terminals. Furthermore, the response characteristics (i.e. whether slowly or rapidly adapting) are dependent upon the position of the ending within the ligament relative to the position of loading (see **414**).

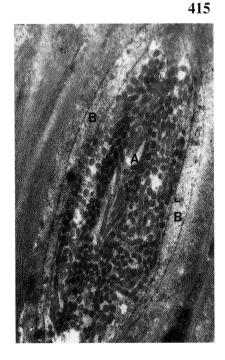

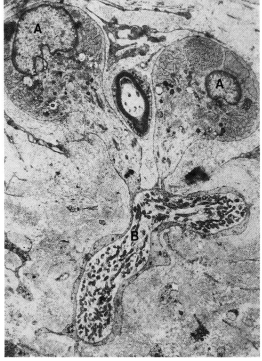

415 The putative nerve endings (A) which may represent mechanoreceptors are characterised by the very large concentrations of mitochondria in the unmyelinated terminations of myelinated nerves. Note the surrounding process of the ensheathing Schwann-type cell (**B**). This type of ending is regarded as being akin to a Ruffini-like nerve terminal. (TEM; ×5,700)

416 The cell bodies of the ensheathing Schwann-type cells contain rough endoplasmic reticulum and the nucleus (**A**) may be indented. Numerous vesicles may be observed within, and forming on, both the inner and outer surfaces of the ensheathing cells. These vesicles may be associated with rapid transport of materials to and from the nerve terminal. The collagen in the immediate vicinity of the nerve ending appears to be arranged in a lamellar pattern. **B**, mitochondria-rich nerve terminal. (TEM; ×5,000)

417

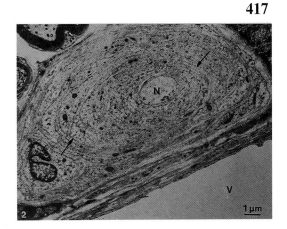

417 Complex putative nerve endings have very occasionally been observed within the periodontal ligament. These are characterised by numerous, circularly arranged cell processes (*arrowed*) surrounding a central structure (**N**) containing microfilaments, microtubules and mitochondria. This central structure is thought to represent a nerve terminal. The morphology of this lamellated structure is reminiscent of cutaneous mechanoreceptors. However, because of their rarity, their significance in the periodontal ligament is unknown. **V**, blood vessel. (TEM; ×4,500)

Little is known about pain fibres within the periodontal ligament, but it is presumed that, as elsewhere in the body, they are represented by fine, unmyelinated fibres terminating as free nerve endings. A similar lack of information exists concerning the fine (0.2–1µm diameter) autonomic fibres. These fibres are important in the control of regional blood flow, having vasoconstrictor activity. Thus, experiments affecting the sympathetic system are seen to produce changes in tooth position (see **660**).

The periodontal ligament as a specialised connective tissue

Although the periodontal ligament has the same components as other soft, fibrous connective tissues (i.e. it is composed essentially of an unmineralised collagen and proteoglycan stroma in which are found connective tissue cells), it has the following features which in combination provide a specialised tissue:

- The principal collagen fibres have a characteristic orientation.
- The types (and amounts) of collagen (Types I and III) and the type of collagen crosslink is unlike those found within most other adult fibrous connective tissues.
- In some species, a pre-elastin-like fibre (oxytalan) is prominent within the periodontal ligament.
- The rate of turnover of the periodontal ligament is very fast.
- The periodontal ligament is remarkably cellular and rich in ground substance.
- The type of proteoglycan in the periodontal ligament (i.e. PG1) is specific to this tissue.
- The tissue hydrostatic pressure may be high.
- The periodontal ligament fibroblasts have features unusual for fibroblasts in adult fibrous connective tissues (e.g. intercellular contacts, cilia).
- The periodontal ligament has cells concerned with the formation of dental tissues.
- The periodontal ligament has a rich vascular and nerve supply.
- The capillaries within the periodontal ligament are fenestrated.

However, the mere listing of these specialised characteristics does not permit inference of the role of these features in the function and pathobiology of the tissue. To do this we need to discover whether there are structural and/or biochemical analogues for the periodontal ligament elsewhere in the body.

Initially, an analogue for the periodontal ligament was sought in mature (adult) fibrous connective tissues with known mechanical demands (i.e. connective tissue placed under either tension or compression). However, such comparisons showed that the periodontal ligament had some characteristics of a tissue under tension whereas others features suggested compression (see page 187). More recently, it has been shown that the periodontal ligament resembles immature, fetal-like connective tissues.

The periodontal ligament and fetal connective tissues (mesenchyme) have the following common features:

1. High rates of turnover.
2. Sharp, unimodal size/frequency distributions of small collagen fibrils.
3. Significant amounts of Type III collagen.
4. The major reducible crosslink is the collagen dehydrodihydroxylisinonorlucene.
5. Changes in collagen fibrils with lathyrogens.
6. Large volumes of ground substance.
7. High content of glucoronate-rich proteoglycans.
8. High contents of the glycoproteins tenascin and fibronectin.
9. Presence of pre-elastin fibres (oxytalan in the periodontal ligament).
10. High cellularity, the fibroblast-like cells passing numerous intercellular contacts.
11. Similar biomechanical properties.

The functional significance of the periodontal ligament being fetal-like relates to the fact that the structural, ultrastructural and biochemical features of the tissue do not depend primarily upon mechanical demands. Indeed, the high rates of turnover may have as great a role in determining the characteristics of the periodontal ligament.

The fetal-like characteristics of the periodontal ligament also may aid our understanding of inflammatory periodontal disease. First, it is well known that processes involved in wound healing in fetal connective tissues differ markedly from those in adult tissues. Consequently, our understanding of repair/periodontal reattachment may benefit from an appreciation of the mode of repair of fetal wounds. Second, it has been proposed that periodontal defects produced by inflammatory periodontal disease may be corrected by grafting of connective tissues. At present, adult-type connective tissues have been tried with varying success. Perhaps grafting of fetal-like connective tissues may be more appropriate.

The tooth support mechanism

The tooth support mechanism describes the manner whereby the periodontal ligament resists the axially directed intrusive loads which occur during biting.

It is still frequently stated that the periodontal ligament behaves as a suspensory ligament during masticatory loading. Accordingly, loads on the tissue are dissipated to the alveolar bone primarily through the oblique principal fibres of the ligament which, being placed in tension, are analogous to the guy-ropes of a tent. On release of the load, there is elastic recoil of the tissue which thus enables the tooth to recover its resting position. The essentially elastic responses of the periodontal ligament during both loading and recovery thus imply that the tissue obeys Hooke's Law. However, tooth mobility studies, surgical studies, and morphological and biochemical studies have provided evidence against the notion that the periodontal ligament is a suspensory ligament.

Physiological tooth mobility studies provide information concerning the basic biomechanical properties of the periodontal ligament. They rely upon analysis of the patterns of mobility when loading teeth whose periodontal tissues have not been altered experimentally. These studies show that the ligament: (a) does not obey Hooke's law during loading and recovery, (b) shows the property of hysteresis, and (c) exhibits responses whose time dependency suggests that the tissue has visco-elastic properties. Furthermore, the patterns of loading are not dependent on the direction of the load relative to the orientation of the principal fibres in the periodontal ligament and, for loads of similar magnitude, the amount of displacement for an axially directed intrusive load is greater than for an extrusive load.

418

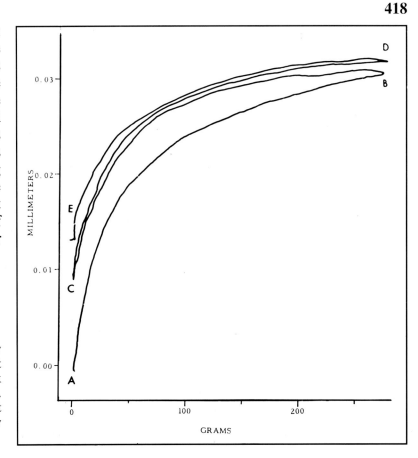

418 Axial load/mobility curve for a human maxillary incisor to show hysteresis. A, initial position of tooth; **B**, position at peak force on the first application of load; **C**, return point on removal of load; **D**, position at peak force on second application; **E**, return point after second removal of load. Note the lack of a straight-line relationship between load and displacement (expected for elastic responses) and also that successive loads and recovery cycles pass along different paths (i.e. there are hysteresis loops).

419 The visco-elastic responses of a tooth observed with an axially directed intrusive load. This is a pen recorder trace of tooth position which shows the effect of applying a load and then sustaining the load for a period of 5 minutes. Note the time dependency of the response, which is biphasic. The first phase is an elastic phase, the more gradual second phase is indicative of the property of creep (i.e. a viscous phase). The recovery responses are also biphasic and suggestive of visco-elasticity.

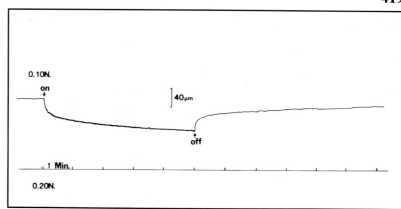

Experimental tooth mobility studies rely upon investigating the effects on the patterns of mobility obtained following alterations to a specific component of the periodontal ligament. Indeed, experiments with lathyrogens (drugs which specifically inhibit the formation of collagen crosslinks and disrupt the fibrous network of the periodontal ligament), with vasoactive drugs, and following surgical disruption of the periodontal ligament indicate that both the periodontal collagen fibres and the periodontal vasculature are involved in tooth support.

420 The effects of lathyrogens on tooth support. This experiment assesses the effects of the drug on axially directed extrusive loads. Note the significant increase in mobility for the tooth in the lathyritic animal, which suggests a role for the periodontal collagen in tooth support. However, the precise mechanism of action remains elusive since the patterns of mobility are the same for normal and lathyritic animals.

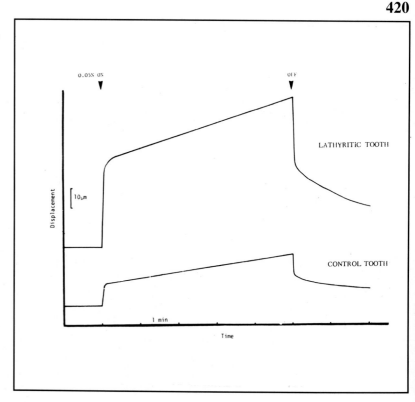

Experiments have been conducted where the apical half of the periodontal ligament was removed and the tooth loaded to assess the effects on its mobility. No effects were observed and consequently it was argued that the ligament did not behave as a compressive structure since it was presumed that only the tissue around the root apex could behave in this manner. Subsequent experiments were performed to assess the role of tension in the more cervically situated principal fibres of the ligament. However, these have shown that the periodontal ligament around the alveolar crest could also be removed without major changes in tooth mobility. These experiments therefore do not provide definitive evidence for or against tension or compression in the periodontal ligament but do suggest that, even where there is marked trauma to a region of the ligament, the remaining tissue can still perform a supporting function in the short term.

Some morphological evidence suggesting that the periodontal collagen is placed in tension during masticatory loading comes from study of the Sharpey's fibre attachments and from the collagen crimps. As mentioned previously (see **380**), the Sharpey's fibres appear as mineralised stubs projecting into the periodontal ligament from the wall of the alveolus. The occurrence of mineralisation at approximately right angles to the long axes of the fibres has been adduced as evidence that the fibres are under tension. However, even if this were indeed the case, the distribution of Sharpey's fibres along the alveolus indicates that they are limited mainly to the region of the alveolar crest (see **381**). The crimping of collagen in the periodontal ligament was described on page 169. Evidence

from connective tissues elsewhere in the body (particularly from tendons) suggests that the crimps are involved in the initial stages of loading, allowing some degree of movement before the tissue is placed under tension.

Morphological and biochemical comparisons between the periodontal ligament and other connective tissues known to be under tension or compression have been undertaken to throw some light on the role of the periodontal ligament in tooth support. This has been undertaken on the assumption that the structure of a connective tissue is dictated by the mechanical demands placed upon it. The table below shows the results of such a comparison.

Table 16: Relationship between the ultrastructural features of the periodontal ligament and mechanical properties.

Features of the periodontal ligament suggesting tension	Features of the periodontal ligament suggesting compression
Sharpey's fibre structure (**380**)	Small collagen fibril diameters (**365**)
The flattened, disc shape of the fibroblasts	Unimodal collagen size/frequency distribution (**366**)
Dermatan sulphate-rich composition of ground substance (see page 172)	Distribution of Sharpey's fibres to socket (**381**)
	Smooth surface of fibroblast membrane
	Large amounts of ground substance (see page 172)

Table 16 shows that whereas some features of the periodontal ligament suggest a tensional mode of activity, many of the features indicate a compressive mode. Indeed, experiments involving relatively long-term changes in the mechanical demands placed upon the tissue (e.g. pinning a tooth to completely prevent tooth movements) produced no major changes in the structure of the periodontal ligament and provided evidence for the view that the ligament is not as affected by the mechanical demands placed upon it as some other tissues elsewhere in the body.

Recent biochemical analysis of the proteoglycans within the periodontal ligament and under different loading regimes show that the degree of aggregation/disaggregation of the ground substance may have a role in tooth support.

There is thus evidence that the collagen fibres, vasculature and ground substance of the periodontal ligament are all involved in tooth support. Consequently, the mechanism of tooth support should not be regarded as a property of a single component of the periodontal ligament, but appears to be a function of the tissue as a whole.

Comparative aspects of tooth attachment

The attachment of teeth to the jaws may be accomplished either by means of a fibrous ligament or by direct union (ankylosis) of the tooth to bone.

A variety of fibrous tooth attachments have been described, and these may be conveniently classified according to whether or not the teeth are socketed:

1. Teeth without sockets
   (a) Continuous fibrous attachment
   (b) Local fibrous attachment
   (c) Hinged attachment.
2. Teeth with sockets
   (a) Thecodont gomphosis
   (b) Gomphosis.

421

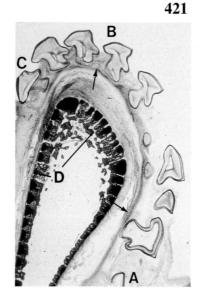

421 Ground, transverse section through the jaw of a thornback ray (*Raia clavata*) demonstrating the continuous fibrous attachment of the teeth typical of elasmobranch fish. The bases of the teeth are attached to a sheet of connective tissue (*arrowed*) which overlies the jaw cartilages (**D**). The teeth are continuously replaced, being generated from a persistent dental lamina low down on the inner aspect of the jaw (immediately below **A**). From this site they migrate around the jaw to become functional at or about position **B**. The teeth are shed at the front of the jaw (**C**). (× 16)

422

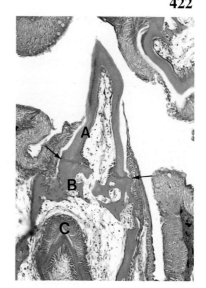

422 Decalcified, longitudinal section through the tooth of a piranha (*Serrasalmus rhombeus*) showing a local fibrous attachment. In this bony fish, each tooth is connected separately to the bone of the jaws by a narrow ring of fibrous tissue (*arrowed*) which here stains a darker green than either the dentine (**A**) or bone (**B**). The tip of a replacing tooth (**C**) is seen below the functional tooth. (Masson's trichrome; × 80)

423

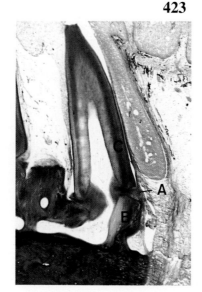

423 Decalcified, longitudinal section through a tooth in an eel (*Anguilla anguilla*). In this bony fish, instead of the fibrous attachment (**A**) of the tooth being inserted directly into the bone of the jaw, there is an intervening cell-free pedicle (**B**) composed of calcified collagen whose matrix is secreted by the odontoblasts (**C**, dentine; **D**, bone of jaw). (Berenbaum's Sudan black; × 80)

The degree of movement during feeding associated with fibrous attachments of teeth will depend, in part, on the length, distribution and elasticity of the fibres. In the above examples, there is relatively little movement of the teeth. However, in a number of carnivorous fishes, modification of the fibrous attachment may produce a hinged attachment which allows a greater range of movement.

424 **425**

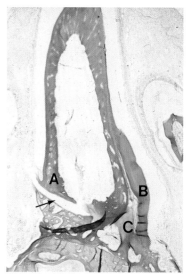 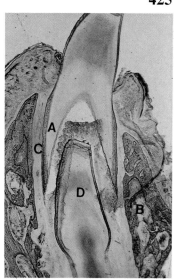

425 Section of a caiman (*Caiman sclerops*) lower jaw showing a thecodont attachment. The Crocodilia are unique amongst the non-mammalian vertebrates in having roots (**A**) situated in deep sockets (**B**) to which they are attached by a periodontal ligament (**C**). The root surfaces of the teeth are covered with a layer of cementum. The socket in this thecodont condition differs from the gomphosis associated with mammalian teeth in that it is permanent and does not undergo significant remodelling, successive replacing teeth (**D**) occupying the same socket. (Ground longitudinal section; × 5)

424 Decalcified, longitudinal section of a hake's tooth (*Merluccius merluccius*) showing an example of a hinged attachment. Prey entering the mouth will depress and pass over the hinged teeth which will subsequently spring upright should the prey try to leave the mouth to make its escape. The base of the outer part of the tooth (**A**) lies above the base of the inner part. The fibrous attachment between the base of the outer surface of the tooth and the jaw prevents lateral displacement. As shown in this section, there is a small, midline region (*arrowed*) which lacks such a fibrous attachment. The attachment between the base of the inner surface of the tooth and the jaw is in two parts: an outer, stiffened portion (**B**), apparently of unmineralised dentine which is elastic, and an inner fibrous portion (**C**). When the tooth is pushed back, the outer band buckles, its subsequent recoil returning the tooth to the upright position when the load is removed. (Picro-indigo-carmine; × 32)

426

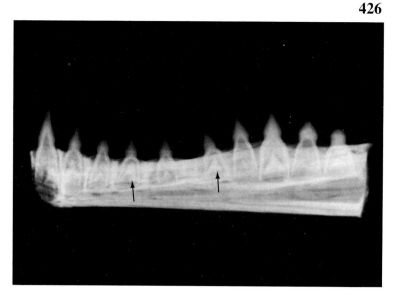

Bony attachment or ankylosis occurs commonly throughout the non-mammalian vertebrates.

426 Radiograph of a crocodile (*Crocodilus niloticus*). Lower jaw showing a thecodont gomphosis. Arrows indicate successional teeth.

427 **428**

427 Decalcified, longitudinal section of a trout tooth (*Salmo gairdneri*) illustrating attachment by ankylosis. Note the attachment of dentine (**A**) directly to the bone of the jaw (**B**), without the intervention of fibrous tissue. (Masson's trichrome; × 32)

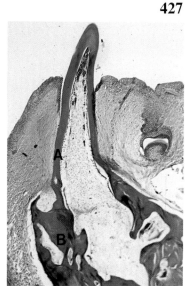

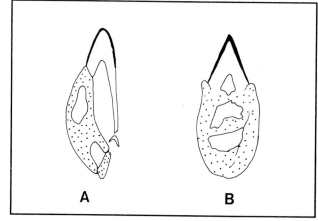

428 In reptiles, two basic types of ankylosis may be recognised. Pleurodont ankylosis (**A**) refers to the attachment of a tooth to the inner margin of the bone of the jaw. Acrodont ankylosis (**B**) refers to an attachment to the crest of the bone. Acrodont teeth are not replaced; pleurodont teeth are replaced.

Alveolar bone

That part of the maxilla or mandible which supports and protects the teeth is known as alveolar bone. An arbitrary boundary at the level of the root apices of the teeth separates the alveolar processes from the body of the mandible or the maxilla. Among its other functions, alveolar bone gives attachment to muscles, provides a framework for bone marrow, and acts as a reservoir for ions (especially calcium). Alveolar bone is dependent on the presence of teeth for its development and maintenance. Where teeth are congenitally absent (as in anodontia), alveolar bone is poorly developed. Following tooth extraction, it atrophies.

Bone is a mineralised connective tissue. About 60% of its wet weight is inorganic material, about 25% organic material and about 15% water. By volume, about 36% is inorganic, 36% is organic and 28% is water. The mineral phase is hydroxyapatite, in the form of needle-like crystallites or thin plates about 8nm thick and of variable length. About 90% of the organic material is present as Type I collagen. In addition, there are small amounts of other proteins (e.g. osteocalcin, osteonectin, osteopontin and proteoglycans) whose biological functions remain largely unknown.

Apart from its obvious strength, one of the most important biological properties of bone is its 'plasticity', allowing it to remodel according to the functional demands placed upon it. That cementum is less readily resorbed than bone under similar continuous pressures allows for orthodontic tooth movement.

The gross morphology and radiographic appearance of the alveolus and tooth sockets are described on pages 21–23 and 66.

429 Ground, longitudinal section of a mandibular tooth *in situ*. Macroscopically, bone can be classified as compact (cortical) or spongy (cancellous). As the names suggest, compact bone forms a dense, solid mass, while in spongy bone there is a lattice arrangement of the individual bony trabeculae which surround soft tissue. Internally, a thin layer of compact bone (**A**) lines the socket, and gives attachment to some of the principal fibres of the periodontal ligament. Externally, on the vestibular and lingual–palatal surfaces, are thicker layers of compact bone (**B**), forming the external and internal alveolar plates. Between these plates of compact bone are variable amounts of spongy bone, depending on site (see page 23). The arbitrary boundary between the alveolar bone and the body of the jaw is indicated by the broken line (**C**). (× 2)

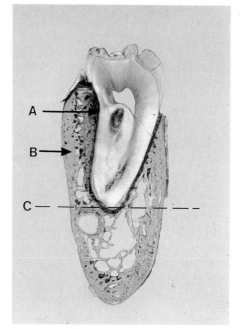

429

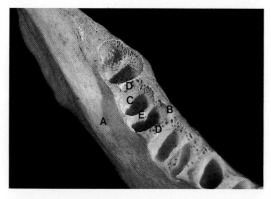

430

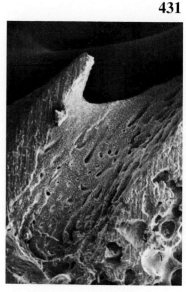

431

430 The morphology of the sockets in the molar region of the mandible. This shows the outer (**A**) and inner (**B**) alveolar plates, the cribriform plate (**C**) lining the sockets and the interdental (**D**) and interradicular (**E**) septa. The compact layer of bone lining the tooth socket has been given various names. It has been referred to as the cribriform plate to describe the sieve-like appearance (as illustrated here) produced by the numerous vascular canals (Volkmann's canals) passing from the alveolar bone into the periodontal ligament. It has also been called bundle bone because numerous bundles of Sharpey's fibres pass into it from the periodontal ligament. In clinical radiographs, the bone lining the alveolus commonly appears as a dense white line and is given the name lamina dura, which is often used synonymously with cribriform plate, although, paradoxically, they are almost etymological opposites. The X-ray appearance derives from the beam passing tangentially through the socket wall. The dense appearance derives from the quantity of bone the beam passes through and not from any greater degree of mineralisation, compared with adjacent bone. Superimposition also obscures the Volkmann's canals.

431 A fractured tooth socket showing the cribriform nature of the cribriform plate. (SEM; × 5)

190

432 Microradiograph of the lamina dura/cribriform plate. High resolution radiography of ground sections of the socket reveals the presence of the vascular canals in the cribriform plate (*arrowed*). The cribriform plate varies in thickness between 0.1 and 0.5mm. The external alveolar plate is usually about 1.5–3mm thick over posterior teeth but is highly variable around anterior teeth, depending on tooth position and inclination. Spongy bone separates the internal and external cortical plates. (× 7)

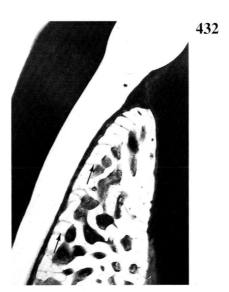

432

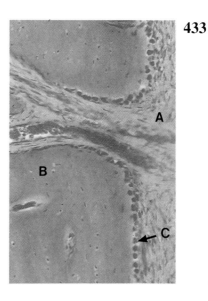

433

433 A Volkmann's canal. A capillary is seen entering the periodontal ligament (**A**) from the supporting bone (**B**). It may be accompanied by nerve fibres. **C**, osteoblast layer. (Demineralised section, H & E; × 230)

The basic unit of bone is the lamella, which is a layer about 5μm thick. Lamellae are demarcated from each other by bands of interlamellar cement approximately 0.1μm thick. The collagen fibres within each lamella are parallel with each other, but have a different orientation to those in the adjacent lamella.

434

434 Compact bone. In compact bone the lamellae are arranged in two major patterns. At periosteal or endosteal surfaces, they are arranged in layers surrounding the bony surface as circumferential lamellae. Alternatively, as illustrated here, they may be arranged as small concentric layers around a central vascular canal (**A**). The vascular (Haversian) canal, together with concentric lamellae (which may comprise between 4–20 layers) is known as an Haversian system or osteon. A cement line of mineralised matrix (about 1μm thick) delineates the Haversian system (*arrowed*). The longitudinally running Haversian canals are connected by transversely running Volkmann's canals. As a result of remodelling, fragments of previous Haversian systems may be present and are known as interstitial lamellae (**B**). (Ground transverse section; × 100)

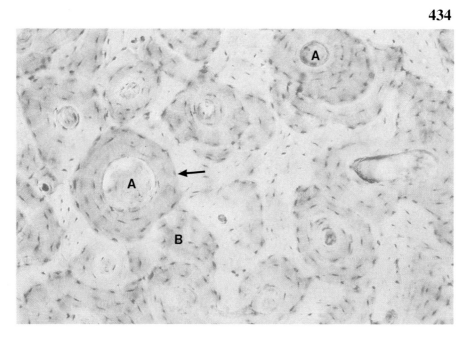

In spongy bone, the lamellae are apposed to each other to form trabeculae about 50μm thick. The trabeculae are not arranged randomly but aligned along lines of stress so as best to withstand the forces applied to the bone while adding minimally to its mass.

Cell types in bone

Five cell types can be distinguished in bone. The bone-forming cells are termed osteoblasts and are found on the surface. They become trapped in their own secretion and subsequently become incorporated into the matrix as osteocytes. Large multinucleated cells are responsible for resorbing bone and are called osteoclasts. In addition to these three principal cell types, osteoprogenitor and bone-lining cells can be identified. Osteoprogenitor cells are mesenchymal, fibroblast-like cells, regarded as forming a stem cell population to generate osteoblasts. They are situated in the vicinity of the blood vessels of the periodontal ligament. When alveolar bone is not being deposited or resorbed (which is probably the case throughout a considerable part of adult life), its quiescent surface is lined by relatively undifferentiated, flattened cells termed bone-lining cells. They may represent inactive osteoblasts, but little is known about them. By providing a lining to the bone surface, they may have important functions, perhaps related to ion exchange and the process of osteoblasis and osteoclasis.

435

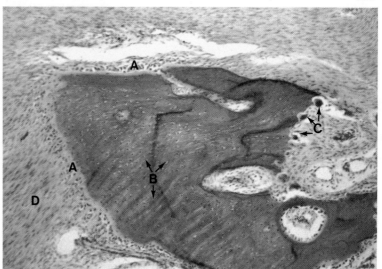

435 Three main cell types in alveolar bone. In this section, bone deposition (osteoblasis) and bone resorption (osteoclasis) are occurring. At the left surface of the bone, osteoblasts (**A**) form a layer of cuboidal cells which are separated from the darker mineralised matrix by a paler zone of unmineralised matrix (the osteoid). Mineralisation of the newly synthesised osteoid takes place after a lag phase of about 5 days. Within the bone, numerous osteocytes (**B**) lying in spaces termed lacunae can be seen. Resorption is occurring on the right surface of the bone as evidenced by large multinucleated cells, the osteoclasts (**C**), lying in concavities on the surface termed Howship's lacunae. The distribution of the cells illustrates a fundamental property of the growth and remodelling of bone; it is a surface phenomenon. Unlike cartilage, which grows interstitially, bone can only be deposited or resorbed at surfaces. However, these surfaces are widespread and incorporate the periosteal and endosteal surfaces, the lining of the Haversian canals and the surfaces of bony trabeculae in spongy bone. **D**, periodontal ligament. (Decalcified section; H & E; × 75)

436

436 A layer of osteoblasts (*arrowed*) **lining the alveolar bone.** Osteoblasts are specialised fibroblast-like cells of mesenchymal origin. A layer of these cells is only prominent where there is active bone formation. Each osteoblast appears cuboidal and exhibits a basophilic cytoplasm which is related to the extensive endoplasmic reticulum within the cell. The prominent, round nucleus tends to lie towards the basal end of the cell. A pale, juxtanuclear area indicates the site of the Golgi material. Note the Sharpey's fibres passing into the bone and the paler staining osteoid layer. Alkaline phosphatase is a useful marker to help identify cells at bony surfaces. (Decalcified, longitudinal section of periodontal ligament; H & E; × 400)

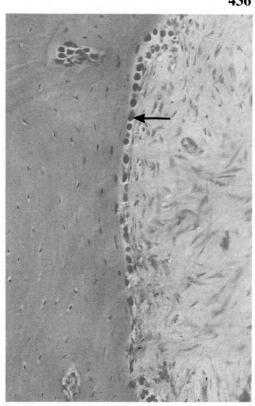

437 Ultrastructural features of the osteoblast. Like the periodontal fibroblasts, active osteoblasts contain an extensive rough endoplasmic reticulum and numerous mitochondria and vesicles. However, their Golgi material appears more localised and extensive. Microfilaments are prominent beneath the cell membrane at the secreting surface. The cells contact one another by means of desmosomes and gap junctions. These provide for cell-to-cell communication. The cell surface adjacent to the demineralised bone (**A**) has many fine cytoplasmic processes, some of which contact underlying osteocytes by gap junctions (TEM; × 6,000)

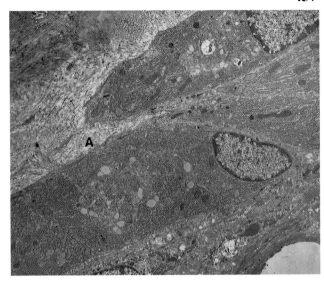

438 Osteocytes. In ground sections of bone, the osteocytes themselves are lost, but the lacunae they occupy appear black in routine transmitted light sections. The lacunae are regularly distributed, and numerous fine canals called canaliculi radiate from them in all directions. The canaliculi allow the diffusion of substances through the bone. Cell processes from the osteocytes run in the canaliculi. Osteocytes thus differ from cementocytes in that they are more regularly distributed and their canaliculi show no preferential orientation. (Ground section; × 260)

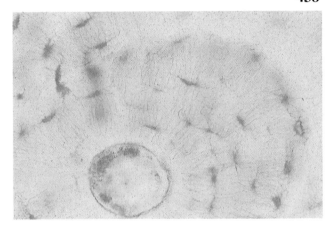

439 Ultrastructural appearance of an osteocyte. The cell has a nucleus and a thin ring of cytoplasm containing few organelles and showing little sign of cellular activity. Slender processes from the osteocyte extend into narrow canals (canaliculi, *arrowed*) in the matrix. The processes of one cell are joined to those of another by gap junctions, which presumably allow cell-to-cell communication and coordination of activity. Osteocytes are thought to play a role in calcium homeostasis. There is also evidence to suggest that they are responsive to mechanical forces, and it has been hypothesised that these cells mediate mechanically adaptive bone remodelling by acting as strain receptors. (TEM; × 5,300)

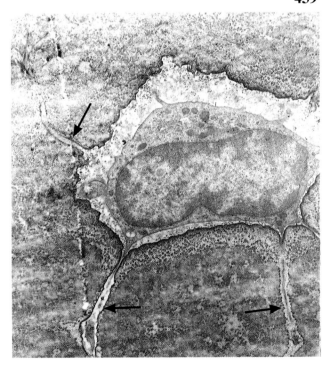

440 Resorbing alveolar bone and the osteo-clast. The surface of the alveolar bone shows resorption concavities (Howship's lacunae), in which lie the osteoclasts (*arrowed*). Osteoclasts show considerable variation in size and shape, ranging from smaller mononuclear cells to large multinucleated cells over 100μm in diameter. The part of the cell which lies adjacent to bone often has a foamy, striated appearance (the so-called brush border). The presence of tartrate-resistant acid phosphatase is used as a marker to help identify these cells. Osteoclasts are thought to arise as the result of fusion of blood cells of the myelo–monocyte cell line, the precursors being disseminated via the vascular system. (Decalcified, longitudinal section of the periodontal ligament; H & E; × 250)

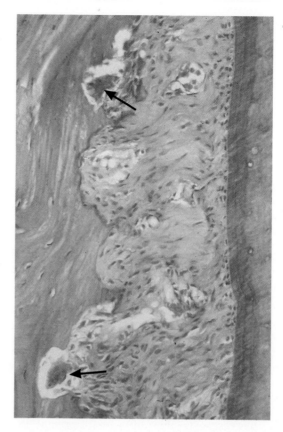

440

441 Ultrastructural features of a multinucleated osteoclast. The brush border (**A**) is comprised of many tightly packed microvilli adjacent to the bone surface. These may be coated with fine, bristle-like structures. At the circumference of the brush border (**B**), the plasma membrane tends to become smooth and the cytoplasm beneath it contains numerous microfilaments. It has been suggested that this modified annular zone may serve to limit the diffusion of hydrolytic enzymes, thereby creating an isolated microenvironment in which resorption can take place. The osteoclast contains many mitochondria distributed throughout the cytoplasm (except for the region immediately beneath the brush border). The rough endoplasmic reticulum is less conspicuous than in osteoblasts, but Golgi material (*arrowed*) is prominent (especially in juxtanuclear areas). Most of the remaining cytoplasm contains large numbers of vesicles of different sizes and types, some containing acid phosphatase. Tissue culture studies indicate osteoclasts are highly motile. Resorption appears to occur in two stages. Initially, the mineral phase is removed, and later the organic matrix. Intracellular collagen profiles have not been observed in normal osteoclasts. (Decalcified; TEM; × 4,400)

441

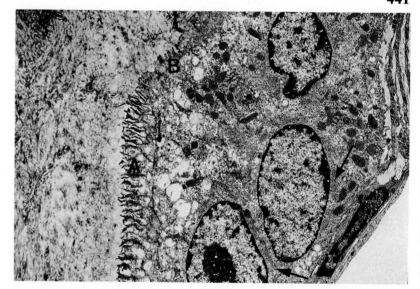

Scanning electron microscope appearances of bone surfaces

442 An alveolar bone surface on which bone formation is occuring is characterised by the presence of numerous small, calcific nodules within and around collagen fibrils. A standard procedure for visualising the mineralising front is shown in **442a** and entails removing all the exposed organic material in the osteoid layer (by means of substances such as sodium hypochlorite), producing an anorganic preparation. The presence of Sharpey's fibres (small, dark, circular areas) bordering the lacunae account for the irregularity of lacunae. **442b** represents a forming alveolar bone surface only partially rendered anorganic to show the smallest calcific nodules (lower and left part of the field) being deposited in relation to the collagen fibrils (upper and right part of the field). (**442a**, anorganic specimen; SEM; × 550; **442b**, SEM; × 650)

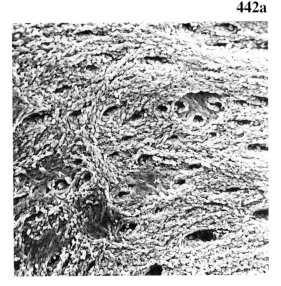

442a

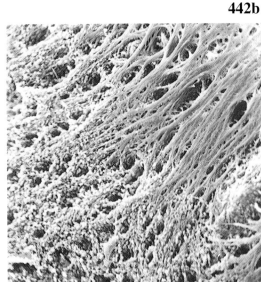

442b

443 An alveolar bone surface on which bone resorption is occuring is characterised by the presence of resorption lacunae. **443a** represents the periostial aspect and hence there are no Sharpey's fibres. In addition to pit-like resorption lacunae (**A**), bone may also exhibit longer 'snail track' resorption lacunae (**B**). In **443b**, the appearance of an area of bone resorption (**A**) in bundle bone is contrasted with the appearance of an adjacent area of bone formation (**B**). Compared with **443a**, note the presence of Sharpey's fibres in the resorbing areas (*arrowed*). (anorganic preparation; SEM; **443a**, × 300; **443b**, × 650)

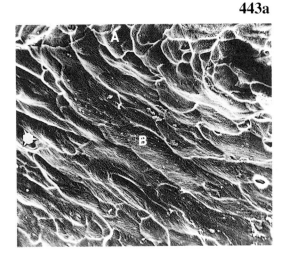

443a

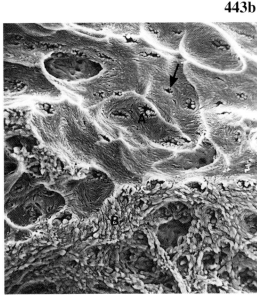

443b

444 A resting alveolar bone surface. When neither bone deposition nor resorption are occuring, the surface of the bone is described as a resting surface. The resting surface (lower left part of field) is characterised by projections marking the sites of extrinsic fibres separated by smooth areas, which contrasts with the granular appearance of the mineral of the intrinsic fibres of the adjacent forming surface (upper right part of field, where the extrinsic fibre positions are seen as holes. (anorganic preparation; SEM; × 500)

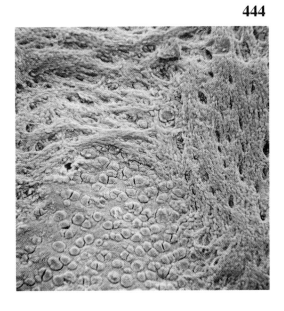

444

195

Radiographic techniques can readily demonstrate that bone is continually turning over, newly-forming bone appearing less dense (and therefore more radiolucent) than mature bone.

445 Alveolar bone (A) near the crest region. B, periodontal space; **C**, root. (Ground, longitudinal section; × 16)

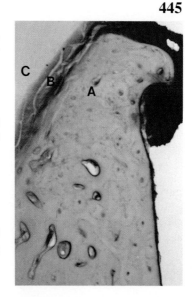

446 Microradiograph of section shown in 445. The varying densities of alveolar bone indicate that it is turning over. (× 16)

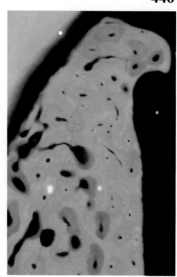

Some of the complexities concerning the control of bone remodelling are indicated in Table 17, which lists factors affecting bone resorption and formation.

Table 17:   Factors affecting bone resorption (R) and formation (F).

Systemic hormones	PTH	R+	F +/ −
	$1,25(OH)_2D_3$	R+	F +/ −
	Calcitonin	R−	? F +
	Sex steroids	R−	F +/ −
	Glucocorticoids	R+	F +/ −
	Growth hormone		F +
	Thyroid hormone	R+	F +/ −
Local factors:	Prostaglandins	R+/ −	F +
	Interleukin-1	R+	F +
	Tumour necrosis factors α, β	R+	? F +
	Interferon-Y	R−	F −
	Insulin-like growth factors		F +
	Transforming growth factor α	R+	F ?
	Epidermal growth factor	R+	F ?
	Transforming growth factor β	R+/ −	F +
	Bone morphogenic proteins	R?	F +
	Platelet-derived growth factor	R+	? F +
	Fibroblast growth factors		F +/ −
	Vasoactive intestinal peptide	R+	
	PTH-related peptide	R+	F +/ −
	Calcitonin gene-related peptide	R−	
Miscellaneous agents:	Immobilisation, weightlessness	R+	F −
	Stress/exercise	R+/ −	F +
	Protons	R+	? F −
	Calcium	R−	F +
	Phosphate	R+	? F +
	Flouride	R−	F +
	Bisphosphonates	R−	
	Alcohol, tobacco		F −

Because many of the receptors to substances resulting in bone resorption are located on osteoblasts (rather than osteoclasts), osteoblasts have been implicated in the control of bone resorption (in addition to their obvious role in osteogenesis). There are two processes whereby the osteoblast could promote osteoclasis. By the local release of substances such as cytokines, osteoblasts could stimulate the production of osteoclasts. By releasing enzymes (e.g. metalloproteins) to degrade the unmineralised osteoid layer covering bone, osteoblasts could help expose mineralised matrix on which osteoclasts could then commence resorption (as osteoclasts are unable to resorb unmineralised matrix). Substances present within bone (e.g. growth factors) could be activated during osteoclasis and subsequently have an effect on remodelling.

Sharpey's fibres

In addition to intrinsic fibres secreted by osteoblasts, alveolar bone also contains extrinsic fibres. Extrinsic fibres, inserting into the cribriform plate as Sharpey's fibres, are derived from the principal fibres of the periodontal ligament. Most Sharpey's fibres appear in the cervical portion (alveolar crest region) of the cribriform plate.

447

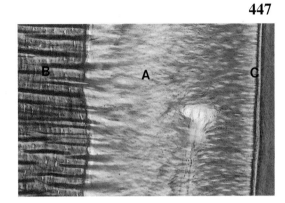

447 Tooth *in situ* showing principal fibres of periodontal ligament. Sharpey's fibres from the periodontal ligament (**A**) entering alveolar bone (**B**). Note that the Sharpey's fibres in bone are less numerous, but thicker, than those at the cementum surface (**C**). Because of the attachments of numerous bundles of collagen fibres, the cribriform plate has also been called bundle bone. Bundle bone usually comprises thin lamellae running parallel to each other and to the root surface. (Decalcified section; van Gieson; × 250)

448

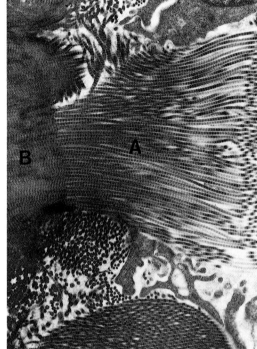

448 Insertion of a principal collagen fibre bundle (A) from the periodontal ligament as a Sharpey's fibre into alveolar bone (B). (Decalcified section; TEM; × 10,500)

449 Periodontal surface of the cribriform plate. In these preparations the organic material has been dissolved in hypochlorite. In the region shown in **449a**, the embedded fibres have remained unmineralised at their centres. Removal of the organic material results in a series of depressions. Conversely, in **449b** the inserting fibres were mineralised beyond the surface of the bone and remain as small, calcified prominences projecting into the periodontal ligament. (SEM; × 300)

449a

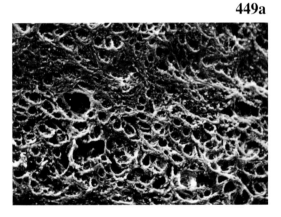

449b

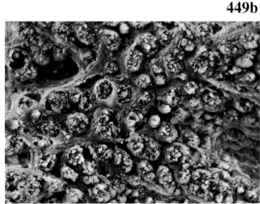

In the cervical part of the interdental septum, where the bone type is mainly compact, Sharpey's fibres entering the bone in the mesiodistal plane may pass straight through to become continuous with similar fibres from the root of the adjacent tooth. These are called transalveolar fibres. A similar pattern exists in the interradicular bone, although in this situation the fibres link roots of the same tooth. Transalveolar fibres also pass through the entire thickness of the alveolar bone in the buccal and lingual planes, intermingling with the overlying periosteum or with the lamina propria of the gingiva. However, where the alveolar bone is cancellous, no transalveolar fibres are seen. In cervical regions, transalveolar and transseptal fibres (see **489**) form a band of connective tissue which interconnects every tooth in the dental arch.

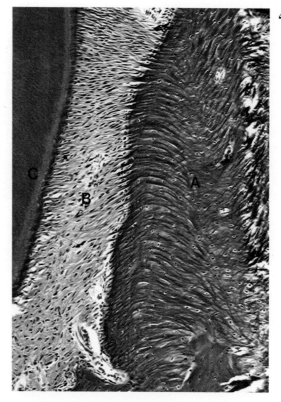

450

450 Transalveolar fibres in interdental alveolar bone. Transalveolar fibres appear to pass completely through the bone at the crest of interdental and interradicular septa. **A**, interdental bone; **B**, periodontal ligament; **C**, root. (Decalcified longitudinal section; Masson's trichrome; × 100)

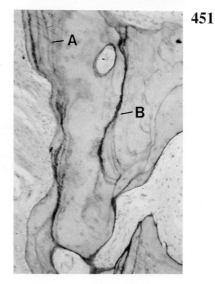

451

451 Resting and reversal lines in bone. Bone is laid down rhythmically and results in the formation of regular parallel lines (**A**) which, because they are formed in periods of relative quiescence, are termed resting lines. These lines are prominent in bundle bone during drift of the teeth. Reversal lines (**B**) mark the position where the activity has changed from deposition to resorption. They are irregular, being composed of a series of concavities which were once the sites of the resorptive Howship's lacunae (H & E; × 80)

The ability of alveolar bone to form throughout life is of obvious clinical importance. Fractures involving the face are among the most common type of fracture encountered. Following immobilisation and approximation of the affected fragments, healing will occur. Following tooth extraction, the socket will subsequently fill in with bone. Initially, immature or woven bone will be formed. This is characterised by coarser and more irregularly disposed collagen fibres, but will be subsequently remodelled to form mature, fine-fibred bone.

Oral mucosa

Whereas the skin is dry and provides the covering for the external surface of the body, the alimentary tract is lined with a moist mucosa (mucous membrane). The mucosa is specialised in each region of the tract but the basic pattern of an epithelium with an underlying connective tissue (the lamina propria) is maintained and is analogous to the epidermis and dermis of the skin. In many regions, a third layer called the submucosa is found between the lamina propria and the underlying bone or muscle.

The oral mucosa shows specialisations which allow it to fulfil several roles. It is protective mechanically against both compressive and shearing forces. It provides a barrier to micro-organisms, toxins and various antigens. It has a role in immunological defence, both humoral and cell-mediated. Minor glands within the oral mucosa provide lubrication and buffering as well as secretion of some antibodies. The mucosa is richly innervated, providing input for touch, proprioception, pain and taste.

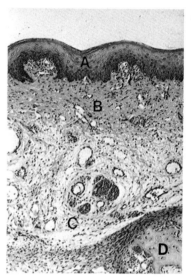

452 Basic morphology of the oral mucosa. Two distinct layers are readily recognised in the oral mucosa for all regions of the mouth. The outer layer is a stratified squamous epithelium that in some areas is keratinised (**A**). The epithelium is derived either from ectoderm or endoderm. Beneath the epithelium is the lamina propria (**B**), a connective tissue. A third layer, the submucosa (**C**), is present in some areas only and consists of a looser connective tissue containing fat deposits and glands. Larger nerves and blood vessels run in the submucosa. The boundary between the connective tissues of the lamina propria and the submucosa is often indistinct. **D**, bone. (Masson's trichrome; × 35)

The epithelium

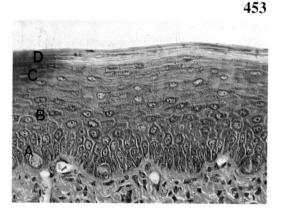

453 Layers of the keratinised oral epithelium. Several layers having distinct morphologies may be recognised in the oral epithelium. A variety of terms have been used to identify the layers, the more common being:

- Stratum germinativum (or stratum basale, **A**)
- Stratum spinosum (or prickle cell layer, **B**)
- Stratum granulosum (or granular layer, **C**)
- Stratum corneum (the keratinised or cornified layer, **D**).

Note that, unlike skin, the oral mucosa does not have a stratum lucidum (clear layer) between the stratum granulosum and stratum corneum.

The different layers of the oral epithelium represent a progressive maturation process. Cells from the most superficial layer (i.e. the stratum corneum) are continuously being shed and replaced from below. Turnover time is fastest in the region of the junctional and sulcular epithelia (about 5 days) which are located immediately adjacent to the tooth surface. This is probably about twice as fast as that seen in lining mucosa

such as the cheek. Turnover time in lining mucosa appears to be a little faster than that in masticatory mucosa.

Cells from the stratum germinativum are the progenitors. Whether all the cells are stem cells is uncertain. There are indications that germinative cells are heterogeneous and that only a minority are true stem cells, the remainder being committed 'transit' cells undergoing a limited number of amplifying divisions before succumbing to terminal differentiation. Mitosis only occurs in this layer. Daughter cells pass towards the surface and, during the process of maturation, take on the appearance characteristic of the various layers.

All epithelial cells have intermediate filaments (10nm) made of keratins. However, there are at least 27 types of keratin, coded by different genes. It is not known why there are so many keratins, but they are expressed in different cell types. Keratin 14 is present throughout the oral epithelium. Keratin 19 is present only in the stratum germinativum. Keratins 1 and 10 are found

suprabasally in keratinised epithelia, and keratins 4 and 13 in non-keratinised epithelia. When the cells leave the stratum germinativum, they switch on the synthesis of an entirely new set of keratins. The old set probably remains but is soon swamped by the massive accumulation of the new set, which may come to represent about 40% of total cell protein. (Masson's trichrome; × 140)

454 The stratum germinativum. This single layer adjacent to the lamina propria consists of cuboidal cells which, being progenitor cells, give rise to the cells in the remaining epithelial layers above. The cells of the stratum germinativum are the least differentiated within the oral epithelium and contain the usual variety of organelles, including a nucleolus, mitochondria, ribosomes, endoplasmic reticulum, Golgi material, and tonofilaments and desmosomes (characteristic features of epithelial cells). The stem cells within the stratum germinativum are thought to lie in the epithelial ridges which project into the lamina propria. Maturing cells are believed to produce growth inhibitors which restrict further cell division by negative feedback. The precise mechanism of inhibitor release is not known but, as the mitotic rate shows diurnal variation, systemic factors may be implicated. There is also evidence for a role for polypeptide growth factors (e.g. epidermal growth factor, trans-forming growth factor α) in promoting prolif-eration and possibly differentiation.

It is not known what triggers differentiation. It does not appear to be simply a matter of displace-ment away from the basal layer; tissue culture studies indicate that, if cells are prevented from migrating away from the basal lamina, differ-entiation still occurs. Rather, the onset of differ-entiation seems to change the adhesive properties of the cell which leads to its 'expulsion' from the stratum germinativum.

Non-keratinocytes may be found in the stratum germinativum. In this particular micro-graph, a lymphocyte (*arrowed*) is present. These are only occasionally seen in healthy mucosa but increase substantially in many diseased conditions. Other non-keratinocytes which may be found in this layer are melanocytes (see **459, 460**), Langerhans cells (see **461, 462**) and Merkel cells (see **463**). (TEM; × 2,800)

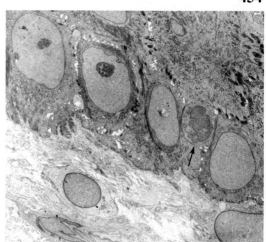

455 The stratum spinosum. Above the stratum germinativum, round or ovoid cells form a layer several cells thick. These cells show the first stages of maturation. The cells are larger and rounder than those in the stratum germin-ativum. The transition from stratum germin-ativum to stratum spinosum is characterised by the appearance of new keratin types. They con-tribute to the formation of the tonofilaments, which become thicker and more conspicuous. Involucrin (the soluble precursor protein of the cornified envelope eventually found in the cornified layer) appears in the stratum spinosum. There is a progressive decrease in synthetic activity through the layer.

In the upper part of the stratum spinosum appear small, intracellular membrane-coating granules (Odland bodies) which are rich in phospholipids. These granules are approximately 0.25μm in length and, in keratinised epithelium, consist of a series of parallel lamellae. They probably originate from the Golgi apparatus. In the more superficial layers of the stratum spinosum the granules come to lie close to the cell membrane.

Within the stratum spinosum, desmosomes increase in number and become more obvious than in the stratum germinativum. The slight shrinkage that occurs in most histological preparations causes the cells to separate at all points where desmosomes do not anchor them together. This gives the cells their spiny appearance. (TEM; × 3,000)

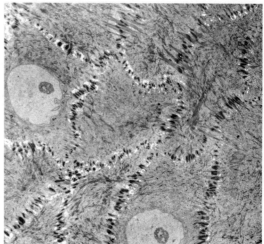

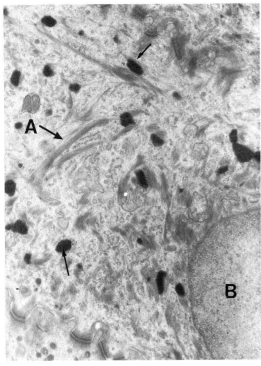

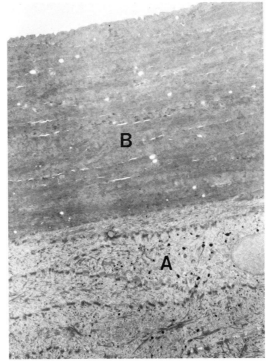

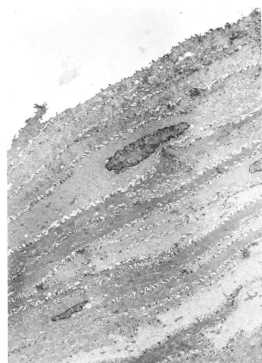

456 The stratum granulosum. The cells in this layer (see also **457**) show a further increase in maturation compared with the strata germinativum and spinosum. Many organelles are reduced or lost, such that the cytoplasm is predominantly occupied by the tonofilaments and tonofibrils (**A**). The cells are larger and flatter but most significantly they now contain large numbers of small granules called keratohyaline granules (*arrowed*). These contain the precursor to filaggrin (profilaggrin). The granules are 0.5–1.0μm in length and form the matrix in which the tonofilaments are embedded. The membrane-coating granules discharge into the extracellular space. This is associated with the development of a barrier in the epithelium which limits the movement of substances between the cells (**B**, nucleus). (TEM; × 12,000)

457 The junction between the stratum granulosum (A) and the stratum corneum (B). The final stage in the maturation of the epithelial cells is the loss of all organelles (including nuclei and keratohyaline granules). Indeed, the cells of the stratum corneum become filled entirely with closely packed tonofilaments surrounded by a matrix protein, filaggrin. This mixture is keratin.

The cells of the stratum corneum may be termed epithelial squames; it is these cells that are shed (the process of desquamation), necessitating the constant turnover of epithelial cells. Desmosomes weaken and disappear to allow for this desquamation.

The stratum corneum provides the mechanical protective function to the mucosa. It varies in thickness (up to 20 cells) and is thicker for the oral mucosa than for most areas of skin (except for the palms of the hands and the soles of the feet). In some areas such as the gingiva, the nuclei may be retained, although small and shrunken. These cells are described as parakeratinised (in contrast to the more usual orthokeratinised cells without nuclei).

In the cornified layer, involucrin becomes crosslinked (by the enzyme transglutaminase) to form a thin (10nm), highly resistant, electron-dense, cornified envelope just beneath the plasma membrane. The trigger for this is probably cell death and the influx of calcium ions. The keratin is also strongly crosslinked by disulphide bonds, contributing to the mechanical and chemical resistance of the layer. (TEM; × 2,800)

458 Surface cells of non-keratinised epithelium. The non-keratinised epithelial cells of the oral mucosa differ from the cells of keratinised epithelia in that they show less developed and dispersed tonofilaments, and lack keratohyaline granules. There are also more organelles in the surface layers than in keratinised cells, although there is still considerable reduction compared with the stratum germinativum. Above the stratum spinosum, the layers are not as clearly defined as in a keratinised epithelium. The outer layers are usually termed the stratum intermedium and the stratum superficiale. Nuclei persist within the surface layers. (TEM; × 2,000)

Non-keratinocytes

As many as 10% of the cells in the oral epithelium are non-keratinocytes, and include melanocytes, Langerhans cells, and Merkel cells. All lack the tonofilaments and desmosomes characteristic of keratinocytes (except for the Merkel cells).

Non-keratinocytes may appear as clear cells in sections stained with haematoxylin and eosin (see **472**). Some non-keratinocytes are inflammatory cells (e.g. the lymphocyte seen in **454**).

459 The melanocyte (*arrowed*). Melanocytes are pigment-producing cells located in the stratum germinativum. They are derived from the neural crest but, once located in the epithelium, are self-replicating. The melanocytes have long processes which extend in several directions and across several epithelial layers. As suggested by their name, melanocytes produce the pigment melanin. The number of melanocytes varies in different regions but the difference in the degree of pigmentation between races is due to differences in the amount of pigment produced rather than the number of cells. (Masson's Fontana; × 280)

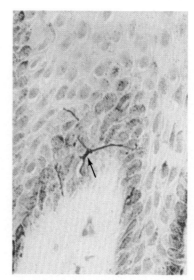

459

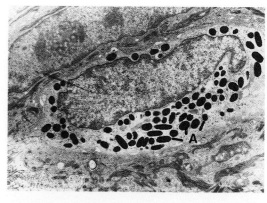

460 Ultrastructure of the melanocyte. The pigment in melanocytes is packaged in small granules termed melanosomes (**A**). The long processes of the melanocyte which extend between other cells permit the transfer of pigment to these cells. Melanin pigmentation is usually not pronounced in the buccal mucosa, tongue, hard palate or gingiva. (TEM; × 60,000)

461 Langerhans cells (*arrowed*) are dendritic cells that appear in routine sections stained with haematoxylin and eosin as clear cells in the layers above the stratum germinativum. The section shows them stained with a lead capture histochemical technique which detects ATPase on the cell membrane. They are derived from the bone marrow and act as part of the immune system as antigen-presenting cells. (× 200)

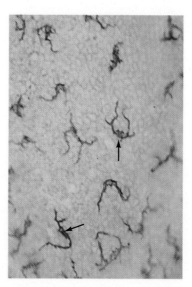

461

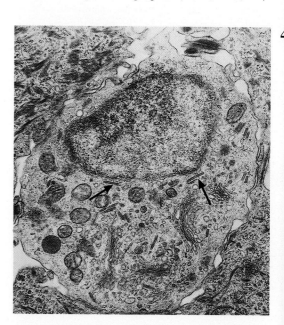

462 Ultrastructure of the Langerhans cell. The cells contain characteristic rod-shaped granules called Birbeck granules (*arrowed*). Foreign antigens penetrate the superficial layers and bind to dendritic antigen-presenting cells such as Langerhans cells, which stimulate helper T-lymphocytes, and Granstein cells, which stimulate specific suppressor T-lymphocytes. T-cells also receive a signal in the form of a cytokine (interleukin-1) from both keratinocytes and dendritic cells. The T-cells then secrete a lymphokine (interleukin-2) which causes the proliferation of T-cells. (TEM; × 15,000)

463 The Merkel cell is thought to act as a receptor and is derived from the neural crest. It is found in the stratum germinativum and is often closely apposed to nerve fibres. The nucleus of the Merkel cell is deeply invaginated and may contain a characteristic rodlet. The cytoplasm contains numerous mitochondria, abundant free ribosomes, and a collection of electron-dense granules (80–180nm in diameter) whose function is unknown. The Merkel cell contains some keratin filaments, but of the simple type (Types 8, 17 and 18), and many small vesicles in the region adjacent to the nerve terminal. Note that free nerve endings not associated with a Merkel cell are also found within the epithelium. These are nociceptors. (TEM; × 16,000)

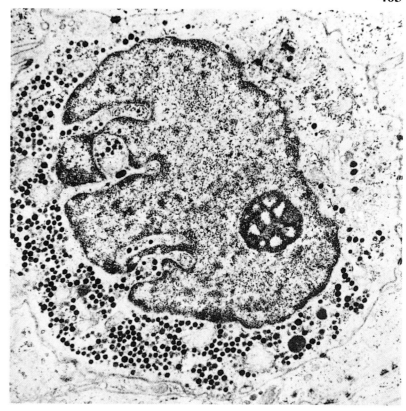

The lamina propria

The connective tissue underlying the oral epithelium can be described as having two layers: a superficial, papillary layer between the epithelial ridges, in which the collagen fibres are thin and loosely arranged; and, beneath this, a deep, reticular layer dominated by thick, parallel bundles of collagen fibres.

464 Fibroblasts of the lamina propria. The fibroblasts of the lamina propria are typical of those found in loose connective tissues. They are spindle-shaped with arms of cytoplasm supported internally by microtubules and microfilaments. They contain the full complement of synthetic organelles consistent with their role in the production and secretion of extracellular fibres and ground substance for the lamina propria. (TEM; × 11,000)

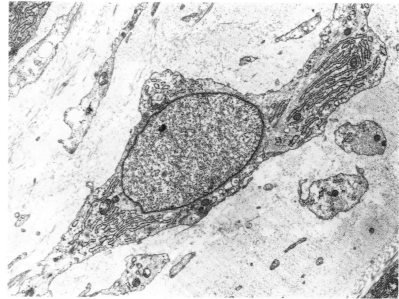

The ground substance of the lamina propria consists of an hydrated gel of glycosaminoglycans. Embedded in the ground substance are collagen fibres (mainly Type I, with a little Type III), elastic fibres and fibronectin. Fibronectin is a fibre-forming glycoprotein that is thought to form a link between intracellular and extracellular fibre systems. Small quantities of fibronectin are bound to the surface of fibroblasts. Thin oxytalan fibres (see page 171) have also been described in the lamina propria. They resemble immature elastic fibres but are not removed by elastase unless previously oxidised.

465 Macrophage in the lamina propria.
Occasional macrophages are seen in the lamina propria. In their fixed, inactive stage, they are known as histiocytes and are difficult to distinguish from fibroblasts. They have a smaller, darker nucleus than fibroblasts and contain lysosomes but little endoplasmic reticulum. As well as having a phagocytic role, macrophages act as antigen-presenting cells. Lymphocytes are also found in small numbers in healthy mucosa, but increase dramatically in inflammation. (TEM; × 10,000)

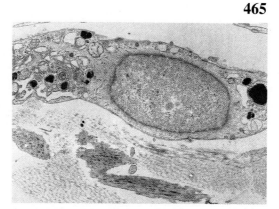

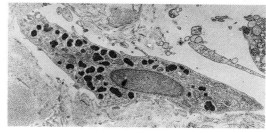

466 Mast cell in the lamina propria. Mast cells are mononuclear, spherical or elliptical in shape, and contain histamine and heparin intracellular granules. They play a role in vascular homeostasis, in inflammation, and in cell-mediated immunity. They are responsible for anaphylactic (Type I) hypersensitivity. (TEM; × 5,000)

Epithelial–connective tissue interface

467a & b The basement membrane and basal lamina of the oral mucosa. A complex arrangement links epithelial and connective tissue components of the oral mucosa. In the light microscope, a layer 1–2μm thick is seen on the lamina propria side of the junction. This is termed the basement membrane. In the electron microscope, the layer appears much thinner and is then termed the basal lamina. The thicker appearance in the light microscope is probably due to the inclusion of some of the subepithelial collagen fibres, which in this region have similar staining properties to the basal lamina.

Ultrastructurally, the basal lamina is found to consist of a complex of fibrils and ground substance. Two zones are seen. The electron-lucent lamina lucida is 20–40nm thick and lies immediately under the epithelium. The thicker (20–120nm) lamina densa is deep to this. The lamina lucida consists of a glycoprotein called laminin which cements non-fibrillar Type IV collagen in the lamina densa to the epithelial cells. The lamina densa consists of the Type IV collagen coated on each side by a glycosaminoglycan — heparan sulphate. Thick collagen fibrils attach onto the lamina densa with finer fibrils running through these to link the whole complex mechanically to the connective tissue. Fibronectin has sometimes been found in the lamina densa and may play a role in adhering fibroblasts and proteoglycans to it. The cell side of the basal lamina consists of hemidesmosomes.

The basal lamina provides mechanical adhesion between the oral epithelium and the lamina propria, acts as a molecular barrier, and plays a role in the response to tissue injury. All the products of the basal lamina appear to be synthesised by the epithelial cells. (TEM; × 34,000)

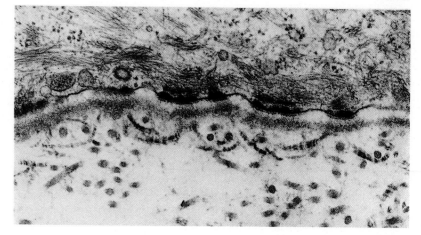

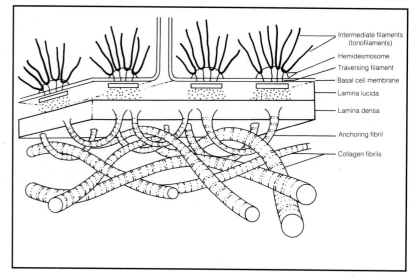

Intermediate filaments (tonofilaments)
Hemidesmosome
Traversing filament
Basal cell membrane
Lamina lucida
Lamina densa
Anchoring fibril
Collagen fibrils

The submucosa

468 Contents of the submucosa. For intestinal mucosa, a thin layer of muscle (the muscularis mucosa) separates the lamina propria from the underlying submucosa. This muscle layer is absent in oral mucosa, and the boundary between the two connective tissue layers comprising the submucosa and the lamina propria is indistinct. In many regions of the mouth, the submucosa is absent. When present, it is a loose connective tissue containing some fat cells and a variable number of minor salivary glands. The submucosa is tightly bound down to underlying bone or muscle by collagen and elastic fibres. (Masson's trichrome; × 15)

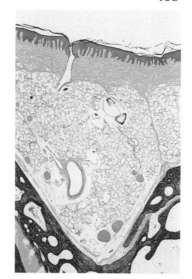

468

Regional variations in the structure of the oral mucosa

469

In different parts of the mouth, the mucosa has different roles and experiences different degrees and types of stress during mastication, speech and facial expression. As a consequence, the structure of the oral mucosa varies in terms of the thickness of the epithelium, the degree of keratinisation, the complexity of the connective tissue–epithelium interface, the composition of the lamina propria, and the presence or absence of the submucosa.

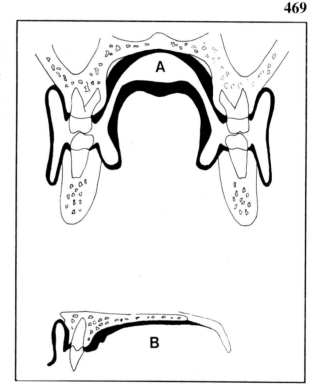

469 Regional variations in the thickness of the oral epithelium. A, coronal section through molar region; **B,** mid-sagittal section through palate. The thickness is not always related to keratinisation. In some areas, non-keratinised epithelium is thicker than keratinised epithelium.

There are three types of oral mucosa: masticatory, lining, and specialised mucosa. Masticatory mucosa is found where there is high compression and friction, and it is characterised by a keratinised epithelium and a thick lamina propria, which is usually bound down directly and tightly to underlying bone (mucoperiosteum). Lining mucosa is not subject to high levels of friction but must be mobile and distensible. It is thus non-keratinised and has a loose lamina propria. Within the lamina propria, the collagen fibres are arranged as a network to allow free movement, and the elastic fibres allow recoil to prevent the mucosa being chewed. Commonly, lining mucosa also has a submucosa. The mucosa of the gingiva and palate is masticatory; that of the lips, cheeks, alveolus, floor of the mouth, ventral surface of the tongue and soft palate is lining. Two areas of specialised mucosa occur. One is the specialised gustatory mucosa of the dorsum of the tongue and the other is where the vermilion zone forms a transition between the skin and the oral mucosa.

Regional variations of the oral mucosa are summarised in Table 18 (page 216).

The lip and cheek

470 The lip has skin (**A**) on its outer surface and oral mucosa (**B**) on its inner surface. Between these two tissues lies the vermilion zone (**C**, also known as the red or transitional zone of the lip). The lips have striated muscles (**D**) in their core which are part of the muscles of facial expression. Substantial amounts of minor salivary glands (**E**) are present in the submucosa beneath the oral mucosa. (H & E; × 2)

470

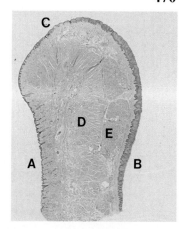

471

471 The skin on the outer surface of the lip shows all the features of skin elsewhere. A keratinised epithelium lies on a bed of connective tissue, the dermis. The border between the two in this area is not markedly folded. The connective tissue contains sweat glands; sebaceous glands and the bases of hair follicles (**A**) pass through the epithelium. The epithelium is, in fact, continuous around the bases of the follicles and is responsible for producing the keratin of which the hair is formed. Sebaceous glands (**B**) drain either into the hair follicles or occasionally directly onto the skin surface. (H & E; × 25)

472

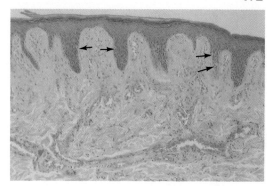

472 The vermilion zone lacks the appendages of skin. However, very occasional sebaceous glands may be found, especially at the angles of the mouth. As the vermilion zone also lacks mucous glands, it requires constant moistening with saliva by the tongue to prevent drying. The epithelium of the vermilion zone is keratinised, but thin and translucent. The connective tissue papillae of the lamina propria are relatively long and narrow, and contain capillary loops. The proximity of these vessels to the surface, combined with the translucency of the epithelium, gives the surface a red appearance and hence its name. This red appearance is a human characteristic. The junctional region between the vermilion zone and the oral mucosa is sometimes known as the intermediate zone and is parakeratinised. In infants, this becomes thickened and forms the suckling pad. Arrows indicate 'clear cells' (non-keratinocytes; see pages 202–203). (H & E; × 65)

473 The oral mucosa of the lip. This is covered by a relatively thick, non-keratinised epithelium. The lamina propria is also wide but the papillae are short and irregular. A submucosa containing many minor salivary glands is present. Strands of dense connective tissue bind the mucosa down to the underlying muscle. (H & E; × 15)

474 The buccal mucosa. The mucosa lining the cheeks is, like the labial mucosa, a lining mucosa. The epithelium is non-keratinised and the lamina propria is dense with short, irregular papillae. A submucosa is present with many minor salivary glands. Sometimes, along a line coincident with the occlusal plane, the epithelium becomes keratinised, forming a white line (the linea alba). Sebaceous glands are sometimes present and seen to become more obvious after puberty in the male and after menopause in the female, when they appear as small yellow patches. These patches are termed Fordyce spots. The role, if any, of sebaceous glands in this location is unknown, although it is important to differentiate them from pathological changes. **A**, fibres of buccinator muscle. (H & E; × 15)

473

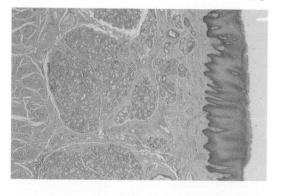

474

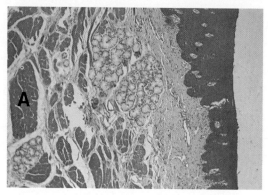

The gingiva, the gingival sulcus and the junctional epithelium

The gingiva is that portion of the oral mucosa which surrounds, and is attached to, the teeth and the alveolar bone.

475 The components of the gingiva as seen in buccolingual section. The gingiva has three recognised regions. The main component is the attached gingiva (**A**) which is directly bound down to the underlying alveolar bone and tooth. The second component, the alveolar mucosa (**B**) meets the attached gingiva at the mucogingival junction. Note that the alveolar mucosa has a submucosa (**C**) before the alveolar bone is reached. Coronal to the attached gingiva is the free gingiva (**D**) which is the narrow rim of mucosa that is not bound down to underlying hard tissue. Its junction with the attached gingiva is sometimes demarcated by a shallow groove, the free gingival groove (**E**). Its coronal limit is the gingival margin (**F**). The unattached region between the free gingiva and the tooth is the gingival sulcus (**G**). The region apical to this, where the gingiva is bound to the underlying tooth, is the junctional epithelium (**H**).

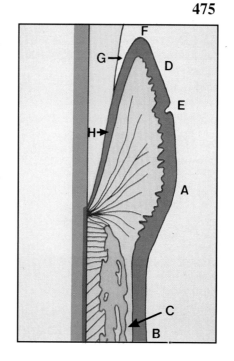

476 The gingiva *in vivo*. The alveolar mucosa (**A**) lines the lower part of the alveolus. It has a loose submucosa which allows for wide degrees of movement. The submucosa on its deep aspect is firmly attached to the underlying periosteum. The mucogingival junction (or health line, **C**) demarcates the boundary between attached gingiva (**D**) and alveolar mucosa. The difference in appearance between the alveolar mucosa and the attached gingiva is due to differences in keratinisation and translucency. The alveolar mucosa epithelium is translucent and the blood vessels lie superficially. Small blood vessels are clearly seen. The junction is scalloped, paralleling the contours of the gingival margin. The free gingival groove that separates the attached gingiva (**D**) from the free gingiva (**E**) is only apparent in about 40% of teeth. It follows the contours of the cement–enamel junction. The groove may be produced by the bundles of principal collagen fibres which run from the cervical cementum to the gingiva, or possibly the groove corresponds to a heavy epithelial ridge. When present, the free gingival groove reflects approximately the location of the bottom of the gingival sulcus. Healthy attached gingiva often shows surface stippling, which corresponds to sites of intersecting epithelial ridges. In some cases, when the free gingival groove is absent, an irregularly aligned line of stipples marks the junction between attached and free gingiva. The free gingiva is smooth. The width of both the free and attached gingivae vary regionally.

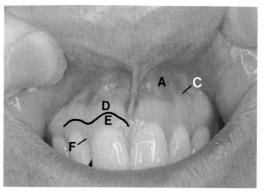

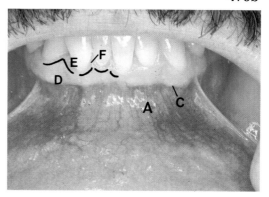

The interdental papilla (**F**) is that part of the gingiva which fills the space between the teeth. Its shape in three dimensions, and its histological appearance, depend on the shape and nature of contact between the apposed teeth.

On the palatal surface of the maxillary teeth, there is no alveolar mucosa. Here, the attached gingiva merges with the palatal mucosa, with no clearly demarcated boundary (see **8**).

477 The alveolar mucosa. A thin, non-keratinised epithelium overlies a lamina propria which shows poorly developed papillae. Underlying blood vessels are near the surface. The extensive submucosa allows free movement and houses numerous minor salivary glands. (H & E; × 15)

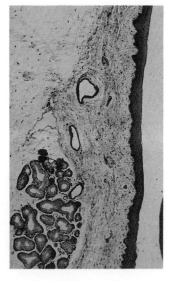

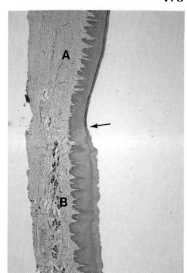

478 The mucogingival junction. The alveolar mucosa (**B**) that adjoins the attached gingiva (**A**) is thicker than elsewhere (and indeed commonly thicker than the adjacent keratinised epithelium). The demarcation between keratinised and non-keratinised epithelium is sharp (*arrowed*), and submucosal vessels and glands are limited to the alveolar component. (Papanicolaou; × 20)

479 The attached gingiva. The mucosa of the attached gingiva is a masticatory mucosa. It is keratinised, but the degree and extent vary considerably between and within individuals. Orthokeratinisation is the norm in mucosa unimpeded by inflammation. However, as much as 75% of the surface may be parakeratinised and as much as 10% non-keratinised. Papillation is variable, the papillae often being aligned in rows (especially at the margin). As little as 0.08mm may separate the tips of some papillae from the surface. The surface is stippled (*arrowed*), the stipples arising from intersecting epithelial ridges. There is no submucosa, the lamina propria being bound directly to bone (**A**) forming a mucoperiosteum. (H & E; × 75)

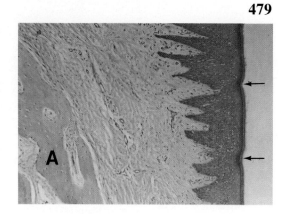

480 The gingival sulcus and junctional epithelium. The mucosa of the free gingiva is indistinguishable from that of the attached gingiva, but may be demarcated from it by the free gingival groove (or a line of stipples). The gingival margin marks the boundary with the gingival sulcus. In germ-free mammals, and in strictly healthy, mechanically-stimulated human gingiva, the sulcus is absent and the gingival margin corresponds to the apical extent of the junctional epithelium. In clinically healthy mouths, the sulcus is 0.5–2.0mm deep. Sulci deeper than 3mm are generally accepted as diseased and are described as 'periodontal pockets'. In this decalcified, buccolingual section, the enamel outline prior to decalcification has been indicated by the black line. The epithelia of the attached (**A**) and free (**B**) gingiva and the gingival sulcus (**C**) as well as the junctional epithelium (**D**) are indicated.

The gingival sulcus is bounded by the gingival margin above and the junctional epithelium below. The epithelium is non-keratinised and thinner, but otherwise similar to the epithelium of the attached gingiva. The sulcular epithelium merges with the junctional epithelium and a distinct boundary is not seen. Externally, the base of the sulcus corresponds approximately with the free gingival groove when present.

The junctional epithelium forms a firm, direct mechanical junction with the underlying tooth structure (be it enamel, cementum or dentine).

An infiltrate of inflammatory cells is present in this specimen beneath the junctional and sulcular epithelium. Even in perfectly healthy gingiva, a few inflammatory cells are present and evidence of some inflammation is common in apparently clinically normal gingiva. (H & E; × 30)

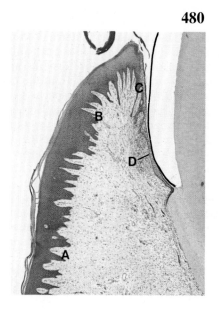

481 The junctional epithelium. The junctional (or attached) epithelium is an epithelial collar which surrounds the tooth and extends from the region of the cement–enamel junction to the bottom of the gingival sulcus (or to the gingival margin if no sulcus is present). Apically, it is 1–3 cells thick; coronally, 15–30 cells. It consists of two zones: a single cell layer of cuboidal cells (the stratum germinativum), overlying several layers of flattened cells equivalent to a stratum spinosum. There is no stratum granulosum or corneum. The junctional epithelium has a high rate of turnover and many cells are exfoliated coronally. It is derived from the reduced enamel epithelium (probably from the stratum intermedium component of that tissue). The cells of the stratum germinativum rest on a typical lamina propria, which shows many capillaries and appears to be more cellular than other parts of the gingiva. The connective tissue interface is smooth. **A**, enamel space. (Demineralised section; H & E; × 150)

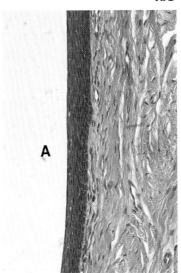

482 The attachment of the junctional epithelium to the tooth. The cells of the junctional epithelium immediately adjacent to the tooth attach themselves to the tooth in the same way as cells of the stratum germinativum elsewhere attach themselves to the lamina propria (i.e. by hemidesmosomes within the cell and a basal lamina produced by the cell beyond the cell). The combination of the hemidesmosomes and basal lamina is known as the attachment apparatus or epithelial attachment. The basal lamina in contact with the tooth is termed the internal basal lamina. On the other surface of the junctional epithelium in contact with the lamina propria is another basal lamina (the external basal lamina). The cells of the junctional epithelium are joined by desmosomes and gap junctions; tight junctions are rare. Note that the size of the intercellular space varies. Occasional neutrophils and mononuclear leukocytes migrate through this space. All cells of the junctional epithelium contain a nucleus.

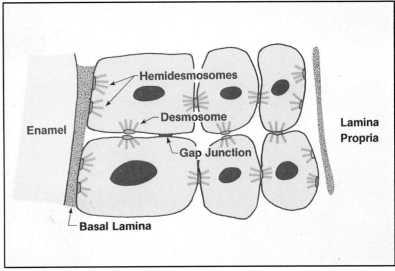

483 Segment of a junctional epithelial cell facing the enamel surface. The attachment of the cell to the enamel (**A**) is mediated by hemidesmosomes (*arrowed*) and a basal lamina (**B**). The cytoplasm of the cell contains numerous free ribosomes, cisternae of endoplasmic reticulum and a prominent Golgi apparatus (**C**), which is probably involved in the synthesis and transport of basal lamina components. Small bundles of poorly developed tonofilaments (**D**) are also present. The basal lamina is seen to contain two zones, an electron-lucent zone adjacent to the cell, and an electron-dense layer against the tooth surface. The pattern of a lamina densa and lamina lucida is not as clear as in other basal laminae, but the combined thickness is similar (100–140nm). The basement membrane, seen in light microscopy adjacent to the connective tissue, would appear much thicker due to a reticular component derived from the connective tissue (which is not discernible in an electron micrograph). The hemidesmosomes consist of thickenings of the inner leaflet of the plasma membrane (called the attachment plaque). Opposite the attachment plaque at the enamel surface, there is a peripheral dense line comparable to that seen in the lamina lucida of the basal lamina between epithelium and connective tissue. Note the absence of both membrane-coating granules and keratinohyaline granules. (Demineralised section; TEM; × 70,000)

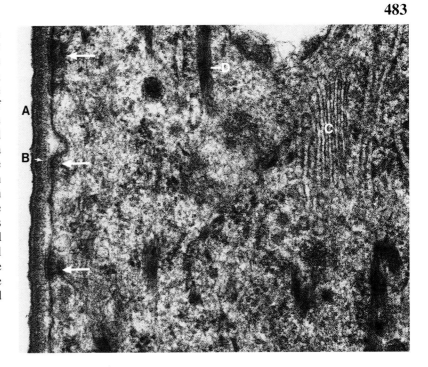

An element not visible in decalcified preparations is the dental cuticle. This cuticle is a non-mineralised structure interposed between the junctional epithelium and the underlying hard tissue. It varies in extent and is not always seen. When present, it is patchy and most prominent when filling depressions in the calcified surface. The cuticle is ultrastructurally amorphous and biochemically distinct from the basal lamina. It is probably proteinaceous and may be derived from serum.

The length of the junctional epithelium attached to the enamel surface varies according to the stage of eruption (see **646**). When the tooth first erupts into the oral cavity, most of the enamel will be covered by junctional epithelium. By the time the tooth reaches the occlusal plane, about one-quarter of the enamel surface is still covered by junctional epithelium. With time, the junctional epithelium proliferates apically and as a consequence may establish a firm union with the surface of the cementum.

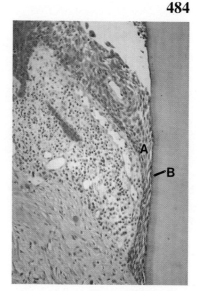

484

484 Junctional epithelium (A) on cementum (B). The apical migration of the junctional epithelium may either be a response to inflammatory disease or it may be related to a physiological process called passive eruption, which is an element of ageing. The migration results in the removal of gingival fibres and alveolar bone, and the exposure of cervical root tissue into the oral cavity. (H & E; × 60)

The dento-gingival junction seals the underlying connective tissue of the periodontium from the oral environment. The strength of the seal is thought not only to be dependent upon the attachment of the junctional epithelium to the tooth but also upon the pressure exerted by the fibres and tissue fluid of the underlying connective tissue. The weakness of the dento-gingival junction derives from its situation, the gingival crevice being a stagnation site. The epithelium provides little resistance against toxic products emanating from the consequent bacterial accumulation. The epithelium of the gingival sulcus is permeable. Indeed, tissue fluid and cells (as well as experimental substances such as dyes, carbon particles and horseradish peroxidase) pass readily through the epithelium from the connective tissue into the sulcus. The permeability of the junctional epithelium may be related to the presence of particularly wide intercellular spaces.

A fluid containing material of low molecular weight, called gingival or crevicular fluid, is said to pass continuously from the subepithelial tissue into the gingival crevice. Other oral epithelial surfaces do not show such exudation of tissue fluid. Since gingival fluid contains gamma globulins and polymorpho-nucleocytes, it has been suggested that the immunological and phagocytic properties of the fluid are important in the defence mechanism of the dento–gingival junction. It is thought by some, however, that gingival fluid only passes into the crevice as a response to pathological stimuli and is absent from perfectly healthy gingiva. Recent investigations suggest that the composition of the gingival fluid provides an indicator of the state of health of the underlying periodontium and may indeed enable the development of a diagnostic marker for the severity of inflammatory periodontal disease.

The turnover of the junctional epithelium is rapid. The epithelial cells migrate in a coronal direction, to be shed into the oral cavity via the gingival crevice. The continual breakdown and reformation of lamina densa, hemidesmosomes and desmosomes allows cells to alter their relationship as they migrate through the junctional epithelium. The rate of turnover is dependent on the demands placed upon the tissue and appears to be directly related to the degree of inflammation. Following the surgical removal of gingiva, a new junctional epithelium rapidly forms that has all the original characteristics.

The interdental gingiva

The shape and arrangement of the gingival tissues between the teeth depend on the shape of the contact between the teeth (although free and attached gingivae are always present). The interdental gingiva occupies the space between the teeth and conforms to its shape. From the buccal or lingual aspects, the gingiva has a wedge-shaped appearance. Between teeth which only contact at a small point, the interdental gingiva would appear similarly 'pointed' when viewed in a buccolingual plane. In a posterior tooth with a broad area of contact, the appearance in the buccolingual plane would be of two peaks on the buccal and lingual aspects with a curved depression between them (the interdental col). When there is no tooth contact, a rounded extension of the attached gingiva is present.

485

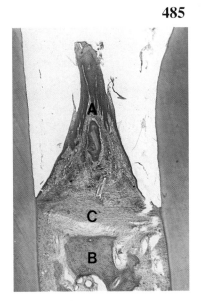

485 The interdental papilla. Viewed from buccal or lingual aspects, the papilla (**A**) appears wedge-shaped. Fibres (**C**) running from one tooth to another above the interdental bone (**B**) belong to the transseptal group of gingival fibres. (H & E; × 20)

486

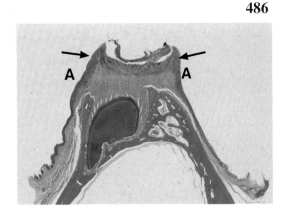

486 Buccolingual section through an interdental papilla. The buccal and lingual margins (*arrowed*) are raised above a central concavity called the interdental col (of Cohen). The col lies directly below the contact points of the teeth. The epithelium of the col is continuous with the junctional epithelium on each side of it and is similarly derived from the reduced enamel epithelium. When teeth are spaced, the col does not exist and a dome-shaped gingiva is seen which is covered by a keratinised epithelium. **A**, attached gingiva. (H & E; × 4)

487

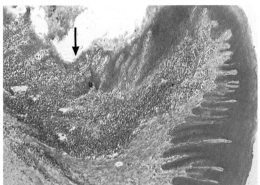

487 The interdental col (*arrowed*). The thinness of the epithelium and its similarity to junctional epithelium may be seen. In this specimen, there is a substantial infiltrate of inflammatory cells. The thinness of the epithelium and its potential as a stagnation site make it highly susceptible to inflammatory disease. (H & E; × 40)

The supra-alveolar fibre apparatus

Many of the collagen fibrils of the gingival lamina propria are grouped into bundles whose functions include the support of the free gingiva, the binding of the attached gingiva to alveolar bone, and the linkage of teeth one to another. These principal fibre groups have been given names based upon their orientation and attachments.

211

488 Arrangement of the principal collagen fibre groups of the gingiva: 488a, Buccolingual section; **488b**, Mesiodistal section; **488c**, Horizontal section; **488d**, Buccolingual section through interdental col.

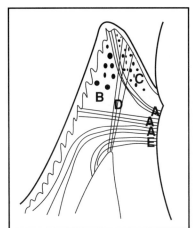

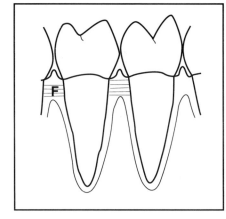

A dentogingival fibres — arise from the root surface above the alveolar crest and radiate to insert into the lamina propria of the gingiva. The most superficial fibres lie beneath the sulcular epithelium, a middle group lies almost horizontally and the deepest group courses between the gingiva and the alveolar bone.

B longitudinal fibres — extend for long distances within the free gingiva, some possibly for the whole length of the arch.

C circular fibres — encircle each tooth within the marginal and interdental gingiva coronal to the transseptal fibres (**f**). Some attach to cementum, some to alveolar bone. Some cross interdentally to join the fibre group of the adjacent tooth.

D alveologingival fibres — run from the crest of the alveolar bone and interdental septum, radiating coronally into the overlying lamina propria of the gingiva.

E dentoperiosteal fibres — only occur in vestibular and lingual gingiva. They arise from cementum and pass over the alveolar crest to insert into the periosteum.

F transseptal fibres — pass horizontally from the root of one tooth, above the alveolar crest, to be inserted into the root of the adjacent tooth.

G semicircular fibres — emanate from cementum near the cement-enamel junction, cross the free marginal gingiva, and insert into a similar position on the opposite side of the tooth.

H transgingival fibres — reinforce the circular and semicircular fibres. The fibres arise from the cervical cementum and extend into the marginal gingiva of the adjacent tooth, merging with the circular fibres.

I interdental fibres — pass through the coronal portion of the interdental gingiva in the buccolingual direction, connecting buccal and lingual papillae.

J vertical fibres — arise in alveolar mucosa or attached gingiva and pass coronally towards the marginal gingiva and interdental papilla.

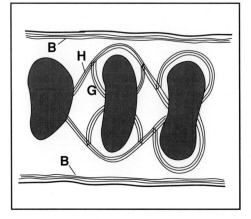

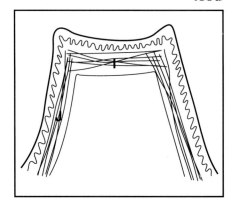

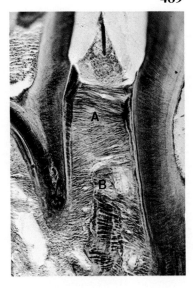

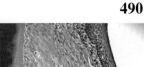

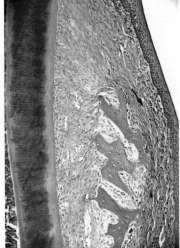

489 Transseptal fibres. In this decalcified longitudinal section, transseptal fibres (**A**) pass from the cementum of one tooth to attach into the cementum of its neighbour. **B**, alveolar crest. (Silver stain; × 85)

490 Dentogingival fibres (*arrowed*). Fibres arising from the root surface on the left pass over the alveolar crest. They insert into the lamina propria of the attached gingiva. (Masson's trichrome; × 80)

The palate

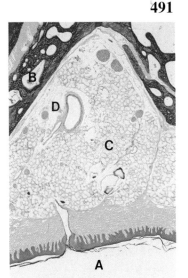

491

491 Hard palate in coronal section. A, oral cavity; **B**, palatal process of maxilla. The mucosa of the hard palate is a typical masticatory mucosa with a keratinised epithelium in all areas. In much of the central region, there is no submucosa and the lamina propria binds down directly to bone (mucoperiosteum, **492**). The same arrangement is seen in much of the attached gingiva (**479**). Where the palate joins the alveolus, however, a submucosa (**C**) is present and contains the main neurovascular bundles (**D**). There are also minor mucous glands (predominantly posteriorly) and adipose tissue (predominantly anteriorly). The nasal surface of the hard palate is lined by a respiratory mucosa of ciliated columnar epithelial cells. (Masson's trichrome; × 15)

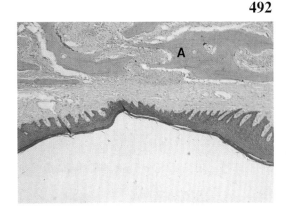

492

492 Mucosa of the hard palate near the mid-line. The heavily keratinised epithelium forms deep epithelial papillae, which are arranged in rows. The lamina propria contains thick collagen bundles and relatively little ground substance. A submucosa is absent. **A**, bone of hard palate. (H & E; × 20)

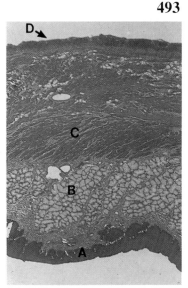

493

493 Mucosa of the soft palate. A non-keratinised lining mucosa (**A**) covers the oral surface of the soft palate. The connective tissue papillae are short and broad. The lamina propria contains many elastic fibres and its collagen bundles are relatively thin. There is a broad submucosa containing many small mucous glands (**B**). The submucosa attaches into the palatal muscles (**C**). The nasal surface of the soft palate is lined by a pseudostratified ciliated columnar epithelium (**D**). (H & E; × 20)

The tongue and the floor of the mouth

494 The ventral surface of the tongue (A) and the floor of the mouth (B). The mucosae in these regions are typical lining mucosae. There is little wear and tear but a need for considerable mobility. The epithelium is thin, non-keratinised and shows short papillae. The submucosa is extensive on the floor of the mouth but indistinct (if not absent) on the ventral surface of the tongue where the mucosa binds down to the tongue muscles (**C**). The thinness of the epithelium and vascularity of the connective tissue make this a route by which some drugs can rapidly reach the blood stream. (H & E; × 20)

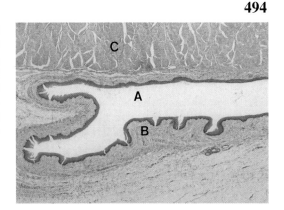

494

The lingual mucosa on the dorsum of the tongue is a masticatory mucosa that is specialised to fulfil sensory as well as mechanical functions. An indistinct groove, the sulcus terminalis (see **12**) divides the tongue into an anterior two-thirds (palatal surface) and a posterior one-third (pharyngeal surface). The anterior two-thirds of the palate is covered with numerous papillae which can be classified into four types: filiform, fungiform, foliate and circumvallate papillae. The posterior one-third of the tongue is studded with small, lymphatic nodules (or follicles).

495 Filiform papillae. Each filiform papilla consists of a central core of lamina propria with smaller, secondary papillae branching from it. The overlying stratified squamous epithelium is keratinised and forms hair-like tufts. The filiform papillae are highly abrasive during mastication when the bolus is compressed against the palate. (H & E; × 40)

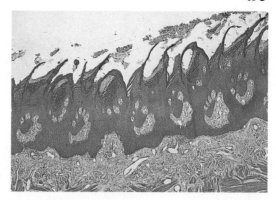

The simplest model of homeostasis in stratified epithelia is that all basal epithelial cells divide in a fairly homogeneous manner, and that increased basal cell 'pressure' generated by dividing cells results in an upward random migration of keratinocytes destined for desquamation. However, it is now clear that many renewing tissues (including oral epithelium) are organised in a much more complicated way, as reference to the mouse filiform papilla shows (see **496**).

496a Each mouse filiform papilla comprises several columns of cells (boundaries arrowed) around a central connective tissue core. The anterior column (**A**) is two cells wide and has well-defined boundaries that result from the difference in cell size and differentiation on either side of each boundary. The posterior column (**P**) of 16–20 cells piled one on top of another gradually inclines as cells move upwards so that the top cell desquamates backwards (towards the pharynx). The buttress column (**B**) appears to fill in the rear of the papilla structure to 'buttress' the posterior column. Note the maturity of basal cells over the apex of the connective tissue core and the method used to number individual cell positions within each column (Longitudinal section; Masson's trichrome; × 120).

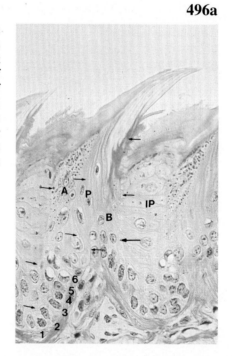

496b Schematic representation of column boundaries and cell migration patterns in the mouse filiform papilla. The stem cell population is at position 1, next to column boundaries. As cells move bodily along the basement membrane, their capacity for proliferation decreases so that by the time they reach the highest cell position number, they are post-mitotic, differentiating cells. This model implies that, because of rapid desquamation of cells, 4–5 cells per day in the posterior column are the stem cells. There is some suprabasal migration in the anterior column in addition to migration along the basement membrane. The posterior column is derived from lateral cell migration and the buttress column from suprabasal migration from the stem cell population at the rear of the papilla. Thus, each of these columns is one cell wide whereas the anterior column is two cells wide. **IP**, interpapillary epithelium.

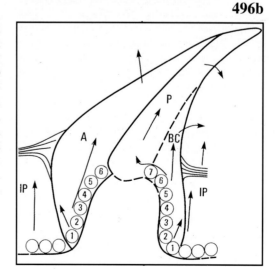

214

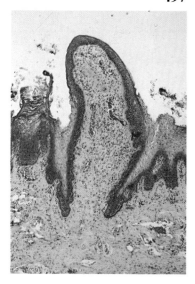

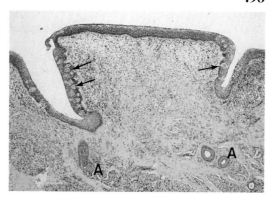

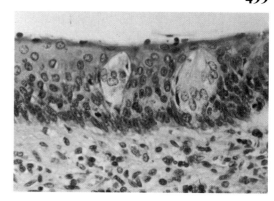

497 Fungiform papillae are isolated, elevated mushroom-shaped papillae and are approximately 150–400μm in diameter. They are covered by a relatively thin, non-keratinised epithelium. Occasional taste buds are found on the surface. (Masson's trichrome; × 40)

498 A circumvallate papillae in longitudinal section. The papilla is covered by a non-keratinised epithelium. Taste buds (*arrowed*) predominate on the internal wall of the trench in the epithelium. Small serous glands (of von Ebner, **A**) empty into the base of the trench. (Masson's trichrome; × 40)

499 The taste bud, the special chemoreceptive organ responsible for taste, is located particularly within the epithelium around the walls of the circumvallate papillae, but also in small numbers on the upper surface of fungiform papillae, in the lateral walls of foliate papillae, and in the mucosa of the soft palate. Two types of cell are present in the taste bud: the supporting cell and the taste cell. A small pore opens from the surface into the taste bud. (Masson's trichrome; × 300)

500 The cells of a taste bud are clearly demarcated from the adjacent epithelial cells (**A**). The morphology of a taste bud may vary according to species and site. Four distinct cell types have been described — Types I, II, III, and IV. The relatively undifferentiated Type IV cells are distinguished by their basal position and the presence of intermediate filaments. Type I cells (**B**) have a dark appearance, while Type II (**C**) and Type III (**D**) are lighter. Type I and III cells may form synapses with intragemmal nerves (*arrowed*). The taste bud is separated from the underlying connective tissue (**E**) by a basal lamina. **F**, taste pore. (TEM; × 11,000)

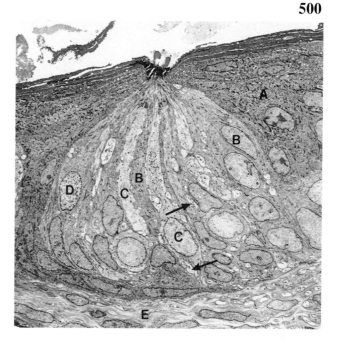

501 Lingual follicles (*arrowed*). The collection of lymphoid follicles on the posterior one-third of the tongue is collectively known as the lingual tonsil and forms a component of Waldeyer's ring, which protects the opening into the pharynx (with the palatine tonsil, and the tubal and pharyngeal tonsils within the nasopharynx). The follicles are deep crypts, lined with epithelium and containing a mass of lymphoid material. The follicles usually open onto the surface of the tongue. The mucosa in this region also contains many mucous glands. Note that some small mucous glands also occasionally occur at the margin and tip of the anterior two-thirds of the tongue. (H & E; × 40)

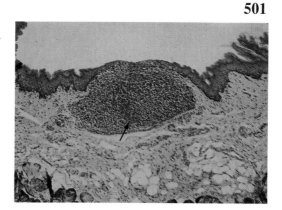

215

Table 18: Principal features and regional variations of the oral mucosa.

Region	Epithelium		Lamina propria		Submucosa		Type of mucosa
	Thickness	*Keratinisation*	*Papillae*	*Fibre types*	*Density*	*Attachment*	
Labial and buccal mucosa	Thick	Non-keratinised	Short and irregular	Collagen and some elastic fibres	Dense	Firmly to under-lying muscle	Lining
Vermilion (red) zone of lip	Thin	Keratinised	Long and narrow	Collagen and some elastic fibres	Dense	Firmly to under-lying muscle	Specialised
Alveolar mucosa	Thin	Non-keratinised	Short or absent	Many elastic fibres	Loose	Loose attachment to periosteum	Lining
Attached gingiva	Thick	Keratinised and parakeratinised	Long and narrow	Dense collagen firmly attached to underlying periosteum	No distinct submucosa		Masticatory
Floor of mouth	Thin	Non-keratinised	Short and broad	Collagen and some elastic fibres	Loose	Loose attachment to underlying muscle	Lining
Ventral surface of tongue	Thin	Non-keratinised	Short and numerous	Collagen and some elastic fibres	Not very distinct layer; attached to underlying muscle		Lining
Dorsum of tongue (anterior two-thirds)	Thick	Primarily keratinised	Long	Collagen and some elastic fibres	Not very distinct layer; attached to underlying muscle		Specialised gustatory
Dorsum of tongue (posterior one-third)	Variable	Generally non-keratinised	Short or absent	Collagen and some elastic fibres	Not very distinct layer; attached to underlying muscle		Lining gustatory
Hard palate	Thick	Keratinised	Long	Dense collagen in submucosa laterally, but lamina propria firmly bound to periosteum without submucosa in midline			Masticatory
Soft palate	Thick	Non-keratinised	Short	Many elastic fibres	Loose	Loose attachment to underlying tissues	Lining

The temporomandibular joint

The temporomandibular joint (TMJ) is the synovial articulation between the mandible and the cranium (the temporal bone). Being a synovial joint, it allows considerable movement and has a joint cavity filled with synovial fluid. The synovial membrane which secretes the synovial fluid lines the internal surface of the joint capsule. Unlike most other synovial joints, the joint space is crossed by an articular disc and the articular surfaces are not comprised of hyaline cartilage but of fibrous tissue (reflecting the joint's intramembranous development; see page 244). The gross anatomy of the temporomandibular joint is described on pages 70–71.

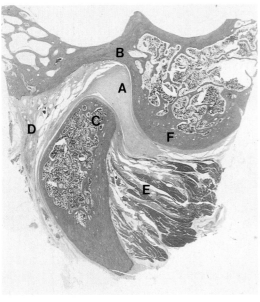

502 The general arrangement of the tissues of the temporomandibular joint. A, articular disc within joint cavity; **B**, mandibular fossa (glenoid fossa) of temporal bone; **C**, condyle of mandible; **D**, capsule of joint; **E**, lateral pterygoid muscle; **F**, articular eminence. (H & E; × 3)

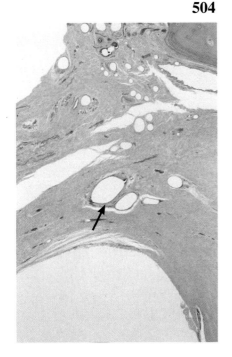

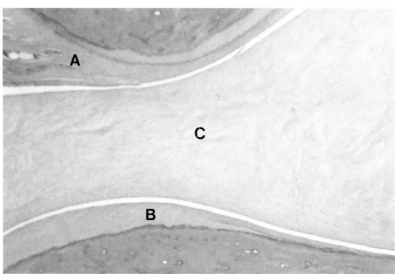

503 The articular surfaces of the mandibular fossa (A) and the mandibular condyle (B) are lined by dense fibrous connective tissues which contain some elastin fibres. The articular layers are thicker over the convexity on the anterior part of the condyle and over the articular eminence of the temporal bone. Beneath each articular layer surface, there is a zone of increased cell density. This represents a proliferative zone, providing a source of fibroblasts to compensate for the slow loss of tissue occurring at the surface. The superficial collagen fibres of the articular layer run parallel to the surface while the deeper fibres are orientated more vertically. The articular disc (**C**) divides the joint into upper and lower joint cavities. The disc is composed of dense fibrous tissue. It is thinnest centrally and thickens at the periphery. Isolated clumps of more rounded, cartilage-like cells have also been described within the disc; the disc has therefore sometimes been described as being fibrocartilaginous. (H & E; × 14)

504 Blood vessels (*arrowed*) in the posterior part of the articular disc. As is evident from **503**, the bulk of the disc is avascular and derives its nutrition by diffusion from the synovial fluid. Blood vessels are localised at the periphery. However, posteriorly (in the bilaminar zone, see **144**) the disc divides into superior and inferior lamellae. The superior lamella possesses numerous blood vessels and elastin fibres. As the disc is pulled forwards by the lateral pterygoid muscle during jaw opening, the tissue of the superior lamella fills the space behind the migrating condyle. As the condyle moves backwards during jaw closure, the disc returns to its original position aided by the elastic recoil of the superior lamella. The inferior lamella is relatively avascular and inelastic. (H & E; × 14)

217

505 Ultrastructural appearance of the articular disc. In common with other fibrous connective tissues, the articular disc consists of cells embedded in an extracellular matrix of collagen and ground substance. The relatively sparsely distributed cells are mainly fibroblasts (*arrowed*). They contain the usual intracellular organelles associated with protein synthesis (e.g. endoplasmic reticulum, Golgi material, mitochondria), indicating that there must be a continuous, albeit slow, turnover of the extracellular matrix. Other more rounded cells having a similar appearance to cartilage cells have also been described. The presence of localised regions of fibrocartilage may be associated with the presence of compressive forces impinging on the articular disc. (TEM; × 2,650)

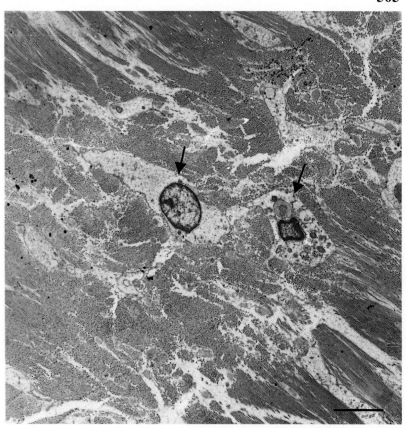

The fibres within the articular disc are principally composed of Type I collagen and comprise about 80% (dry weight) of the disc. In the thinner central region of the disc, the collagen fibres are described as running mainly in an anteroposterior direction. In the thicker anterior and posterior portions of the disc, however, prominent fibre bundles run transversely with a mediolateral orientation. Very small amounts of Type III collagen have been described at the posterior attachment region of the disc. The localised areas of fibrocartilage would be expected to contain small amounts of Type II collagen. Some elastin fibres have also been described in the articular disc. The glycosaminoglycan of the articular disc comprises about 5% of its dry weight. About 80% of the glycosaminoglycan is chondroitin sulphate and about 15% dermatan sulphate. As chondroitin sulphate is also the major proteoglycan present in cartilage, its presence in the articular disc suggests that the disc is subjected to compressional loads. The observation that collagen fibril diameters are small (about 45nm) is further evidence that the disc is subjected to compression.

506

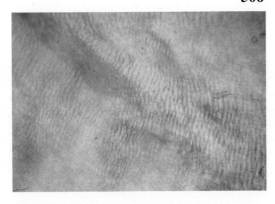

506 Crimping of collagen fibres in the articular disc. When viewed in polarised light, the appearance of lines (in this case, vertically oriented) running across the longitudinal axis of the collagen fibres indicates that the collagen is crimped. This special type of 'folding' (see page 169 for crimps in the periodontal ligament) is presumed to be important when considering the biomechanical properties of the disc. (× 15)

507 The synovial membrane (A) lines the inner surface of the fibrous capsule of the temporomandibular joint and the margins of the articular disc (**B**). However, it does not cover the articular surfaces of the joint. The synovial membrane consists of a layer of flattened, endothelial-like cells resting on a vascular layer. It may be folded at rest, these folds flattening out during movements of the joint. The synovial membrane secretes the synovial fluid which occupies the joint cavities (**C**). The synovial fluid lubricates the joint and presumably also has nutritive functions. Important components of the fluid are the proteoglycans, which aid lubrication. At rest, the hydrostatic pressure of the synovial fluid has been reported as being subatmospheric, but greatly elevated during mastication. **D**, posterior surface of mandibular condyle. (H & E; × 60)

507

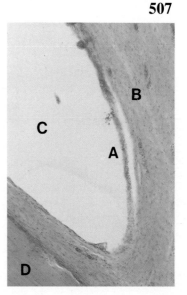

The histological appearance of the mandibular condyle varies according to age. This is due to the presence of the secondary condylar cartilage. This cartilage appears initially at about the tenth week of intrauterine life and remains as a zone of proliferating cartilage until about the end of the second decade of life.

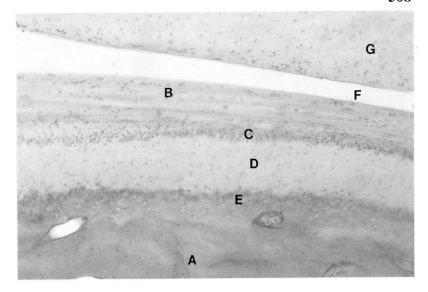

508 **In the adult condyle**, the bony condylar head (**A**) is covered superficially by the fibrous articular zone (**B**). A layer containing an increased number of nuclei can be observed in the lower layers of the covering fibrous layer, indicative of a proliferative zone (**C**). Two additional layers have been described below the proliferative layer. First, a region regarded as being comprised of fibrocartilage (**D**), beneath which is a thin zone of calcified cartilage (**E**), representing the remains of the original secondary condylar cartilage (see page 243). **F**, lower joint space; **G**, articular disc. (H & E; × 100)

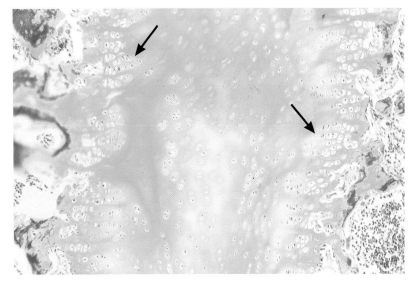

509 **The condyle of a child** is lined by a layer of fibrous tissue (**A**). Beneath this articular layer is a proliferative layer of undifferentiated cells (**B**). Cells from this proliferative layer may pass superficially to replenish the articular layer or pass deeply where they differentiate into chondrocytes (**C**) which form the secondary condylar cartilage. The chondrocytes hypertrophy at the site of endochondral ossification. In brief, the process involves mineralisation of the cartilage matrix. Part of the calcified cartilage is resorbed by large multinucleated osteoclasts (*small arrow*). Subsequently, bone-forming cells, the osteoblasts (*large arrow*) deposit woven bone (**D**) around a template of calcified cartilage (**E**). Eventually, this area will be remodelled to produce mature bone. Note the lack of organisation of the chondrocytes into columns. The role of the condylar cartilage in growth of the mandible is controversial and is discussed on page 245. **F**, marrow space. (H & E; × 130)

510 **The spheno-occipital synchondrosis** is described here to provide a comparison between a primary cartilage and a secondary cartilage as exemplified by the condylar cartilage. Developmentally, the primary cartilage appears first to map out the shape of the future bone. In the case of the condylar cartilage, the ramus has already formed in membrane before this secondary cartilage appears. Primary cartilages have inherent growth potential, as is evidenced when they are transferred to tissue culture. The condylar cartilage has little intrinsic growth potential when tissue-cultured. In the synchondrosis, proliferative zones lie on either side of the central region of the cartilage, and proliferation involves cartilage cells (as opposed to undifferentiated cells in the secondary cartilage). The cells align themselves in columns in the direction of growth on each side of the synchondrosis (*arrowed*), hypertrophy, and undergo endochondral ossification. There is considerable production of extracellular matrix which, together with the original proliferation, is responsible for providing the growth force. In the secondary condylar cartilage, however, there is far less production of extracellular matrix and there is no alignment of the hypertrophic chondrocytes into columns. This might relate to the ability of the secondary cartilage to produce growth in various directions. In the case of an epiphyseal growth plate, columns of cartilage cells are only produced on one side. (H & E; × 100)

Salivary glands

Salivary glands are compound, tubuloacinar, merocrine, exocrine glands whose ducts open into the oral cavity. The term compound refers to the fact that a salivary gland has more than one tubule entering the main duct; tubuloacinar describes the morphology of the secreting cells; merocrine indicates that only the secretion of the cell is released; and exocrine describes a gland which secretes onto a free surface.

Saliva is over 99% water. It contains small quantities of ions and macromolecules that perform many of its important functions. Its major role is as a lubricant during mastication, swallowing and speech. Saliva brings substances into solution so that they can be tasted. It has a protective function, keeping the mucosa moist and limiting bacterial activity by preventing their aggregation and by the presence of antibacterial substances (e.g. lysozyme). Saliva contains minerals and acts as a buffer; both features help to maintain the integrity of the dental enamel. The substances kallikrein, renin and tonin affect local vascularity as well as water and electrolyte balance. Epidermal growth factor and nerve growth factor are produced by the submandibular gland, the former possibly being involved in wound healing. Immunoglobulins (IgA) are produced by plasma cells in the salivary glands, and may be part of a widespread mucosal immune system that includes lymphoid tissue in the gut and bronchi. A carbohydrate-fragmenting enzyme called amylase is present in saliva. Also present in saliva are blood group substances. Saliva may play a role in water balance. If the body is dehydrated, the rate of salivation is reduced. This gives rise to a dry mouth, encouraging the individual to drink.

Salivary glands consist of two main elements: the glandular secretory tissue (the parenchyma) and the supporting connective tissue (the stroma).

511

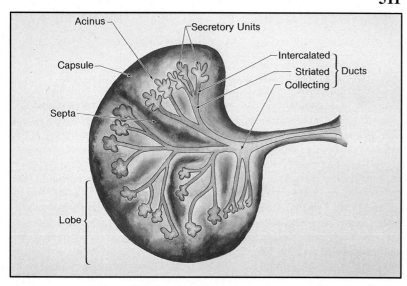

512

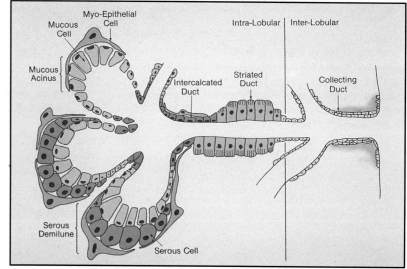

511 General organisation of a salivary gland. From the capsule surrounding and protecting the gland pass septa which subdivide the gland into lobes. Each lobe contains numerous secretory units and each unit consists of a cluster of grape-like structures (the acini) positioned around a lumen. A secretory acinus may be serous, mucous or mixed. It empties into an intercalated duct lined by cuboidal epithelium, which in turn joins a larger striated duct formed of columnar cells. Both the intercalated and striated ducts are intralobular and affect the composition of the secretion passing through them. Plasma cells (which secrete the immunoglobulins) are found around the intralobular ducts. The striated ducts empty into the relatively inert collecting ducts, which carry the saliva to the mucosal surface and which may be lined near their termination by a layer of stratified squamous epithelial cells. The collecting ducts are interlobular. The connective tissue septa carry the blood and nerve supply into the parenchyma. Unlike endocrine glands, whose secretion may be controlled by the activity of hormones, the secretion of salivary glands is under the control of the autonomic nervous system.

512 Secretory elements of the salivary glands. The serous and mucous cells of the parenchyma are responsible for the production of the primary secretion. Saliva is the product of an active secretory process and is not merely an ultrafiltrate of blood. The serous cells produce a watery proteinaceous fluid and are the source of amylase. The secretory product of mucous cells have proteins linked to a greater amount of carbohydrate, forming a more viscous mucin-rich product. Both serous and mucous cells are arranged as acini, although groups of mucous cells may have a more tubular form. Acini may contain either serous or mucous cells, or they may be mixed. When mixed, the serous cells form a cap or demilune outside the mucous cells. The secretions of the demilune pass between the mucous cells through small canaliculi to enter the lumen of the acinus. Sometimes, extensions of the demilune pass between the mucous cells to contact the lumen directly. Outside the acini, contractile cells with several processes are present. These are myoepithelial (basket) cells which, when contracted, expel preformed saliva from the lumina of the acini into the duct system.

Salivary glands may be classified according to size (major and minor) and/or the types of secretion (mucous, serous or mixed). The three paired major salivary glands are the parotid, the submandibular and the sublingual glands. The numerous minor salivary glands are scattered throughout the oral mucosa and include the labial, buccal, palatoglossal, palatal and lingual glands.

Parotid gland

513

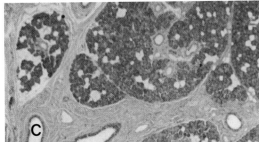

513 The parotid gland is the largest of the salivary glands. It is enclosed within a well-defined capsule. The gland is almost entirely composed of serous acini. The pale-staining stroma of the connective tissue (**B**) can be seen subdividing the secretory parenchyma (**A**) into lobes. The connective tissue contains blood vessels, nerves and collecting ducts (**C**). (H & E; × 36)

514

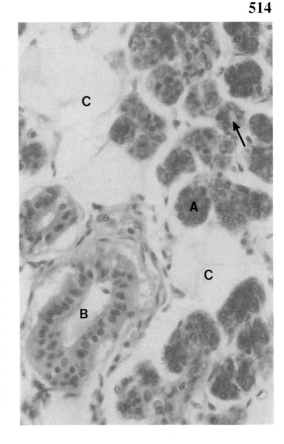

514 Serous acini (A) in the parotid gland. The lumina of the acini are very narrow (*arrowed*), unless distended by the accumulation of secretions. The prominent nuclei are round and located in the basal third of the cell, which is basophilic due to the presence of rough endoplasmic reticulum. The granular appearance of the serous acinar cell results from the numerous refractile eosinophilic granules in the distal portion of the cell (adjacent to the lumen). Intercalated ducts passing from the acini open into striated ducts (**B**). Some fat cells (**C**) are also seen. The number of fat cells increases with age (H & E; × 400)

515

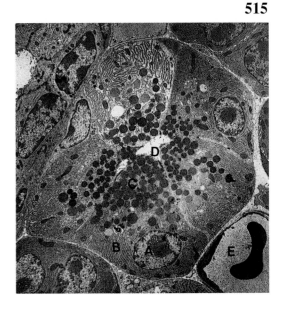

515 A serous acinus. In the serous acinus, wedge-shaped cells surround a central lumen (**D**). The basal part of each serous cell contains a nucleus (**A**) and rough endoplasmic reticulum (**B**). The distal part of the cell adjacent to the lumen contains dense, round zymogen granules (**C**). Many narrow canaliculi run between the cells and join the lumen. Both the canaliculi and the lumen are lined by short microvilli. The presence of an erythrocyte (**E**) in a capillary demonstrates the proximity of the blood supply. Both para-sympathetic and sympathetic fibres innervate the acini. Some nerve endings occur beneath the basal lamina in direct contact with the plasma membrane. Others end outside the basal lamina which delineates the acinus from the surrounding connective tissue. Endings at each site probably affect the cell as transmitter vesicles are present at both locations. Parasympathetic drive causes fluid formation by the secretory units; sympathetic drive usually increases the output of preformed components from the cells. Both pathways cause contraction of the myoepithelial cells, which pushes material in the acini out along the duct system. The role of both components of the autonomic system and of peptidergic fibres, which are also present, is complex, and acts through several effectors, including the secretory cells, myoepithelial cells, intralobular ducts and local blood vessels. (TEM; × 2,000)

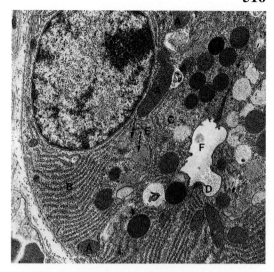

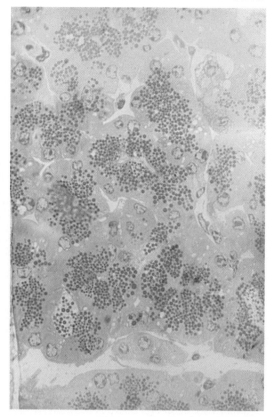

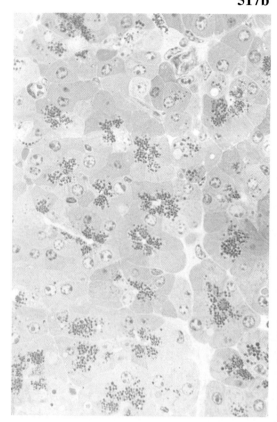

516 Part of a serous cell. Many of the components of the synthetic secretory pathway are seen. Proteins assembled by the ribosomes of the rough endoplasmic reticulum (**B**) move into the cisternae of the reticulum and from there to the Golgi material (**E**). Here the proteins are glycosylated and released in vacuoles as secretory granules (**C**). Initially the granules are of pale electron density (*arrowed*). The granules move to the luminal plasma membrane, become more electron-dense, and are subsequently discharged by exocytosis (**D**). The mitochondria (**A**) supply the energy for the process. **F**, a microvillus on the luminal surface. (TEM; × 6,700)

517 The appearance of serous cells varies with the levels of secretory activity. Following the synthesis of secretory products, resting (unstimulated) serous cells will contain numerous zymogen granules in the distal parts of their cytoplasm (**517a**). Following stimulation, the granules will be depleted after being discharged into the lumen by exocytosis (**517b**). (Toluidine blue; × 600)

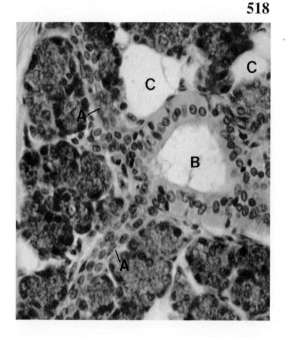

518 The intercalated duct (**A**) leads from the serous acini into the striated duct (**B**) and is usually compressed between the acini. The intercalated duct is lined by cuboidal epithelial cells. The nuclei in the duct cells appear prominent, owing to the relatively scanty cytoplasm. **C**, fat cell. (H & E; × 360)

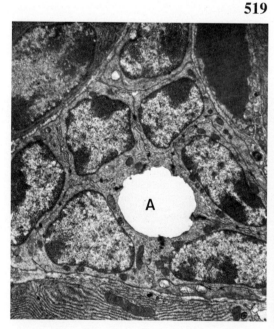

519 An intercalated duct (**A**). Intercalated ducts consist of a simple cuboidal epithelial tube with the processes of myoepithelial cells entwined around it (see **526**). Both luminal and basal surfaces of the duct cells are smooth. Desmosomes unite adjacent cells. The cells have occasional granules and only small amounts of the organelles associated with protein synthesis. It is possible, but unclear, whether the duct cells have any role in modifying the electrolyte composition of the secretion. They might act as stem cells and be able to differentiate into secretory, myoepithelial or striated duct cells.

Several acini drain into each intercalated duct. In the parotid gland, intercalated ducts are characteristically long, narrow, and branching. (TEM; × 5,700)

520 Striated duct cells. The striated ducts form a much longer and more active component of the duct system than the intercalated ducts. The cells of the striated ducts have a large amount of cytoplasm and a large, spherical, centrally positioned nucleus (see also **518**). The ductal surface has short microvilli. The striations of these cells, visualised in the light microscope, are derived from multiple infoldings of the plasma membrane at the base of the cell (*arrowed*). Vertically aligned mitochondria are packed between the infoldings. Adjacent cells are intertwined in a complex pattern and anchored together by desmosomes. This large surface area, supplied with high levels of energy, is clearly involved in active transport. It is thought that the striated ducts are the site of electrolyte reabsorption (especially of sodium and chloride) and secretion (potassium and bicarbonate). As this reabsorption is against a concentration gradient, it requires substantial amounts of energy. The effect on the material in the lumen (**A**) is to convert an isotonic or slightly hypertonic fluid (with concentrations similar to those in the plasma) to a hypotonic fluid. (TEM; × 12,000)

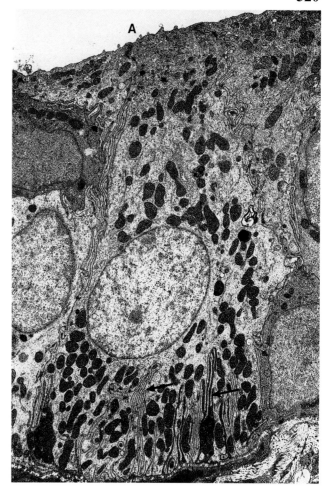

521 A collecting duct (A). The striated duct leads into the collecting duct. In addition to the columnar layer (which now lacks striations), the collecting duct may have an additional layer of basal cells. In the early parts of the collecting duct, partial re-equilibration of saliva with plasma occurs, and concentrations of ions return to more plasma-like levels. As it enlarges, the main parotid duct appears like many excretory passages and contains three layers: mucosa, muscular layer and adventitia. As in other areas, this arrangement probably plays some role in controlling the flow of the saliva along the duct. Near its termination, the lining of the main duct may be composed of stratified squamous epithelium. (H & E; × 60)

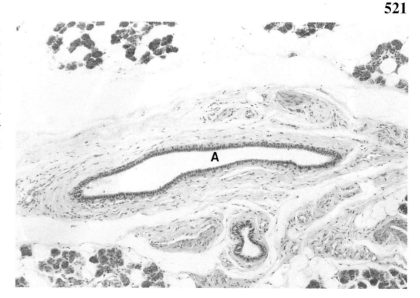

Submandibular gland

The second largest of the salivary glands, the submandibular gland produces a mixed mucous–serous secretion. Serous acini appear to outnumber mucous acini by approximately 10:1. The gland has a well-formed connective tissue capsule.

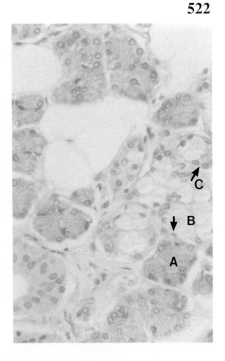

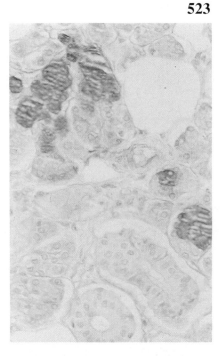

522 Serous and mucous acini in the submandibular gland. Much of the submandibular gland contains serous acini (**A**) similar to those in the parotid gland (see **514**). However, the submandibular gland also contains collections of mucous acini (**B**). These are readily distinguished in the resting gland from the darker staining and granular serous acini, as they are paler and their nuclei (*arrowed*) are compressed against the basal aspect of the cell. The mucous acini are pale because their mucinous content does not readily take up routine stains or is lost during preparation. Small, crescent-shaped collections of serous cells may be found around the mucous acini. **C**, serous demilunes. (H & E; × 330)

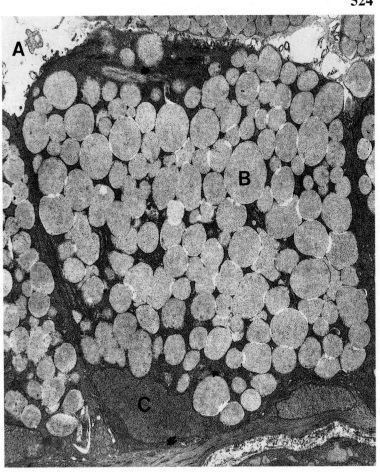

523 Mucous acini can be specifically stained with periodic acid-Schiff stain. This stain gives the mucous acini a purplish colouration. The serous cells, lacking mucosubstance in their cytoplasm, take up the counterstain (in this case yellow). (PAS stain counterstained with tartrazine and iron haematoxylin; × 250)

524 A mucous cell. In the early stages of the synthesis of secretory products, large amounts of rough endoplasmic reticulum are present and few mucous droplets. Compared with serous cells, mucous cells have a more conspicuous Golgi apparatus (because of the greater amount of carbohydrate that is added to the secretory products). The cell illustrated is in a late phase of its secretory cycle. At this point, numerous granules (**B**) occupy almost the entire cell, compressing other organelles (including the nucleus, **C**) to the periphery. The granules discharge into the lumen (**A**) by exocytosis. Following discharge, the nucleus becomes more prominent in the basal part of the cell (see page 225). (TEM; × 5,000)

525 Part of a serous demilune. There are
many serous acini in the submandibular gland.
Some of the serous cells are contained in
demilunes capping mucous acini and emptying
into the lumen through canaliculi between the
mucous cells **A**, lumen of acinus; **B**, mucous
cell; **C**, serous cell. (TEM; × 2,000)

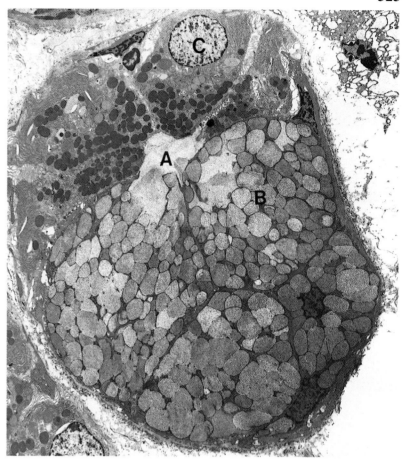

526 Myoepithelial cells are stellate, contractile
cells consisting of a cell body (**A**) and a number
of tapering processes (**B**). They lie between the
basal lamina and the basal membranes of acinar
secretory cells (**C**) and also intercalated duct
cells. The secretory cells illustrated are serous.
Contractile myofilaments, some of which are
aggregated into dense bundles (*arrowed*) are present in the cell process. Pinocytotic vesicles and
dense attachment areas are associated with the
part of the plasma membrane covered by the
basal lamina. On contraction, myoepithelial cells
compress the underlying acinus or intercalated
duct and propel the saliva along the duct system.
Note the variable appearance and density of the
secretory granules in the serous cells. (TEM;
× 6,500)

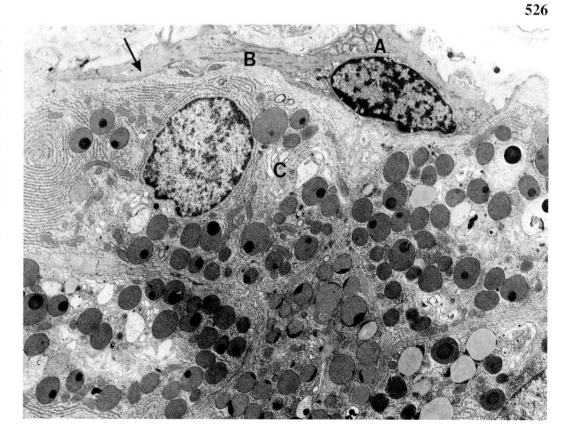

527 A collection of mucous cells in an unstimulated submandibular gland. The mucous cells are filled with secretory granules and consequently their nuclei are compressed into the basal parts of the cells. (TEM; × 1,000)

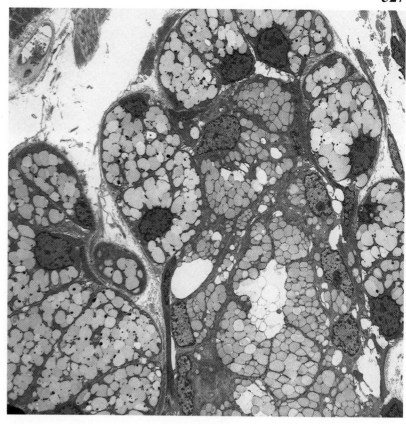

528 A collection of mucous cells in a recently stimulated submandibular gland. The mucous cells have lost their secretory granules and consequently their nuclei are more prominent in the cell. (TEM; × 1,000)

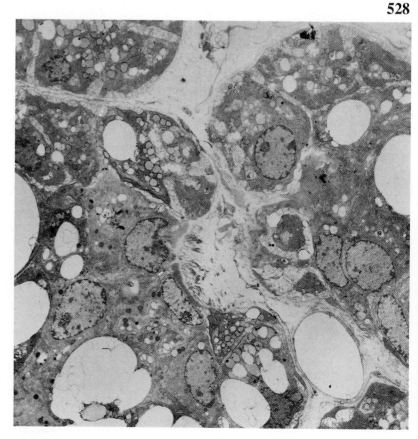

The ductal cells of the submandibular gland are similar to those of the parotid. The intercalated ducts are, however, much shorter, and may be difficult to locate in histological sections, while the striated ducts are longer and more obvious.

Sublingual gland

The human sublingual gland is not a single unit like the parotid and submandibular glands, but is made up of one large segment (the major sublingual gland) and a group of 8–30 minor glands, each having its own duct system emptying into the sublingual fold (see **10**). The major sublingual gland is mixed, with more mucous than serous elements.

529 The sublingual gland. Pale-staining mucous cells predominate in the glandular tissue (**A**). The upper surface in this micrograph is the oral mucosa (**B**). The gland capsule merges imperceptibly with the mucosa. (Masson's trichrome; × 25)

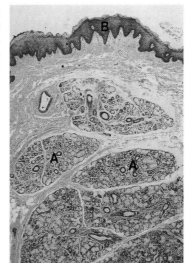

529

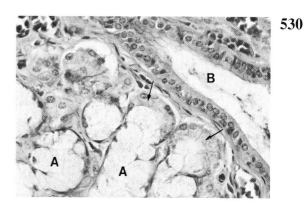

530

530 Glandular tissue of the sublingual gland consists primarily of pale-staining mucous cells (**A**). While there are some serous acini, the majority of serous cells are contained in demilunes (*arrowed*) around mucous acini or tubules. The duct system is much less well-developed than in the other major salivary glands and striated ducts are lacking. The initial duct segments are similar to intercalated ducts elsewhere but are short. The next larger ductal element (**B**), while being rich in mitochondria, lacks the basal striations that characterise striated ducts. This may be related to the formation of a sodium-rich saliva. (Masson's trichrome; × 240)

Minor salivary glands

The minor salivary glands are classified by their anatomical location: buccal, labial, palatal, palatoglossal and lingual. They are primarily mucous. The labial and buccal glands are illustrated on page 206. The palatoglossal glands are located in the region of the pharyngeal isthmus. The palatal glands lie in both the soft and hard palate (page 213). The anterior lingual glands are embedded within muscle near the ventral surface of the tongue, and have short ducts opening near the lingual frenulum. The posterior glands are located in the root of the tongue. Both groups are mucous. The von Ebner glands empty into the trench of the circumvallate papillae and are serous (**498**).

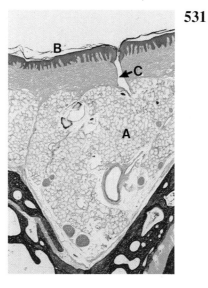

531

531 Minor mucous gland (A) in the submucosa of the hard palate. Note the masticatory mucosa (**B**) at the surface. C, collecting duct. (Masson's trichrome; × 15)

Division of salivary acini into serous and mucous types in routine sections stained with haematoxylin and eosin is clearcut. Ultrastructural and histochemical methods do not contribute further to the ease of separation.

Morphological variations among secretory granules of the same type of cell have been found in secretory acini (as well as ductal cells). Variation is greatest in serous cells (**526**). A possible explanation is that one type of cell may be able to produce a range of secretory products, packaging them variously into secretory granules and thus creating different appearances. Histochemically, there is evidence that serous cells in the parotid gland can secrete neutral mucins, while serous cells in the submandibular gland can secrete acid mucins.

There is a low level of secretion throughout the day, mainly from the minor glands with periodic large additions from the major glands (e.g. at meal times). An average of about 750ml of saliva is secreted each day, with about 90% derived from the major salivary glands. A very small contribution to the pooled saliva is derived from gingival fluid (see page 210).

Development of oro-dental tissues

Development of the face

532 The face of a 4-week-old embryo. This model shows the frontal aspect. During early development, the primitive oral cavity (stomodeum) is bounded by five facial swellings produced by proliferating zones of mesenchyme lying beneath the surface ectoderm. The frontonasal process (**A**) lies above, the two mandibular processes (**B**) lie below, and the maxillary processes (**C**) are located at the sides. The maxillary and mandibular processes are derived from the first branchial arches. The facial processes are demarcated by grooves which, in the course of normal development, become flattened out by the proliferative and migratory activity of the underlying mesenchyme. At this early stage of development, a membrane (the oropharyngeal membrane) separates the primitive oral cavity from the developing pharynx. The oropharyngeal membrane is bilaminar, being composed of an outer ectodermal layer and an inner endodermal layer. This membrane soon breaks down to establish continuity between the ectodermally-lined oral cavity and the endodermally-lined pharynx. Though not detectable in the adult, the demarcation zone between mucosa derived from ectoderm and endoderm corresponds to a region lying just behind the third permanent molar. **D**, pericardial swelling.

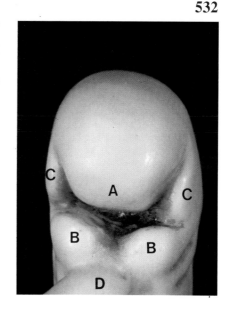

532

533 The face of a 5-week-old embryo. This model shows the lateral aspect. Localised thickenings of ectoderm give rise to the nasal and optic (**A**) placodes. These placodes will form the olfactory epithelium and the lenses of the eyes. The nasal placodes sink into the underlying mesenchyme, forming two blind-ended nasal pits (**B**), the primitive nasal cavities. Proliferation of mesenchyme from the frontonasal process around the openings of the nasal pits produces the medial (**C**) and lateral (**D**) nasal processes. Also shown on the model is a maxillary process (**E**), a mandibular process (**F**) and the second branchial arch (**G**).

The nasal pits continue to deepen until eventually they approach the roof of the primitive oral cavity, being partitioned from it by oronasal membranes. By the end of the fifth week these membranes rupture, thus producing communications between the developing nasal and oral cavities. Before the oronasal membrane ruptures, a sheet of epithelium (the nasal fin) may be seen in front of each nasal pit. The nasal fin does not, as was once thought, form an epithelial partition between the maxillary and medial nasal processes. A bridge of mesenchyme, the maxillary isthmus, joins the two processes in front of the nasal fin.

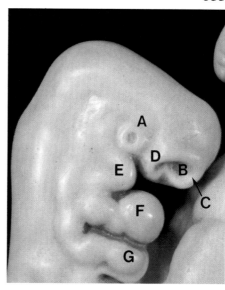

533

534 a & b Sagittal section through the developing nasal (A) and oral (B) cavities. Note the position of the nasal fin (**C**), the oronasal membrane (**D**), and the maxillary isthmus (**E**) at the end of the fifth week of development. The nasal fin is eventually incorporated into either the walls of the nasal pit or the oronasal membrane. However, should the fin become enlarged, it may constitute a line of weakness between the mesenchyme of the maxillary and medial nasal processes and eventually lead to a cleft in this region. **F**, developing tongue. (**534a,** Toluidine blue; × 30)

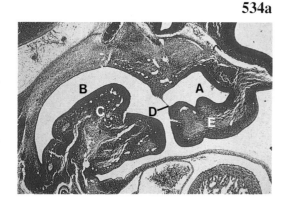

534a

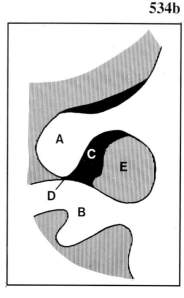

534b

535 The face of a 6-week-old embryo. This model shows the lateral aspect. The two mandibular processes (**A**) fuse in the midline to form the tissues of the lower jaw. Rarely, persistence of a midline groove in this region produces a mandibular cleft. The mandibular processes and maxillary processes (**B**) meet at the angles of the mouth, thus defining its outline. Disturbances in this development may give rise to macrostomia or microstomia, or rarely, an astomia. From the corners of the mouth, the maxillary processes grow inwards beneath the lateral nasal processes (**C**) towards the medial nasal processes (**D**) of the upper lip. Between the merging maxillary and the lateral nasal processes lie the naso-optic furrows (**E**). From each furrow a solid ectodermal rod of cells sinks below the surface and canalises to form the nasolacrimal duct. Persistence of the naso-optic furrow may produce an oblique facial cleft.

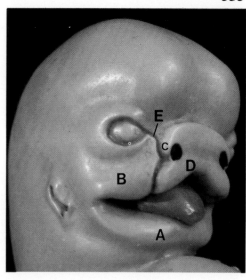

Two differing accounts have been given for the development of the upper lip. One view suggests that the maxillary processes overgrow the medial nasal processes to meet in the midline and thus contribute all the tissue for the upper lip. This is based upon an appreciation of the innervation of the fully formed upper lip (i.e. the infra-orbital branch of the maxillary division of the trigeminal nerve), the maxillary processes being supplied by the maxillary nerve, the frontonasal process by the ophthalmic nerve. Alternatively, it has been suggested that the maxillary processes meet the medial nasal processes without such overgrowth, the middle third of the upper lip being derived from the frontonasal process. While histological evidence favours the latter explanation, at present little is known about the behaviour of the mesenchyme of the facial processes after the initial fusion, thereby not excluding the possibility of subsequent migration of tissue derived from the maxillary processes towards the midline.

536 Contributions to the adult face from the embryonic facial processes.

A Maxillary process.
B Mandibular process.
C Medial nasal process.
D Lateral nasal process.

This diagram is based upon the suggestion that the middle third of the upper lip is derived from the frontonasal process. The facial derivatives shown are therefore at odds with the sensory distribution of the adult face, because (as previously mentioned) the fully developed lip is supplied only by the maxillary division of the trigeminal nerve and has no contribution from the ophthalmic division.

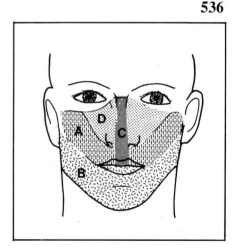

The facial muscles are derived from the mesenchyme of the second branchial arch, and are therefore innervated by the facial nerve.

The cells that make up the mesenchyme of the facial primordia are derived from two main sources: connective tissue cells migrating from the neural crest and muscle cells from the paraxial mesenchyme. Further development involves the four fundamental mechanisms that underlie all embryonic development: growth, morphogenesis, cell differentiation, and pattern formation. The latter mechanism leads to the spatial ordering of cell differentiation. Present research into the development of the face is geared towards understanding the basis of all these mechanisms.

The size of the cell populations is of key importance and is likely to be controlled, at least in part, by growth factors. These may also be of significance in the epithelial–mesenchymal interactions known to induce cartilage, bone and tooth differentiation within facial primordia. Pattern formation in developing limbs is controlled by vitamin A derivatives (retinoids), which form morphogenetic gradients within the limb bud. While such gradients have not yet been demonstrated in the face, a similar mechanism seems likely to be present, as the facial primordia are sensitive to exogenous retinoic acid and the mesenchymal cells contain specific retinoic acid receptors.

It is worth noting that the brain and facial mesenchyme have been shown to express particular genes at key times in their development. These are called homoeobox genes and were discovered in embryos of the fruit fly *Drosophila*. They are responsible for the spatial organisation of the developing *Drosophila* embryo. Similar genes are expected to be of major importance in mammalian development and are the subject of intensive research.

Failure of fusion of the maxillary and medial nasal processes produces the common congenital malformation of cleft lip, which may be unilateral or bilateral. Failure of the medial nasal processes to merge may be responsible for the formation of median cleft lip.

537 Facial clefts.
A = Median cleft lip.
B = Bilateral cleft lip.
C = Oblique facial cleft.
D = Lateral facial cleft.
E = Median mandibular cleft.

537

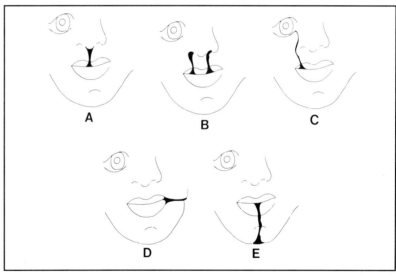

Development of the palate

The definitive palate (or secondary palate) appears in the human foetus between the sixth and eighth week of intra-uterine life. Palatogenesis is a complex event and is often disturbed to produce the congenital defect known as cleft palate. Consequently, the events and mechanisms responsible for the development of the palate have been much studied, although considerable controversy remains.

538

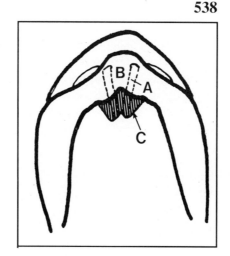

538 By the sixth week of development, the primitive nasal cavities (**A**) are separated by a primary nasal septum (**B**) and are partitioned from the primitive oral cavity by a primary palate (**C**). Both the primary nasal septum and primary palate are derived from the frontonasal process. The stomodeal chamber is divided at this stage into the small primitive oral cavity beneath the primary palate, and the relatively large oronasal cavity behind the primary palate.

539

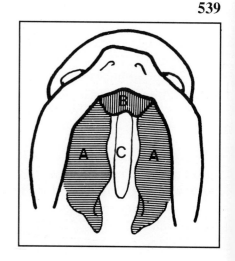

539 During the sixth week of development, two lateral palatal shelves (**A**) develop behind the primary palate (**B**) from the maxillary processes. A secondary nasal septum (**C**) grows down from the roof of the stomodeum behind the primary nasal septum, thus dividing the nasal part of the oronasal cavity into two. It seems that the mesenchyme within the palatal shelves originates from the neural crest.

540

540 Coronal section through the developing head during the seventh week of development showing the palatal shelves (A). Note that the oral part of the oronasal cavity becomes completely filled by the developing tongue (**B**). Growth of the palatal shelves continues such that they come to lie vertically. Two peaks of DNA synthesis occur as the palatal shelves are formed: during initial shelf outgrowth and during vertical shelf elongation. The reason for mammalian shelves forming with a vertical orientation is unknown. It has been suggested that the potential space in the oronasal cavity is insufficient because of the evolution of a large tongue in mammals. (Masson's trichrome; × 30)

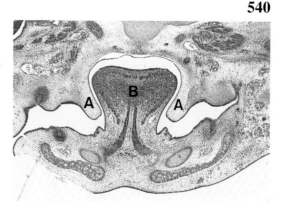

541 During the eighth week of development, the stomodeum enlarges, the tongue 'drops' and the vertically-inclined palatal shelves become horizontal. It has been suggested that the descent of the tongue is related to mandibular growth and/or a change in the shape of the tongue. On becoming horizontal, the palatal shelves contact each other (and the secondary nasal septum) in the midline to form the definitive or secondary palate. The shelves contact the primary palate anteriorly so that the oronasal cavity becomes subdivided into its constituent oral and nasal cavities. **B**, primary palate. **A**, palatal shelves forming secondary palate.

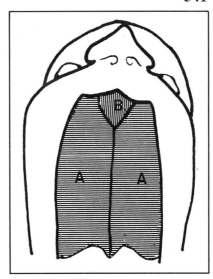

542 Coronal section through developing oronasal regions following contact of the palatal shelves (A) and secondary nasal septum (B). After contact, the medial edge epithelia of the two shelves fuse to form a midline epithelial seam (**C**). Subsequently, this degenerates so that mesenchymal continuity is established across the now intact and horizontal secondary palate. Fusion of the palatal processes is complete by the 12th week of development. Behind the secondary nasal septum, the palatal shelves fuse to form the soft palate and uvula. **D**, developing bone of maxilla. (Masson's trichrome; × 30)

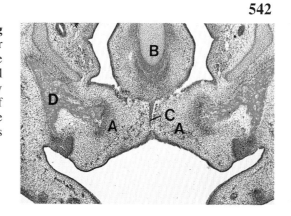

Clefts of the palate, like those of the lip, are multifactorial malformations, involving both genetic (polygenic) and environmental factors. Clefts may result from disturbances of any of the processes involved during palatogenesis (i.e. from defective palatal shelf growth; delayed shelf elevation or failure of elevation; defective shelf fusion or degeneration of the midline epithelial seam; or failure of mesenchymal consolidation and/or differentiation). Recent research on palatogenesis has concentrated on two main events: palatal shelf elevation and the initial stage of fusion of the shelves.

Palatal shelf elevation

Several mechanisms have been proposed to account for the rapid movement of the palatal shelves from the vertical to the horizontal position. Although it was once thought that extrinsic forces might be responsible (e.g. forces derived from the tongue or jaw movements), research has primarily focused on the search for a force intrinsic to the palatal shelf. It has been proposed that the intrinsic shelf elevation force might develop as a result of hydration of ground substance components (principally hyaluronan) in the shelf mesenchyme, or as a result of mesenchymal cell activity. Of course, the intrinsic shelf elevating force might be multifactorial, although there is as yet no experimental evidence to support what otherwise might be considered this common-sense view.

543

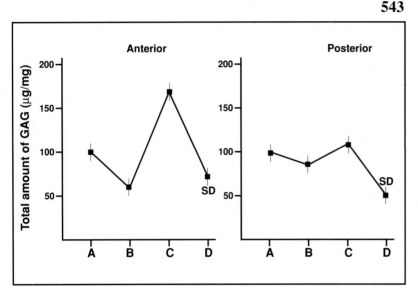

543 Graphs illustrating the changing amounts of glycosaminoglycans (GAG) during development of the anterior (presumptive hard) and posterior (presumptive soft) palates. Stage A is immediately prior to shelf elevation; Stage B is immediately after shelf elevation; Stage C is the stage of shelf fusion and early histogenesis; Stage D represents a stage of marked histogenesis after fusion. Note that the most significant changes occur after elevation and that during the time of elevation there are no differences between the anterior and posterior regions of the shelves even though, in the statistical species studied here, the posterior region of the shelf does not elevate but grows initially with a horizontal disposition.

544

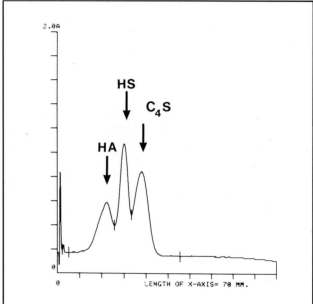

544 Densiometric scan of electrophoretograms showing the GAG within palatal shelves. Three GAG types are found *in vivo*: hyaluronan (**HA**), heparan sulphate (**HS**) and chondroitin 4-sulphate (**C$_4$S**). If palatal shelves are cultured *in vitro*, dermatan sulphate is also present, highlighting the difficulties of extrapolating from the findings of tissue culture to the *in vivo* situation.

545

545 Section through a vertical (pre-elevation) palatal shelf (A) stained using the hyaluronectin/anti-hyaluronectin technique. Note the intense staining for hyaluronan within the palatal shelf mesenchyme. It has been proposed that hyaluronan is a GAG involved in shelf elevation because it is a highly electrostatically charged, open coil molecule which is capable of binding up to 10 times its own weight in water. (× 30)

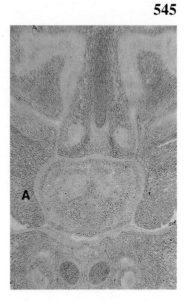

546 Graphs showing the changing concentrations of hyaluronan within the anterior and posterior regions of palatal shelves. The stages of palatogenesis (**A–D**) are the same as those described for **543**. Note that, statistically there is significantly more hyaluronan in the shelves immediately before elevation than immediately after elevation. However, the data does not agree with some reports that there is less hyaluronan posteriorly than anteriorly, and again the pattern of change in hyaluronan is similar both anteriorly and posteriorly even though the posterior region does not undergo elevation to reach the horizontal.

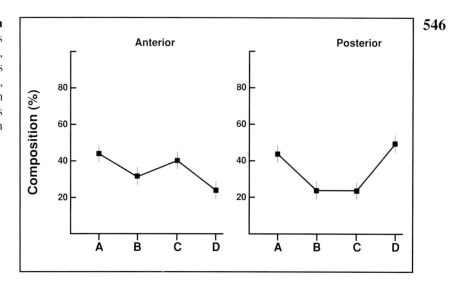

547 Transverse section of a palatal shelf stained immunocyto-chemically with antibodies against Type I collagen. Note the stout bundles of collagen which run down the centre of the shelf (**A**) and which are orientated from the base (**B**) towards the tip (**C**). It has been suggested that the shelf elevation force is directed by these collagen fibres. (× 240)

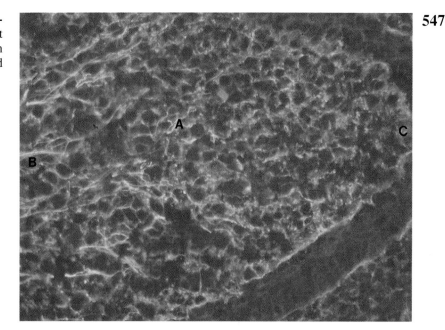

548 Silver staining of the palatal shelves (A) to assess the degree of activity of the mesenchymal cells. It has been reported that a specific number of mesenchymal cells are required within the palatal shelves for elevation to proceed. It has also been proposed that cellular activity (e.g. cell migration and/or contraction) might be responsible for generating the intrinsic shelf elevation force. To assess whether cell activity changes at different stages of palatogenesis, an Ag-NOR staining technique has been employed which produces grains in the nucleolar region (see inset), the number and configuration of which reflect the overall degree of protein synthesis by the cells. This staining procedure confirmed that the rate of protein synthesis during palatogenesis is high, is higher pre-elevation than post-elevation, and is higher still during later stages of histogenesis. It further shows that protein synthesis is severely depressed during cleft formation, but the technique is unable to demonstrate major differences between anterior and posterior regions. (Silver stain; × 45)

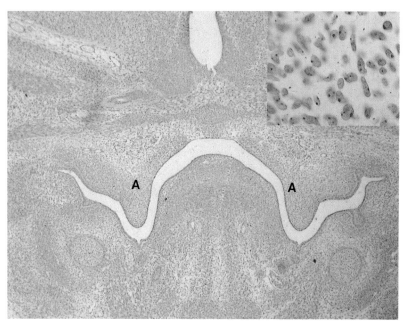

237

Fusion of the palatal shelves

Once the palatal shelves have elevated, they make contact (initially in the middle third of the palate) and adhere by means of a 'sticky' glycoprotein which coats the surface of the medial edge epithelia of the shelves. Additionally, the epithelial cells develop desmosomes and consequently an epithelial seam is formed. The adherence of the medial edge epithelia is specific, as palatal epithelia will not fuse with epithelia from other sites (e.g. the tongue). This may be related to the fact that the proteins associated with the formation of desmosomes (i.e. desmoplakin) appear specifically on the cell membranes of the medial edge epithelia just prior to shelf contact.

549

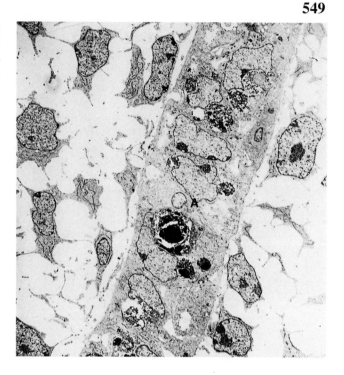

549 The midline epithelial seam for fusing palatal shelves. Within the epithelial cells (**A**) are numerous lysosomes. An intact basal lamina lies on either side of the epithelial seam. (TEM; × 3,900)

550

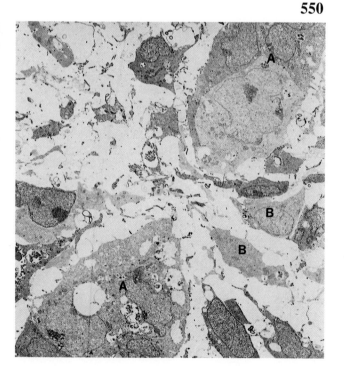

550 Disruption of the epithelial seam (A) with penetration by mesenchymal cells (B). (TEM; × 3,900)

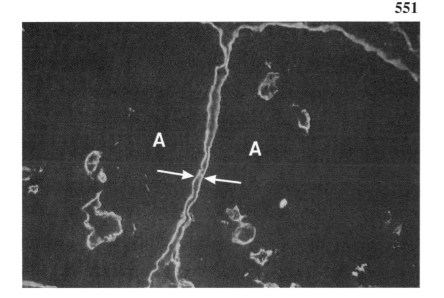

551 Fusing palatal shelves (A) immunocytochemically stained with antibodies against Type IV collagen found in basal lamina (*arrowed*). Note that the lamina remains intact during the early stages of fusion. (× 110)

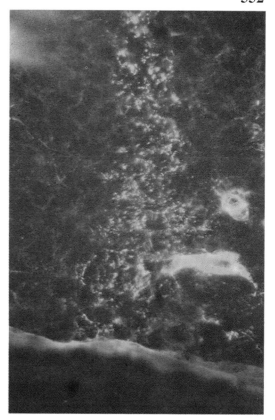

552 A later stage of fusion of the palatal shelves immunocytochemically stained for Type IV collagen showing that, with migration of the epithelial cells into the mesenchyme, the midline epithelial seam is disrupted and the migrating cells initially carry with them fragments of the disrupted basal lamina. Fibrils comprising tenascin and Type III collagen have been shown to run at right angles to the basal lamina and may provide guiding pathways for the migrating epithelial cells. Recent evidence indicates that the events leading to the breakdown of the epithelial seam occur in single isolated palatal shelves and therefore do not depend upon shelf contact. (× 180)

Almost as soon as the epithelial seam is formed, it thins to a layer two or three cells thick. This thinning may be the result of three processes. First, the seam is thinned by growth of the palate (in terms of oronasal height) and by epithelial cell migration from the region of the seam onto the oral and nasal aspects of the palate. Second, there is programmed cell death in the seam. This is shown by the finding that DNA synthesis ceases in the medial edge epithelial cells one day prior to shelf contact. Furthermore, cyclic AMP increases just before shelf fusion and exogenous cyclic AMP is associated with precocious cell death in the medial edge epithelia. It has also been shown that epidermal growth factor inhibits medial edge cell death and that this inhibition is blocked by exogenous cyclic AMP. Care must be taken, however, when interpreting the effects of cyclic AMP since physiologically it is an intracellular messenger and may therefore be mediating differential gene expression triggered by other events occurring at the cell surface. Third, there is good evidence that some of the epithelial cells migrate from the seam into the palatal shelf mesenchyme and differentiate into cells indistinguishable from the mesenchymal cells. Indeed, it is well known that epithelial cells can migrate and differentiate into mesenchymal-like cells in other circumstances during development.

There have been many experiments to help clarify the nature of the epithelial–mesenchymal interactions during fusion of the palatal shelves. In the main, these experiments have involved the separation and then the recombination in culture of the epithelial and mesenchymal components of the shelves.

Overall, these experiments have shown that, as with epithelial–mesenchymal interactions for tooth development (see pages 254–256), it is the mesenchyme that signals epithelial differentiation and behaviour. The nature of this signal is controversial.

553a

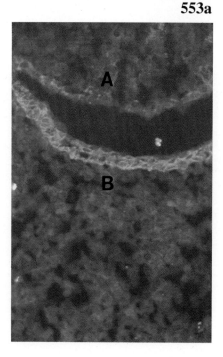

553a The medial edge epithelia of palatal shelves stained immunocytochemically for Type IX collagen before shelf elevation. Although it was once proposed that the palatal mesenchyme could signal epithelial differentiation directly by cell to cell contact, mesenchymal–epithelial cell contacts are very rare during palatogenesis. Recent evidence indicates that extracellular matrix molecules may provide the signal, and work has been undertaken to assess the role of Type IX collagen. This section shows that, at the earliest stages before shelf elevation, the medial edges of the palatal shelves (**A**) stain poorly for Type IX collagen compared with floor of the mouth epithelia (**B**). (× 280)

553b

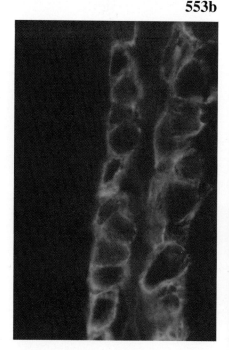

553b The medial edge epithelia of palatal shelves stained immunocytochemically for Type IX collagen at a time when medial edge epithelial differentiation occurs as determined by recombination experiments. Note that at this stage Type IX collagen appears around the surfaces of the medial edge epithelial cells. Present-day thinking suggests that the control of the synthesis of Type IX collagen is influenced by growth factors. (× 280)

554 Immunocytochemical staining with antibodies against epidermal growth factor receptors of the mesenchymal cells adjacent to the midline epithelial seam of fusing palatal shelves. Epidermal growth factor (EGF), or its embryonic homologue known as transforming growth factor α (TGFα) is known to inhibit palatal medial edge epithelial cell death in the presence of mesenchyme. Furthermore, it has been shown that the synthesis of extracellular matrix molecules (including Type IX collagen) is stimulated by factors such as TGFα and TGFβ and is inhibited by fibroblast growth factors (FGF). When palatal shelves are organ-cultured with EGF, the medial edge of the palatal shelf shows a nipple-like bulge, medial edge epithelial cell death is absent, and the mesenchyme possesses increased quantities of extracellular matrix molecules. It has been proposed, therefore, that the palatal shelf mesenchyme produces growth factors which either directly signal epithelial differentiation or, by stimulating extracellular matrix production, indirectly influence differentiation through this matrix. The photomicrograph suggests that EGF receptors (appearing here as white dots, *arrows*) show regional heterogeneity and that the receptors only appear beneath the medial edge of the shelves when the epithelial seam (**A**) is degenerating. (× 85)

554

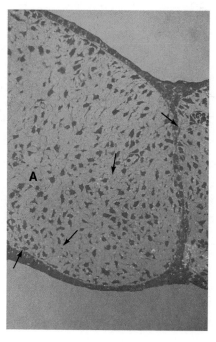

The hard palate ossifies intramembranously from four centres of ossification, one in each developing maxilla and one in each developing palatine bone. The maxillary ossification centre lies above the developing deciduous canine tooth germ and appears in the eighth week of development (**556**). The palatine centres of ossification are situated in the region forming the future perpendicular plate and appear in the eighth week of development. Incomplete ossification of the palate from these centres defines the median and transverse palatine sutures. There does not appear to be a separate centre of ossification for the primary palate (the premaxilla).

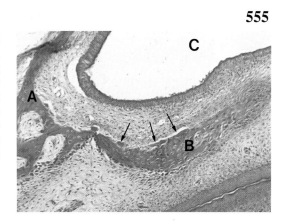

555

555 Coronal section through the developing hard palate showing early ossification. A, developing body of maxilla; **B**, bone extending from body into palate; **C**, nasal cavity. The expansion of the nasal cavities is reflected in resorption of bone at the upper border of the palate and deposition at its lower border. Note the osteoclasts (*arrowed*) on the nasal surface and osteoblasts on the oral surface of the palatal bone. (Masson's trichrome; × 80)

Malformations of palatogenesis may result in the appearance of clefts. The mildest form of cleft is that affecting the uvula, such a disturbance occurring relatively late in the process of palatal fusion. Disturbances occurring during the early phases of palatal fusion can result in a more extensive cleft involving most of the secondary palate. Should the cleft involve the primary palate, it may extend to the right and/or left of the incisive foramen to include the alveolus, passing between the lateral incisor and canine teeth. Cleft palate may be associated with cleft lip, though the two conditions are independently determined. Dental malformations are commonly associated with a cleft involving the alveolus. A submucous cleft describes a condition where the palatal mucosa is intact, but the bone/musculature of the palate is deficient beneath the mucosa.

556a

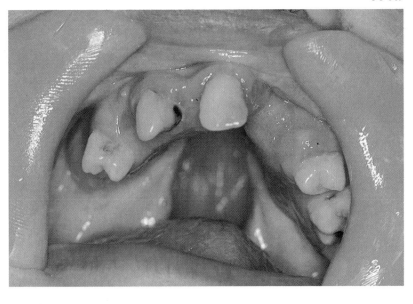

556b

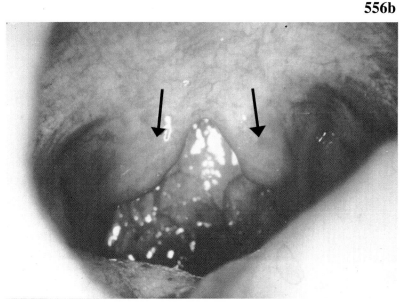

556 Cleft palate (556a) and cleft uvula (556b).

Development of the jaws

The mandible

The mandible initially develops intramembranously but its subsequent growth is related to the appearance of secondary cartilages (the condylar cartilage being the most important).

The developing mandible is preceded by the appearance of a rod of cartilage belonging to the first branchial arch. This is known as Meckel's cartilage and it first appears at about the sixth week of intra-uterine life.

Meckel's cartilage makes little contribution to the adult mandible but provides a framework around which the bone of the mandible forms. The mandible first appears as a band of dense fibrous tissue on the anterolateral aspect of Meckel's cartilage. During the seventh week of intra-uterine life, a centre of ossification appears in this fibrous tissue at a site close to the future mental foramen. Form this centre, bone formation spreads rapidly backwards, forwards and upwards around the inferior alveolar nerve and its terminal branches, the incisive and mental nerves. Further spread of the developing bone in a forward and backward direction produces a plate of bone on the lateral side of Meckel's cartilage which corresponds to the future body of the mandible and which extends towards the midline where it comes to lie in close relationship with the bone forming on the opposite side. However, the two plates of bone remain separated at the mandibular symphysis by fibrous tissue.

557

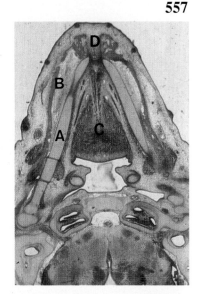

557 Meckel's cartilage (A) around which the bone of the mandible (B) is forming in membrane. This is a horizontal section through the developing mandible during the eighth week of intrauterine life. Meckel's cartilage, the cartilage of the first branchial arch, extends from the cartilaginous otic capsule to a midline symphysis (**D**) where initially it is separated from its fellow of the opposite side by mesenchyme. **C**, tongue. (Masson's trichrome; × 12)

558

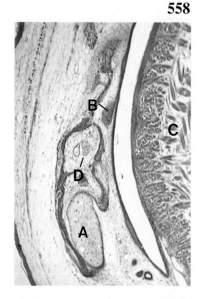

558 Transverse section through the early developing mandible (8th week of development). At this stage, only a small amount of mandibular bone has formed intramembranously on the lateral aspect of Meckel's cartilage (**A**). Note the beginnings of tooth development in this region indicated by the dental lamina (**B**). **C**, tongue. **D**, neurovascular bundle. (Masson's trichrome; × 60)

559

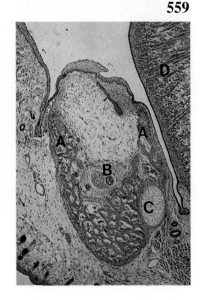

559 A later stage in the development of the body of the mandible. Continued bone formation has increased the size of the mandible. The alveolar process (**A**) grows to surround the developing tooth germ. The developing teeth share the same common crypt as the neurovascular bundle (**B**). Note that Meckel's cartilage (**C**) is now comparatively small, though it still lies medial to the developing mandibular bone. **D**, developing tongue. (Masson's trichrome; × 25)

560

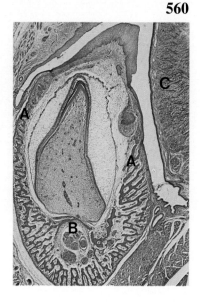

560 Even later stage in the development of the body of the mandible. Meckel's cartilage has been resorbed. The neurovascular bundle (**B**) is now contained within its own bony canal and there has been considerable development of the alveolar process (**A**). **C**, developing tongue. (Masson's trichrome; × 25)

Although Meckel's cartilage contributes no significant tissue to the developing mandible, nodular remnants of cartilage may be seen in the region of the symphysis until birth, and in its most dorsal part Meckel's cartilage ossifies to form the ear ossicles (i.e. the malleus and incus). Behind the body of the mandible, the perichondrium of Meckel's cartilage persists as the sphenomandibular and sphenomalleolar ligaments. The sphenomandibular ligament ossifies at its sites of attachment to form the lingula of the mandible and the spine of the sphenoid bone.

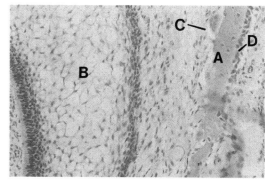

561 Development of the mandibular alveolus (A) in the region of a developing tooth (B). As the developing tooth germ reaches the early bell stage, developing bone becomes closely related to it to form the alveolus. The size of the alveolus is dependent upon the size of the growing tooth germ. Note that resorption is occurring on the inner wall of the alveolus (indicated by osteoclasts lying in Howship's lacunae, **C**) while, on the outer wall of the alveolus, bone is being deposited (indicated by osteoblasts (**D**) lining an osteoid seam). The developing teeth therefore come to lie in a trough of bone. Later the teeth become separated from each other by the development of interdental septa. With the onset of root formation, interradicular bone develops in multirooted teeth. (Decalcified section; Masson's trichrome; × 110)

The ramus of the mandible is first mapped out as a condensation of fibrocellular tissue which, though continuous with the developing body of the mandible, is positioned some way laterally from Meckel's cartilage. Further development of the ramus is associated with a backward spread of ossification from the body and by the appearance of a number of secondary cartilages. Between the 10th and 14th week *in utero*, three secondary cartilages develop within the growing mandible. The largest and most important of these is the condylar cartilage which, as its name suggests, appears beneath the fibrous articular layer of the future condyle (**509** and **563**). By proliferation and subsequent ossification of the cartilage, it is thought to serve as an important centre of growth for the mandible, functioning up to about the 20th year of life. Less important transitory secondary cartilages are seen associated with the coronoid process and in the region of the mandibular symphysis.

562 The appearance of the developing jaws of a human foetus (14 weeks *i.u.*).

A Body of mandible.
B Ramus of mandible.
C Secondary condylar cartilage.
D Secondary coronoid cartilage.
E Frontal bone.
F Parietal bone.
G Occipital bone.
H Squamous portion of temporal bone.
I Maxilla.

(Cleared, alizarin red preparation; × 5)

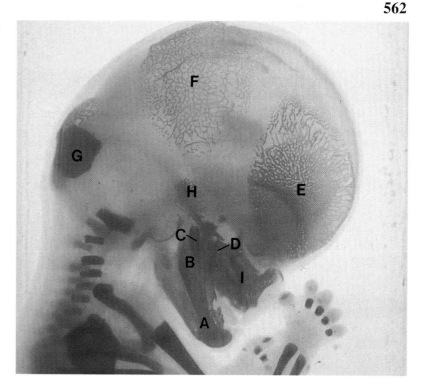

The temporomandibular joint develops from mesenchyme lying between the developing mandibular condyle below and the temporal bone above, which develop intramembranously. During the 12th week of intra-uterine life, two clefts appear in the mesenchyme, producing the upper and lower joint cavities, the remaining intervening mesenchyme becoming the intra-articular disc. The joint capsule develops from a condensation of mesenchyme surrounding the developing joint. At birth the mandibular fossa is flat and there is no articular eminence, the latter only becoming prominent following the eruption of the deciduous dentition.

563

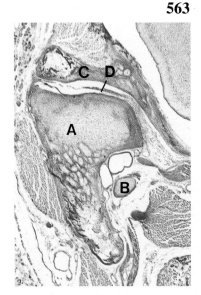

563 The early developing condylar cartilage (A) and temporomandibular joint. B, Meckel's cartilage; **C**, developing bone of mandibular fossa; **D**, part of developing articular disc of temporomandibular joint. (Decalcified section; Masson's trichrome; × 20)

564a

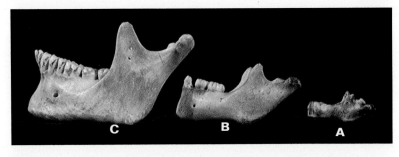

564b

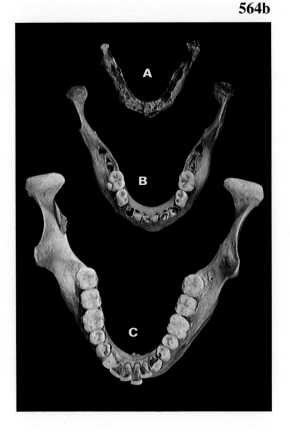

564 The postnatal development of the mandible illustrated by lateral (**564a**) and occlusal (**564b**) views of the mandible at birth (**A**), at 6 years (**B**) and in an adult (**C**). The ratio of body to ramus is greater at birth than in the adult, indicating a proportional increase with time in the development of the ramus. At birth, there is no distinct chin and the two halves of the mandible are separated by the mandibular symphysis. Ossification of the symphysis is complete during the second year, the two halves of the mandible uniting to form a single bone. The chin becomes most prominent after puberty, especially in the male. There is some evidence that the angle of the mandible decreases from birth to adulthood.

Some indication of the directions of growth of the mandible can be obtained by superimposing traces of the neonatal and adult mandibles. Indeed, there is some evidence that the region around the mental foramen is a 'fixed' point for such an endeavour.

565 Superimposed neonatal and adult mandibles. Note that growth of the mandible results in posterior relocation of the ramus of the mandible.

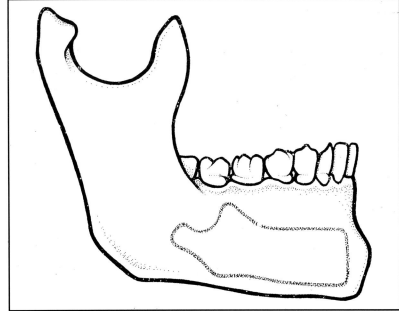

Growth of the mandible occurs by the remodelling of bone. In general terms, increase in the height of the body occurs primarily by formation of alveolar bone, though some bone is also deposited along the lower border of the mandible. Increase in the length of the mandible is accomplished by bone deposition on the posterior surface of the ramus with compensatory resorption on its anterior surface, accompanied by deposition of bone on the posterior surface of the coronoid process and resorption on the anterior surface of the condyle. Increase in width of the mandible is produced by deposition of bone on the outer surface of the mandible and resorption on the inner surface.

There is some controversy concerning the role of the condylar cartilages in mandibular growth. One view states that continued proliferation of this cartilage is primarily responsible for the increase in both the mandibular length and the height of the ramus. Alternatively, it has been suggested that proliferation of the condylar cartilage is a response to growth and not its cause. The latter view has been supported by experiments showing that mandibular growth is relatively unaffected following condylectomy, providing normal mandibular function is maintained.

Although the mandible is a single bone, it may be thought of as a number of skeletal units each associated with one or more soft tissue 'functional matrices'. The behaviour of these matrices primarily determines the growth of each skeletal unit. For example, the coronoid process forms a skeletal unit acted upon by the temporalis muscle. Sectioning of the temporalis muscle during early mandibular development may result in atrophy or complete absence of a coronoid process in the adult mandible. Similarly, the alveolar process is influenced by the teeth, the condyle by the lateral pterygoid muscle, the ramus by the medial pterygoid and masseter muscles and the body by the neurovascular bundle.

The maxilla

As with the mandible, the maxilla develops intramembranously. The centre of ossification appears during the 8th week of intra-uterine life close to the site of the developing deciduous canine tooth. Unlike the mandible, maxillary growth and development is not related to the appearance of secondary cartilages. Because of the maxilla's position in the developing skull, this jaw's growth is influenced by the development of the orbital, nasal, and oral cavities.

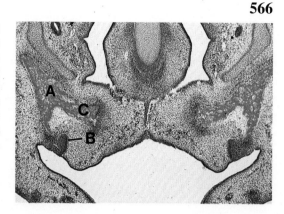

566 The early developing maxilla (A) in the region of the developing deciduous canine (B). From this site, ossification spreads throughout the developing maxilla into its growing processes (i.e. palatine (C), zygomatic, frontal and alveolar processes). See page 241 for the ossification of the palatine processes, and **562** for the appearance of the developing maxilla seen in a cleared alizarin red preparation. (Decalcified section; Masson's trichrome; × 35)

At one time it was thought that the incisor-bearing part of the maxilla, which develops from the frontonasal process, had a separate centre of ossification. It was consequently called the premaxilla. However, it is now clear that ossification spreads from the body of the maxilla into its incisor-bearing component.

Growth of the maxilla occurs by bone remodelling (i.e. surface deposition of bone with associated resorption) and by sutural growth. Among the agents which provide the forces separating the maxilla from the adjacent bones — thus permitting growth at the sutures — are the growing eyeballs, cartilaginous nasal septum and orbital pad of fat. Thus, growth of the maxilla is not an isolated phenomenon but occurs in association with the development of the orbital, nasal and oral cavities. It has been suggested that the growing nasal septum pulls the maxilla forward by means of a septo-premaxillary ligament which runs from the anterior border of the nasal septum postero-inferiorly towards the anterior nasal spine and interpremaxillary suture. As in the lower jaw (page 245), growth in height of the maxilla is related to the development of the alveolar process. It is difficult to determine how much of the adult alveolus is the result of bone deposition and how much is due to bodily displacement of the maxilla. Studies using metal implants suggest that each method of growth contributes equal amounts. Increase in height of the nasal cavity is associated with resorption of bone on the upper surface of the palatine process of the maxilla and deposition of bone on the lower surface (see **555**).

The maxillary sinus appears as an outpocketing of the mucosa of the middle meatus of the nose at the beginning of the fourth month of intra-uterine life. Though small at birth, the maxillary sinus is identifiable radiologically. After birth, the maxillary sinus enlarges with the growing maxilla, though it is only fully developed following the eruption of the permanent dentition. Forward growth of the whole face (including the maxillae) is dependent upon growth of the spheno-occipital synchondrosis (**510**).

Development of the tongue

567 The schema of tongue primordia. 567a shows the ventral wall of the pharynx at the fourth week of intrauterine life. **567b** illustrates the developing tongue at the fifth month *i.u.* The numbers **1–4** indicate the positions of the branchial arches. The anterior two-thirds of the tongue develops from three swellings, the lateral lingual swellings (**A**) and the midline tuberculum impar (**B**). Each is formed by proliferation of mesenchyme beneath the endodermal lining of the first branchial arch. The posterior third of the tongue develops from a single midline swelling, the copula (**C**), which is derived mainly from the third branchial arch with a small contribution from the fourth arch. The copula overgrows the second arch to merge with the first arch swellings.

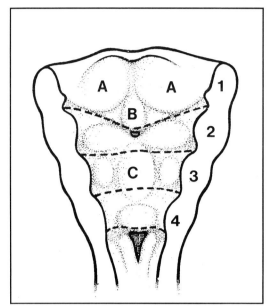

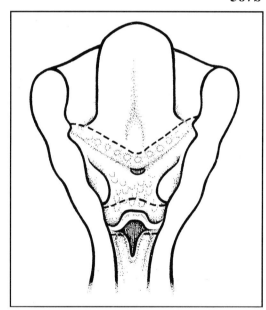

The diverse embryological origin of the tongue explains its diverse sensory supply (**173**). General sensation to the anterior two-thirds of the tongue is supplied by the lingual nerve, a nerve of the first branchial arch. General sensation and taste to the posterior third of the tongue is supplied by the glossopharyngeal and superior laryngeal nerves, the nerves of the third and fourth arches. The perception of taste in the anterior two-thirds of the tongue is associated with the chorda tympani nerve. The chorda tympani is a branch of the facial nerve, the nerve of the second branchial arch. Since this arch does not contribute tissue to the anterior part of the tongue, in this situation it is termed a pretrematic nerve. The muscles of the tongue develop primarily from occipital somites which migrate into the developing tongue carrying their nerve supply, the hypoglossal nerve, with them.

The thyroid gland develops between the tuberculum impar and the copula. On the fully formed tongue, this site is demarcated by a small pit, the foramen caecum (**12**).

Early tooth development

Tooth development can be divided into three overlapping phases: initiation, morphogenesis, and histogenesis. During initiation, the sites of the future teeth are established with the appearance of tooth germs along an invagination of the oral epithelium called the dental lamina. During morphogenesis, the shape of the tooth is determined by a combination of cell proliferation and cell movement. During histogenesis, differentiation of cells (begun during morphogenesis) proceeds to give rise to the fully formed dental tissues, both mineralised (i.e. enamel, dentine and cementum) and unmineralised (i.e. dental pulp and periodontium). Tooth development is characterised by complex interactions between epithelial and mesenchymal tissues.

568

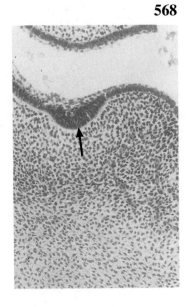

568 Primary epithelial band (*arrowed*). The first histological signs of tooth development are the appearance of a condensation of mesenchymal tissue and of capillary networks beneath the presumptive dental epithelium of the primitive oral cavity. By the sixth week of development, the oral epithelium thickens and invaginates into this mesenchyme to form the primary epithelial band. (H & E; × 115)

There is now experimental evidence that the mesenchymal cells adjacent to the dental lamina are ectomesenchymal (neural crest) in origin, having migrated into the jaws from the margins of the neural tube.

569

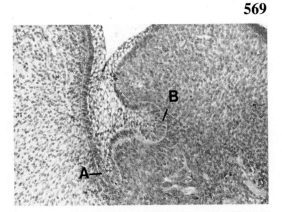

569 By the seventh week, the primary epithelial band divides into two processes: a buccally located vestibular lamina (A) and a lingually situated dental lamina (B). The vestibular lamina contributes to the development of the vestibule, delineating the lips and cheeks from the tooth-bearing regions. The dental lamina contributes to the development of the teeth. (H & E; × 120)

570

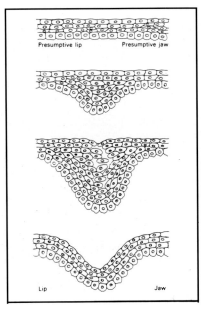

570 Formation of the vestibule of the oral cavity. The cells of the vestibular lamina proliferate. Subsequently, there is degeneration of the central epithelial cells, which results in the formation of a sulcus, the vestibule.

571

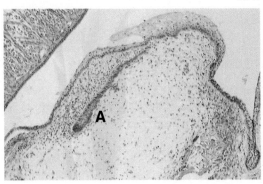

571 Further development of the dental lamina (A) is characterised by an increase in length, although it is not known whether this results from active invagination of the lamina or upward proliferation of the mesenchyme. (Masson's trichrome; × 55)

572 By the 8th week, a series of swellings develop on the deep surface of the dental lamina (*model*). The complete dental lamina of the lower jaw is shown as the green structure and the epithelial swellings indicating early developing tooth germs are arrowed. Note that the dental lamina appears as an arch-shaped band of tissue which follows the line of the vestibular fold (**A**). Although not shown on the model, each epithelial swelling is almost completely surrounded by a mesenchymal condensation.

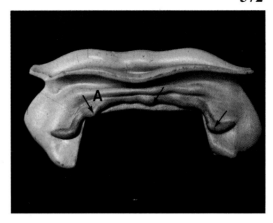

For descriptive purposes, tooth germs are classified into bud, cap and bell stages according to the degree of morphodifferentiation and histodifferentiation of their epithelial components (enamel organs). Leading up to the late bell stage, the tooth germ changes rapidly both in its size and shape; the cells are dividing and morphogenetic processes are taking place. At the late bell stage, hard tissues are forming and further growth of the crown is related mainly to the deposition of enamel, the rate of cell division being reduced.

573 Bud stage. The enamel organ (**A**) in the bud stage appears as a simple, spherical to ovoid, epithelial condensation which is poorly morphodifferentiated and histodifferentiated. Compared with the overlying oral epithelium, however, the cells of the tooth bud have a higher RNA content, a lower glycogen content and an increased oxidative enzyme activity. Note the surrounding mesenchymal condensation (**B**). As yet, it has not been established whether the epithelial bud is induced by the underlying mesenchyme. Nevertheless, the successful development of the tooth germ relies upon a complex interaction of the mesenchymal and epithelial components since, should these be separated and cultured individually, neither component will differentiate further. The epithelial component is separated from the adjacent mesenchyme by a basement membrane. (Masson's trichrome; × 60)

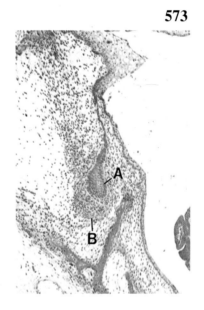

574 Early cap stage. By the 11th week, morphogenesis has progressed, the deeper surface of the enamel organ invaginating to form a cap-shaped structure. In this section, both maxillary and mandibular cap stages are shown (*arrowed*), each enamel organ appearing relatively poorly histodifferentiated. However, a greater distinction develops between the more rounded cells in the central portion of the enamel organ and the peripheral cells which are becoming arranged to form the external and internal enamel epithelia. **A**, Meckel's cartilage; **B**, developing tongue. (Masson's trichrome; × 32)

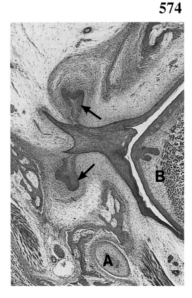

575 Late cap stage. By about 12½ weeks, the central cells of the enlarging enamel organ have become separated though maintaining contact by desmosomes. The resulting intercellular spaces contain significant quantities of glycosaminoglycans. The resulting tissue is termed the stellate reticulum (**A**), although it is not fully developed until the later bell stage. The cells of the external enamel epithelium (**B**) remain cuboidal whereas those of the internal enamel epithelium (**C**) become more columnar. The latter show an increase in RNA content and hydrolytic and oxidative enzyme activity while the mesenchymal cells continue to proliferate and surround the enamel organ. The part of the mesenchyme lying beneath the internal enamel epithelium is termed the dental papilla (**D**) while that surrounding the tooth germ forms the dental follicle (**E**). (H & E; × 75)

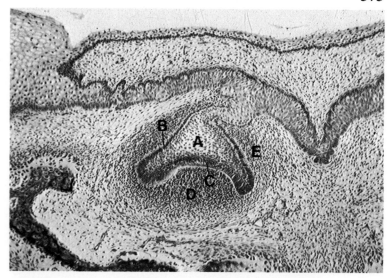

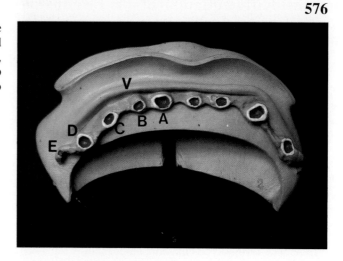

576 The arrangement of deciduous tooth germs at 13 weeks on the dental lamina of the lower jaw (*model*). The dental lamina is represented by the green, arch-shaped band on which the tooth germs (red) are aligned, five in each quadrant. At this time, most of the tooth germs are at the cap stage. The labelling identifies the developing deciduous teeth according to the Zsigmondy system. **V**, vestibular fold.

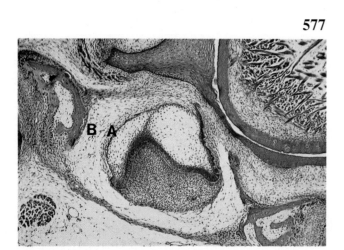

577 Early bell stage. By the 14th week, further morphodifferentiation and histodifferentiation of the tooth germ leads to the early bell stage. The configuration of the internal enamel epithelium broadly maps out the occlusal pattern of the tooth. This folding is related to differential mitosis along the internal enamel epithelium. The future cusps and incisal margins are sites of precocious cell maturation associated with cessation of mitosis, while areas corresponding to the fissures and margins of the tooth remain mitotically active. Thus, cusp height is related more to continued downward growth at the margins and fissures rather than to upward extension of the cusps.

Interposed between the enamel organ and the wall of the developing bony crypt is the mesenchymal tissue of the dental follicle, which is generally considered to have three layers. The inner investing layer (**A**) is a vascular, fibrocellular condensation, three to four cells thick, immediately surrounding the tooth germ; the nuclei of the cells tend to be elongated circumferentially. The outer layer of the dental follicle (**B**) is represented by a vascular mesenchymal layer which lines the developing alveolus. Between the two layers is loose connective tissue with no marked concentration of blood vessels. There is evidence to suggest that the cells of the inner layer of the dental follicle may be derived from the neural crest. (Masson's trichrome; × 45)

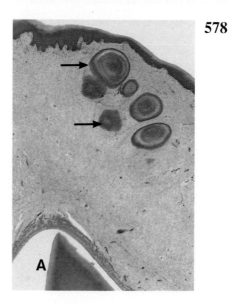

578 Epithelial pearls (of Serres). During the bell stage of development, the enamel organ (**A**) loses its connection with the oral epithelium as the dental lamina breaks down. At the same time, the dental lamina between tooth germs also degenerates. Remnants of the dental lamina (*arrowed*) may remain in the adult mucosa as clumps of resting cells which may contain keratin and can be involved in the aetiology of cysts. (H & E; × 8)

579 A high-power view of the early bell shows the high degree of histodifferentiation which has been achieved. The enamel organ shows four distinct layers:

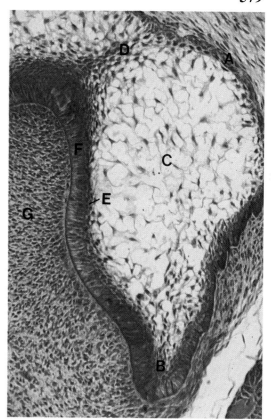

- **External enamel epithelium (A).** As its name suggests, this forms the outer layer of cuboidal cells which limits the enamel organ. It is separated from the surrounding mesenchymal tissue by a basement membrane 1–2μm thick which, at the ultrastructural level, corresponds to the much narrower basal lamina with associated hemidesmosomes (**467**). The external enamel epithelia cells contain large, centrally placed nuclei. Ultrastructurally, they contain relatively small amounts of the intracellular organelles associated with protein synthesis (e.g. endoplasmic reticulum, Golgi material, mitochondria) and they contact each other via desmosomes and gap junctions. The external enamel epithelium is thought to be involved in the maintenance of the shape of the enamel organ and in the exchange of substances between the enamel organ and the environment. The cervical loop (**B**), at which there is considerable mitotic activity, lies where the external enamel epithelium is continuous with the internal enamel epithelium.

- **Stellate reticulum (C).** This tissue is most fully developed at the bell stage. The intercellular spaces become fluid-filled, presumably related to osmotic effects arising from the high concentration of glycosaminoglycans. The cells are star-shaped, with bodies containing conspicuous nuclei and many branching processes. In addition to glycosaminoglycans, the cells also contain alkaline phosphatase but have only small amounts of RNA and glycogen. Within the stellate reticulum can be seen a 'structure' termed the enamel cord (**D**) (see also **585**). The main function ascribed to the stellate reticulum is a mechanical one. This relates to the protection of the underlying dental tissues against physical disturbance and to the maintenance of tooth shape. It has been suggested that the hydrostatic pressure generated within the stellate reticulum is in equilibrium with that of the dental papilla, allowing the proliferative pattern of the intervening internal enamel epithelium to determine crown morphogenesis. However, a change in either of these pressures might lead to a change in the outline of the internal enamel epithelium and this could be important for crown morphogenesis.

- **Stratum intermedium (E).** This first appears at the bell stage and consists of two or three layers of flattened cells lying over the internal enamel epithelium (and its derivatives). The cells of the stratum intermedium resemble the cells of the stellate reticulum, although their intercellular spaces are smaller and the cells contain more alkaline phosphatase. It has been suggested that the stratum intermedium is concerned with the synthesis of proteins, the transport of materials to and from the ameloblasts, and/or the concentration of materials.

- **Internal enamel epithelium (F).** The cells of this layer are columnar at the bell stage but, beginning at the regions associated with the future cusp tips (i.e. the sites of initial enamel formation), the cells become elongated. The internal enamel epithelial cells are rich in RNA but, unlike the stratum intermedium and stellate reticulum, do not contain alkaline phosphatase. Desmosomes connect the internal enamel epithelial cells and also link this layer to the stratum intermedium. The internal enamel epithelium is separated from the peripheral cells of the dental papilla by a basement membrane and a cell-free zone 1–2μm wide.

The differentiation of the dental papilla (**G**) is less striking than that of the enamel organ. Up until the late bell stage, the dental papilla consists of closely packed mesenchymal cells with only a few delicate extracellular fibrils. Histochemically, the dental papilla becomes rich in glycosaminoglycans. (Masson's trichrome; × 120)

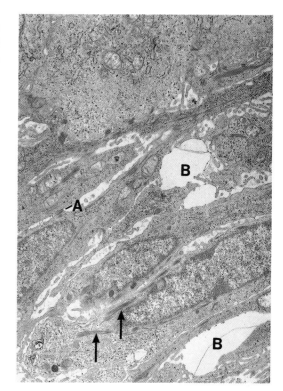

580 Stellate reticulum. Ultrastructurally, the cells of this layer possess little endoplasmic reticulum and few mitochondria. However, there is a relatively well-developed Golgi complex which, together with the presence of microvilli on the cell surface, has been interpreted as indicating that the cells contribute to the secretion of the extracellular material. Numerous tonofilaments (*arrowed*) are present within the cytoplasm, and desmosomes (**A**) and gap junctions are present between the cells. **B**, intercellular space. (TEM; × 6,380)

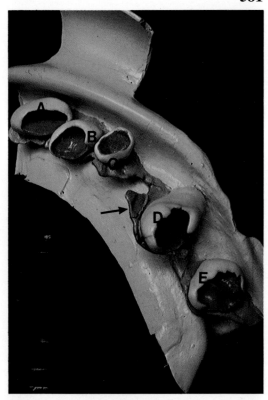

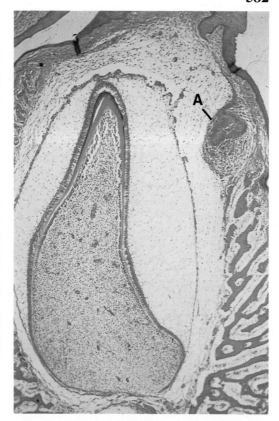

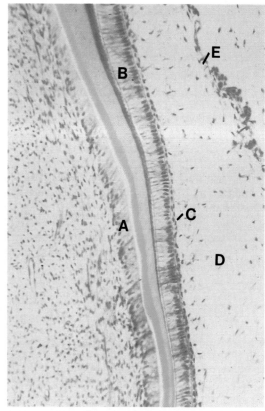

581 The arrangement of deciduous tooth germs at 17 weeks on the dental lamina of a lower jaw quadrant (*model*). The dental lamina is represented in green and is beginning to degenerate. The labelling identifies the developing deciduous teeth, which are at the bell stage according to the Zsigmondy system. Downgrowths on the lingual aspect of the enamel organs (*arrowed*) indicate the early development of the successional (permanent) teeth.

582 Late bell stage (appositional stage). This stage is associated with the formation of the dental hard tissues, commencing at about the 18th week. Dentine formation always precedes enamel formation. Detailed accounts of amelogenesis and dentinogenesis are given on pages 258–269. In the section shown, developing enamel is stained red and dentine blue. Downgrowths of the external enamel epithelium appear from the lingual sides of the enamel organs. In deciduous teeth, these lingual downgrowths give rise to the tooth germs of the permanent successors and first appear alongside the incisors at about 5 months *in utero*. In enamel organs of permanent teeth, however, these downgrowths eventually disappear. In this section, the permanent tooth (**A**) has reached the bud stage of development. Behind the deciduous second molar, the dental lamina grows backwards to bud off successively the permanent molar teeth. The first permanent molar appears at about the 4 months *in utero*. The tooth bud for the second permanent molar appears about 6 months after birth, while that for the third permanent molar appears at about 4–5 years. (Masson's trichrome; × 60)

583 High-power view of a region of a tooth germ at the late bell stage to show enamel and dentine formation. Under the inductive influence of developing ameloblasts (pre-ameloblasts), the adjacent mesenchymal cells of the dental papilla become columnar and differentiate into odontoblasts (**A**). The odontoblasts then become involved in the formation of dentine. In this decalcified section, the matrix of the calcified dentine is stained pale green while the uncalcified predentine nearer the odontoblasts is a darker green. The presence of dentine induces the ameloblasts (**B**) to secrete enamel. The developing enamel is stained red. **C**, stratum intermedium; **D**, stellate reticulum; **E**, external enamel epithelium. (Masson's trichrome; × 130)

252

During the early stages of tooth development, three transitory structures may be seen: the enamel knot, enamel cord and enamel niche.

584 The enamel knot (A) is a localised mass of cells produced by a rapid multiplication of cells in the centre of the internal enamel epithelium. Characteristically, the enamel knot forms a bulge into the dental papilla, at the centre of the enamel organ. It was once thought that the enamel knot played a role in the formation of crown pattern by outlining the central fissure. However, the enamel knot soon disappears and its role is unknown, although it appears to contribute cells to the enamel cord. (H & E; × 120)

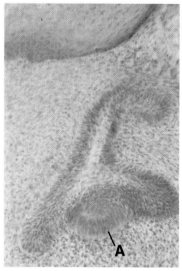

585 The enamel cord (A) is a strand of cells seen at the early bell stage of development, extending from the stratum intermedium into the stellate reticulum. When present, the enamel cord overlies the incisal margin of a tooth or the apex of the first cusp to develop (primary cusp). When it completely divides the stellate reticulum into two parts, reaching the external enamel epithelium, it is termed the enamel septum. Where the enamel cord meets the external enamel epithelium, a small invagination termed the enamel navel (B) may be seen. The cells of the enamel cord are distinguished from their surrounding stellate reticulum cells by their elongated nuclei. It has been suggested that the enamel cord may be involved in the process by which the cap stage is transformed into the bell stage (acting as a mechanical tie) and/or that it is a focus for the origin of stellate reticulum cells. (Masson's trichrome; × 120)

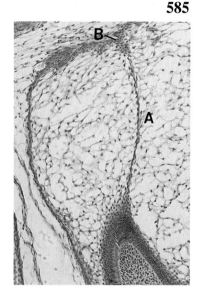

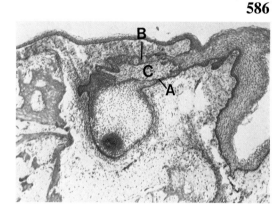

586 Enamel niche. The tooth germ may appear to have a double attachment to the dental lamina, the lateral (A) and medial (B) enamel strands. These strands enclose a funnel-shaped depression containing connective tissue, which is termed the enamel niche (C). Its significance is unknown. (H & E; × 40)

The enamel cord and the double attachment of the tooth germ were once regarded as evidence supporting the view that the complex crown form of mammalian teeth evolved from fusion of a number of individual, simpler elements. However, this view is not now generally accepted.

There is conflicting evidence as to when and where nerve fibres first appear during tooth development. It has been reported that nerve fibres are present in the immediate vicinity of presumptive dental epithelium at the very earliest stage of tooth induction. Subsequently, the nerves form a plexus below the dental papilla at the cap stage. From such plexuses, the nerves spread into the dental follicle as it develops. Penetration of nerves into the dental papilla occurs with the onset of dentinogenesis. The nerve fibres associated with blood vessels are presumed to be autonomic; others lying free within the papilla are presumed to be sensory. However, the innervation of the dental papilla remains rudimentary until after birth and may only be fully developed after the tooth has erupted.

Small blood vessels invade the dental papilla at the early bell stage. They are also evident in the dental follicle in close association with the external enamel epithelium. Although vessels may lie in invaginations of the external enamel epithelium, they never penetrate the stellate reticulum.

Epithelial–mesenchymal interactions during tooth development

The development of the tooth germ into the fully formed tooth involves many reciprocal interactions between the epithelium of the enamel organ and the mesenchyme of the dental papilla. These interactions are termed epithelial–mesenchymal interactions and involve changes resulting in increasing complexity in shape (morphodifferentiation) followed by increasing complexity in structure (histodifferentiation). That both tissues are required for development to occur has been established by experiments in which very early tooth germs are obtained and separated into their two components using trypsin. When grown separately (either *in vivo* or *in vitro*), neither the enamel organ nor the dental papilla undergoes further differentiation. Following recombination, however, normal development occurs.

The nature of the inductive message

During tooth development, 'messages' pass between the epithelium and mesenchyme to produce changes of increasing complexity (i.e. differentiation) within the cell layers. The term induction is used to describe the effect that one cell layer has on another.

Three main hypotheses have been put forward to explain how information leading to induction may be transferred between epithelium and mesenchyme:

1. A chemical substance (short-range hormone) is produced by one cell layer and diffuses across the narrow intervening space to be taken up and cause induction in the other cell layer.
2. Induction is triggered by direct cell-to-cell contact and does not involve a diffusible molecule.
3. Induction is due to the presence of the initial extracellular matrix (ECM), a thin layer situated between the epithelium and mesenchyme and comprising the basal lamina and adjacent region. The extracellular matrix has a complex composition, consisting of collagen (mainly Type IV, but possibly some Type I and III), proteoglycans and glycoproteins.

To assess which of the three hypotheses is likely to provide the correct explanation for reciprocal control of differentiation, experiments have been undertaken in which the epithelial and mesenchymal components are dissected out and separated at the early bell stage, prior to any significant degree of cytodifferentiation. They are then recombined for tissue culture, but with a porous membrane placed between; the size of the pores in the membrane can be varied to ascertain the point at which both ameloblasts and odontoblasts differentiate.

587

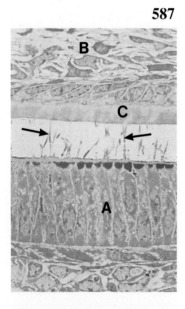

587 The enamel organ (A) and dental papilla mesenchyme (B) cultured on either side of a porous membrane. The pore size is 0.6μm and differentiation of the cells has occurred with the formation of predentine (**C**). Cell processes (*arrowed*) from odontoblast cells can be seen passing through pores in the membrane. (Mallory's; × 45)

588

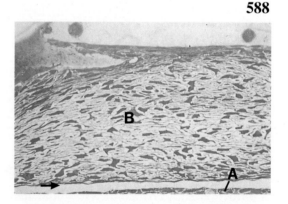

588 The enamel organ (A) and dental papilla mesenchyme (B) cultured on either side of a porous membrane (*arrowed*). The pore size is 0.1μm. No differentiation has occurred and cell processes do not pass through the membrane. (Toluidine blue; × 70)

As molecules can readily diffuse through a pore size just less than 0.2μm, the absence of differentiation seen in **588** argues against hypothesis 1 above (a diffusible chemical substance). The lack of differentiation with pores less than 0.2μm coincides with both the absence of the extracellular matrix and with the absence of cell processes invading the porous membrane. Thus, either cell-to-cell contact or the extracellular matrix could be implicated in differentiation. However, as *in vivo* direct cell-to-cell contact does not appear to occur (although the processes do come very close together), it is the extracellular matrix which may be most important in induction. The extracellular matrix itself is a product of both the epithelial and the mesenchymal cells.

Evidence indicating the importance of the extracellular matrix in the inductive process can be obtained from the following experiments:

● Drugs are available which can inhibit the formation of specific components of the extracellular matrix. For example, lathyrogens are drugs which interfere with cross linking of collagen. When added to tissue culture medium, these drugs inhibit differentiation of the tooth germ.

● Isolated pieces of extracellular matrix will produce histological signs of differentiation in internal enamel epithelial cells of the enamel organ.

Until very recently, technical considerations limited transplantation experiments on tooth differentiation to the early cap stage. At this stage, little differentiation is evident, and the question posed by investigators was: 'Which of the two components is more important for inducing morphogenesis and histogenesis — the enamel organ or the dental papilla?' A series of experiments was undertaken involving the interchange of epithelial and mesenchymal components between different developing teeth (i.e. incisors and molars) and between tissues from non-dental regions. The results indicate that, at the cap-stage of tooth development, the principal organiser is the dental papilla, both in terms of morphogenesis and histogenesis.

589

590

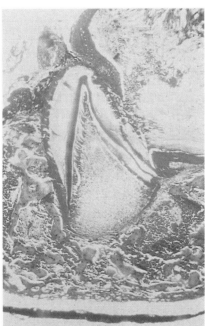

589 The result of culturing dental papilla mesenchyme with epithelium from the developing foot pad. Normal tooth development occurs, illustrating the importance of the dental papilla. (Masson's trichrome; × 300)

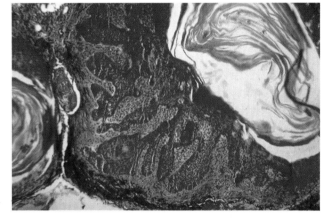

590 The result of culturing the enamel organ of a tooth with mesenchyme from the developing foot pad. Tooth development does not occur. (Masson's trichrome; × 750)

Techniques have recently been developed whereby it is possible to dissect out and recombine mammalian epithelium and mesenchyme in different combinations before there are any signs of tooth development. Thus, neural crest material (which gives rise to the bulk of the future dental papilla) can be obtained from the region of the developing brain before it actually migrates into the developing jaws, and challenged with epithelium from different sites.

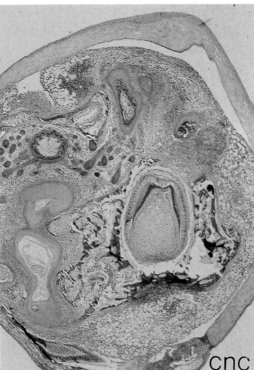

591 The result of culturing premigratory cranial neural crest with oral epithelium. A developing tooth (*arrowed*) is seen in the middle of the section. (Masson's trichrome; × 65)

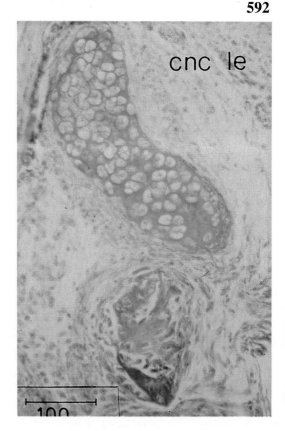

cnc le

cnc
me

592 The result of culturing premigratory neural crest with limb epithelium. Teeth do not develop, only islands of bone and cartilage. (Masson's trichrome; × 200)

100

The most important conclusion to be derived from the results illustrated in **591** and **592** is that premigratory neural crest will only form teeth when associated with oral epithelium. From this it is reasonable to infer that during normal development the neural crest that enters the mandibular arch is odontologically unspecified before or during migration, and that the oral epithelium is the earliest known site of tooth pattern.

The question arises as to whether the local environment of the jaws provides signals important for the initiation and development of the teeth (i.e. field theory). One way in which the possible contribution of the jaw environment can be assessed is to remove the dental lamina in the developing molar region together with the surrounding mesenchyme, which subsequently gives rise to the first molar tooth germ. This very early and undifferentiated tooth germ is then cultured in a totally different site away from the jaws.

593 A tooth germ of the first molar at the cap stage of development has been removed from an embryo and transplanted for culture in a different site. Not only does the first molar continue to develop normally, but the remaining second and third molars have also developed. This finding is consistent with the idea that a series of related structures can form by budding off from a single precursor (clone theory) and that the differences between the individual structures (e.g. size and crown complexity) result from the increasing age of the tooth-budding region as it grows distally from the jaw. (Alizarin red whole-mount)

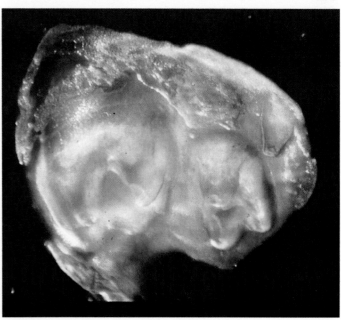

Mineralisation of dental hard tissues

The production of mineralised tissues involves two major processes. Initially, there is the extracellular secretion of an organic matrix. This is followed by the deposition of mineral (primarily in the form of calcium hydroxyapatite crystals) within the organic matrix. For dentine, cementum and bone, the organic material is collagenous and a lag period between matrix formation and mineralisation results in the presence of a layer of unmineralised organic matrix a few micrometres thick, which is visible at the light microscope level. For enamel, however, the organic matrix is not collagenous but is comprised mainly of unique proteins, reflecting the tissue's epithelial origin. In addition, initial mineralisation of enamel matrix takes place almost simultaneously with organic matrix production, such that an unmineralised layer of organic matrix is not found. Whereas the organic matrix of dentine, cementum and bone forms a substantial part of the mineralised tissue, the organic matrix of enamel is removed during the final mineralisation phase (called maturation), leaving less than 1% by weight of organic matrix in fully formed enamel.

The mechanisms involved in mineralisation are incompletely understood. The most difficult step to explain in biological mineralisation is the formation of the first crystals. Blood plasma (and presumably extracellular fluid) in most tissues is supersaturated with calcium and phosphate ions and thus mineralisation is not limited by the overall supply or control of basic ions. Therefore, any tissue could, under appropriate conditions, calcify once crystal formation is initiated. Indeed, pathological calcification does occur in soft tissues (e.g. muscle and tendon). Local conditions will determine whether and when a tissue will calcify. Precisely what these conditions are remains the subject of some controversy.

One mechanism, best established in calcifying cartilage (but possibly also occurring in the initial formation of dentine and bone), involves direct control by the cells. The cells form small 'matrix vesicles' which contain calcium and phosphate ions, alkaline phosphatase and calcium-binding lipids. These vesicles bud off from the cells and separate from them. Conditions within the vesicles permit the formation of hydroxyapatite crystals, and these can be seen within the matrix vesicles (see **612**). Once crystals are formed, the membrane around the vesicle disappears, the crystals grow and more crystals form around them, enlarging into islands of calcification that ultimately fuse. Most of the steps in this process have been described and there is little doubt that matrix vesicles exist, although their contribution to nucleation remains controversial. During mineralisation of all connective tissues, crystals are found widely distributed at many different sites in collagen fibre bundles, and it seems that collagen can provide sites for the initiation of crystal formation. The presence of collagen alone cannot determine that mineralisation will commence as, of course, much collagenous connective tissue is unmineralised. Phosphoproteins are thought to work in concert with collagen by acting as nucleating agents, with the collagen fibrils providing a template (specifically at the gap zones associated with the quarter stagger). In dentine, a specific phosphoprotein (phosphoporyn) has been identified with this role. Other phosphoproteins may act similarly in other calcifying tissues. In non-mineralising tissues, inhibitory factors may prevent calcification. A dermatan sulphate proteoglycan has been implicated in this activity.

In the developing tooth, mineralisation begins in the dentine and follows in the enamel. Matrix vesicles are found in dentine but are absent from enamel. It has been suggested that mineralisation spreads by crystal growth across the future enamel–dentine junction and that the crystals of the enamel take on their very different size as a result of the unique matrix in which they form. In some areas, enamel mineralisation seems to begin at some considerable distance from the dentinal crystals. Thus, it seems possible that mineralisation in enamel, while following chronologically that of dentine, may be initiated separately and by a different, non-matrix vesicle mechanism that is as yet unknown. Non-amelogenins (enamelins — see page 259) are anionic (negatively charged) proteins which may have properties similar to phosphoproteins; it is possible, but not established, that they may be involved in the nucleation process, although obviously without the presence of a collagen template.

The structural unit of mineral in calcified tissues is the crystal (or crystallite) and it differs in size but not in basic shape in all four calcified tissues. Factors unique to the tissue must determine its size and also its distribution and orientation within the tissue. Once a crystal is formed within a supersaturated solution, it will grow even under test tube conditions, but in the test tube no limits on growth are imposed. The factors that limit crystal growth to the size characteristic for the particular tissue are unknown. The fact that calcified tissues are made up of many small crystals suggests that there are multiple nucleation sites, one per crystal. This would seem to indicate that matrix vesicles, if responsible for nucleation, are only so at some limited sites.

Amelogenesis

The deposition of enamel begins at the late bell stage, immediately after dentinogenesis has commenced. Although differentiated before the odontoblasts (and supplying the message to determine their differentiation), the ameloblasts require the signal of dentine formation to initiate their secretory activities. Amelogenesis consists of three main phases:

- *Presecretory*, when the cells differentiate in cohorts of similar chronological age and align themselves into rows with older cells cuspally and younger cells cervically.
- *Secretory*, when the rows of ameloblasts retreat from the dentine in unison and lay down enamel. The enamel is laid down mineralised with no 'pre-enamel' layer analogous to predentine or osteoid. The whole cell retreats and no process is left embedded in the matrix. The matrix begins to degrade at this stage and starts to be replaced by water.
- *Maturation*, when the full thickness of enamel has been formed and is morphologically complete. The remaining protein and water are removed and mineral ions added. Growing crystals in turn displace the water, resulting in fully calcified, native enamel.

594

Legend:
— Basement lamina
Endoplasmic reticulum
Mitochondria
Golgi material
○ Secretory vesicles
○ Absorption granules
||||||| Primary enamel cuticle
▦ Dentine
∷∷∷ Enamel

1 2 3 4a 4b 5a 5b 6

594 Life cycle of the ameloblast. An understanding of amelogenesis is best approached by outlining the life cycle of the ameloblast. The cells of the internal enamel epithelium (**1**) start to differentiate, beginning at the future enamel–dentine junction of the cusp tip. The differentiating cell (**2**) is characterised by a reversed polarity; the cell becomes columnar and the nucleus moves to that part of the cell furthest from the dentine. Secreting organelles are formed and that end of the cell adjacent to the dentine becomes the site for secretion. At the next stage (**3**), the cell secretes the initial enamel component of the enamel–dentine junction. This thin layer will be continuous with the inter-rod enamel of the later formed tissue. As the cell retreats, the secreting pole becomes morphologically distinct as a pyramidal Tomes process (**4a**). Crystals are formed at both surfaces of the process. The proximal region between two processes, deep in the junctional regions, always secretes ahead of the more distal region so that pits surrounded by inter-rod enamel are formed. These are then filled, giving the 'rod' (or prism) configuration to the tissue (see page 113). Simultaneous secretion of both organic material and mineral continues until the full thickness of the tissue is formed. During this secreting phase, two appearances of ameloblasts can be distinguished by the position of the nuclei within the cell; high (**4a**) and low (**4b**). At the beginning of secretion, half the cells are in each form. Towards the end of secretion, most of the high nuclei have moved to a low position, effectively increasing the areas of the internal enamel epithelium as the surface of forming enamel increases. When the full thickness of enamel has formed, ameloblasts lose the secretory extension, the Tomes process (**5a**). 25% of the cells die and are phagocytosed by others in the layer. The maturation phase is two to three times longer than the secretory phase. During the maturation phase there is a regular, repetitive modulation of cell morphology between a ruffled (**5a**) and a smooth (**5b**) surface apposed to the enamel. Once the maturation changes are complete, the cells regress in height and appear to resemble gingival epithelium (**6**). At this stage, they serve to protect the surface during eruption and later will contribute to form the junctional epithelium.

595 The distal cytoplasm of an early differentiating ameloblast. Internal enamel epithelial cells and early differentiating ameloblasts possess a large ovoid nucleus (**A**) and a small Golgi complex lying in the basal end of the cell adjacent to the stratum intermedium. In the distal cytoplasm neighbouring the dental papilla, there are a few organised membranous structures, but large numbers of free ribosomes (**B**). Numerous vesicles (**C**) are present, and the surface membrane shows invaginations (**D**) typical of pinocytosis. **E**, rough endoplasmic reticulum; **F**, mitochondria; **G**, gap junction; **H**, dental papilla. The differentiating ameloblasts induce the adjacent mesenchymal cells of the dental papilla to differentiate into odontoblasts. There is a basal lamina separating the two layers and preventing direct cell contact. (TEM; × 21,000)

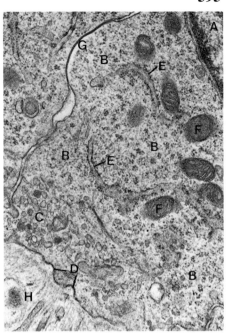

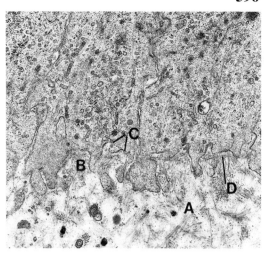

596 The distal cytoplasm of late differentiating ameloblasts. Following the onset of dentine formation (**A**) and immediately prior to the onset of amelogenesis, the distal plasma membrane of the differentiating ameloblasts exhibits undulations and shows invaginations (**B**) and projections. Coated pits (**C**) are present at the base of some invaginations. The basal lamina undergoes degeneration and remnants can be identified (**D**). The distal cytoplasm contains many small vesicles and vacuoles, which may be elongated or rounded, with contents of varying electron-opacity. Large multivesicular bodies are also present. Some of the vesicles may represent an endosomal system associated with the removal of the basal lamina. (TEM; × 15,600)

597 The distal ends of early secretory ameloblasts. Immediately prior to the onset of amelogenesis, there is a marked aggregation of vesicles (some containing stippled material) at the distal end of the ameloblast. **A**, secretory vesicles. The material contained within the vesicles is thought to be the organic matrix of enamel. By reverse pinocytosis, the contents of the vesicles are discharged into the extracellular space. Enamel matrix (**B**) can be seen in this section between adjacent ameloblasts. As the enamel matrix is secreted, the ameloblasts are pushed outwards away from the dentine surface (**C**). A distinct zone of uncalcified organic matrix, corresponding to osteoid of bone and predentine of dentine, is never seen since hydroxyapatite crystals begin to form when the enamel matrix is only about 50nm thick. In this illustration, the early calcified enamel (**D**) shows thin, needle-like hydroxyapatite crystals. Recent evidence suggests that the initial foci for enamel crystals may be crystals in the adjacent mantle dentine. Note that, at this early stage of amelogenesis, the distal ends of the ameloblasts form a relatively flat surface and that no prismatic structure can be discerned in the developing enamel. (TEM; × 15,000)

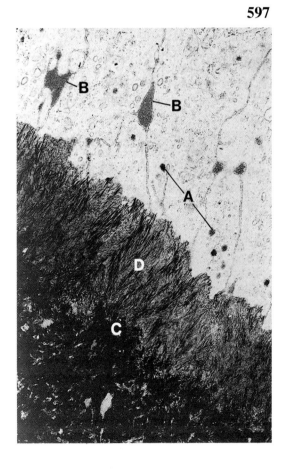

The newly formed enamel is 65% water, 20% organic material and 15% inorganic. The matrix of new enamel consists of two proteins. Most of the protein (95%) consists of amelogenins — hydrophobic, proline-rich molecules, M.W. 25,000. The remaining 5% of the protein consists of non-amelogenins as determined by SDS electrophoresis. Their molecular weights are about 55,000. As deposition continues, the amelogenins break up into units of lower molecular weight. The initial crystals are long, thin plates which increase in thickness as deposition continues, bringing the inorganic content of enamel prior to maturation to 30%.

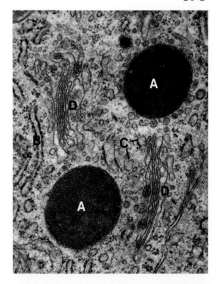

598 Part of a secretory ameloblast showing two large, dense vesicles or secretory granules (A). The stippled material within the vesicles is thought to be the future organic matrix of enamel. **B**, rough endoplasmic reticulum; **C**, Golgi vesicles; **D**, Golgi units. (TEM; × 30,500)

599 Decalcified, longitudinal section through a tooth germ during the initial stages of amelogenesis and dentinogenesis. A, ameloblasts; **B**, odontoblasts; **C**, developing enamel; **D**, developing dentine; **E**, stratum intermedium; **F**, stellate reticulum. The cells of the stratum intermedium and stellate reticulum are believed to play a role in enamel formation. Ameloblasts are rich in RNA and have a high oxidative enzyme activity. However, they lack the enzyme alkaline phosphatase, which is present in large amounts in the cells of the stratum intermedium. It has been suggested that the stratum intermedium may be concerned with the synthesis of proteins, with the transport of materials to and from the ameloblast or with the concentration of materials. The stellate reticulum is rich in glycoaminoglycans, and may have a mechanical function. (Masson's trichrome; × 80)

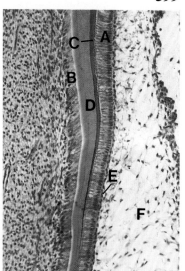

After the initial stages of amelogenesis, the secretory end of the ameloblast becomes pyramidal in shape, forming the so-called Tomes process.

600 Decalcified, longitudinal section through developing enamel showing the cone-shaped Tomes process at the distal end of each ameloblast. A, ameloblasts; **B**, enamel matrix; **C**, dentine; **D**, stratum intermedium. Note that in this section, taken from a developing human tooth, Tomes processes are present only after a small amount of enamel has been laid down. The Tomes processes are demarcated at their bases by junctional complexes. The alignment of these complexes gives the appearance of a terminal bar (**E**) running through the ameloblast layer. At the electron microscope level, the terminal bars appear as desmosomes with associated tonofilaments. The tonofilaments pass only a short distance into the cell to form an incomplete septum between the Tomes process and the rest of the ameloblast. A similar terminal bar apparatus is found at the basal end of the ameloblast. Other desmosomes and tight junctional complexes may be discerned at a variety of sites linking adjacent ameloblasts. The junctional complexes that unite ameloblasts (seen in the light microscope as the terminal bar apparatus) are of the zonular type that completely encircle the cell and prevents the movement of most materials between the cells. They effectively separate the environment of the forming enamel from the interior of the enamel organ such that all secretion and modification of the matrix occurs via Tomes processes. Junctional complexes also join the cells more basally, adjacent to the stratum intermedium. The complexes at this level are of the macular variety and provide mechanical union without limiting the passage of materials. Gap junctions unite adjacent cells as a means of communication. They allow the movement of small molecules, which presumably harmonise the activities of all cells within the same layer. Gap junctions are better developed within, rather than between, rows of ameloblasts. (Toluidine blue; × 1,000)

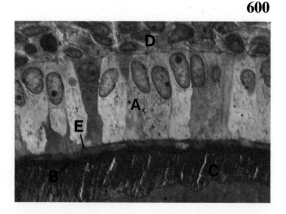

601 Advanced secretory ameloblasts showing Tomes processes (A). B, developing enamel. Note that the Tomes processes fit into pits in the surface of the enamel. (TEM; × 6,000)

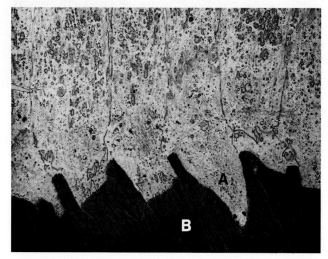

Interprismatic 'prongs' develop between the growing, and elongating, interdigitating portions of Tomes processes. The prongs between the processes form walls that delineate pits or depressions in the interprismatic enamel, which are occupied by Tomes processes. As the ameloblasts have two secretory sites, the pattern followed is of continuous formation of the interprismatic enamel at one site, followed a short time later by the filling in of holes by the secretion of the prisms at the prism secretion sites. The presence of prisms, therefore, is related to the configuration of the Tomes processes.

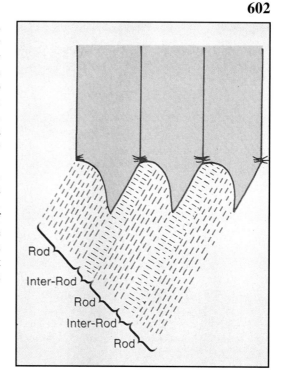

602 The relationship between Tomes processes and enamel prism formation. The enamel of prism and interprismatic areas is identical and only differs in the orientation of the crystals. In human enamel, prisms are clearly distinct from interprismatic enamel on most of their circumference, but at one site the distinction between the two is lost. The 'attachment' between the two enamels has led to the description of human enamel as a 'keyhole' pattern without the need to recognize interprismatic enamel (see pages 113–117). The difference between the two descriptions is slight. Both recognize a homogeneous composition of enamel with a visual difference being due to differing orientations in crystals.

This diagram shows the formation of prismatic and interprismatic enamel. The prism is formed from a single ameloblast, but four ameloblasts (when considered in three dimensions) contribute to the interprismatic region. Interprismatic enamel is formed first, giving a pit-like surface appearance of developing enamel. The side of a completed interprismatic hole and the beginning of the prism are continuous, accounting for the 'tail' which forms first and is then attached to the 'head' which forms last. Thus, it may be that the only difference between the 'keyhole' and 'interprismatic' descriptions is one of semantics.

Various lines and patterns have been described in enamel, and have been attributed to the rhythmic and incremental activity of the ameloblasts. Cross-striations (page 117) are usually seen in ground sections and appear as dark lines about 4μm apart. They are commonly believed to be due to a diurnal rhythm in enamel prism growth. They cannot be seen in ultra-thin sections, nor as variations in prism thickness in fractured enamel. Examination of ground sections in the SEM has suggested that the appearance of cross-striations is a preparatory artifact, related either to rows of cross-cut prisms aligned linearly, or to gouged-out portions of prism crystals that followed a recurring spiralling pattern of the crystals. However, examination using other techniques (including confocal scanning microscopy) indicates cross-striations are not artifactual, as does their relationship with enamel striae, which are also generally regarded as representing growth lines.

The enamel striae (see pages 118–119) follow the contours of the developing crown and have been considered to be incremental (analogous to growth lines in trees), and may result from changes in the direction of enamel prisms. It seems more likely that the striae represent a boundary between groups of prisms formed by different cohorts of ameloblasts. In human enamel, about seven rows of ameloblasts are generated together at the cervical loop and the resulting prisms will extend around the crown. The subsequent group will have a somewhat different orientation and the boundary between the two could constitute a striation. The striae successively outline the position of the mineralising enamel front. They thus do not reach the surface over the tips of the cusps or incisal edges (see **220b**). As the daily increments of enamel are smaller towards the end of enamel formation, the striae are closer together towards the cervical margin. As there are about seven cross-striations between successive striae, the striae are thought to represent approximately weekly incremental lines (circaseptan). One theory to account for their presence suggests that, superimposed on the normal 24 hour daily rhythm, there is another rhythm of about 27 hours. The two would coincide about every 7 days, resulting in the presence of striae.

Hunter–Schreger bands (see page 120) result from optical interference produced by alternating planes of prisms, but the migratory activity of the ameloblasts required to produce these alternating planes has not been fully explained.

Maturation

Once the entire thickness of the enamel has formed it is structurally complete, with all the morphological features of mature enamel. It is, however, only mineralised to 30% of that of the erupted tooth. The process by which the enamel changes into its final form is termed maturation. During maturation, enamel crystals increase in width and thickness with a consequent reduction in the intercrystalline space.

Organic matrix is removed, reducing the protein content of the final tissue to less than 1% (from 30%). There is also a change in the proteins present. Amelogenins are removed, leaving behind small peptides and amino acids, together with larger components (non-amelogenins) bound to the crystals. This accounts for mature enamel having more glycine but less histidine and proline than young, immature enamel. Most of the water remaining is also removed.

The changes during maturation are achieved by (or through) the ameloblasts. The cells themselves change considerably. The Tomes process is lost and the organelle content reduced. The remaining organelles congregate at the distal end of the cell and the plasma membrane infolds to form a striated border. The ameloblast is described as ruffle-ended. This morphology alternates with that of the smooth-ended ameloblast, in which the striated border is absent. Modulation between the two forms occurs between five and seven times during maturation. The modulation may alternate between resorptive and secretory phases. The removal of matrix occurs when the crystals are expanding from their early dimensions of 1.5nm thick to their mature thickness of 25nm. The degradation of the enamel matrix by serine proteases from the enamel organ seems to precede mineral gain, matrix degradation and removal being essential to facilitate crystal growth.

603

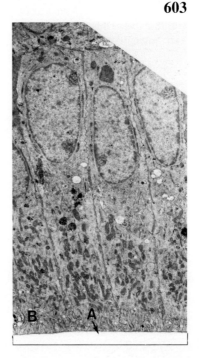

603 Decalcified section showing ameloblasts at the early maturation stage. A, enamel space. Compared with the ameloblast during its secretory phase, the cell shortens and loses its Tomes process which is replaced by a striated border (**B**) consisting of an infolded cell membrane. Mitochondria, though scattered throughout the cell, are arranged in two major clusters, one at the basal end of the cell, the other at the distal end near the striated border. There is a great reduction in the amount of rough endoplasmic reticulum. Associated with the loss of the Tomes processes, the surface layer of enamel may be prism-free (**246**). (TEM; × 2,700)

604

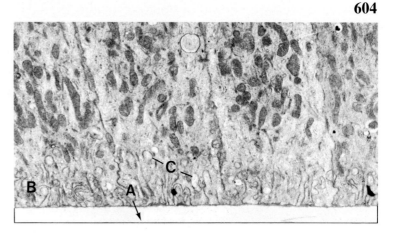

604 High-power view of 603, showing striated border (B). A, enamel space. In undermineralised material the projections from the distal end of the cell are separated from the mineralised mass of the enamel by a narrow interval containing dense, finely granular material. It is assumed that such material is being absorbed into the ameloblast within absorption granules (**C**) shown here in a demineralised section. Within the cell, there is increased acid phosphatase and aminopeptidase activity. (TEM; × 6,700)

605 Pattern of mineralisation in a molar tooth during maturation. Stippled areas represent initial enamel deposition. Black areas show the pattern that increased mineralisation follows during maturation. Once the full thickness of enamel is formed in any area, maturation commences. Initial deposition and maturation can thus occur at the same time in a developing tooth. The mineralisation during maturation follows a different pattern than initial deposition. Commencing at cusps, it passes to the enamel–dentine junction and along the junction before continuing throughout the more superficial regions.

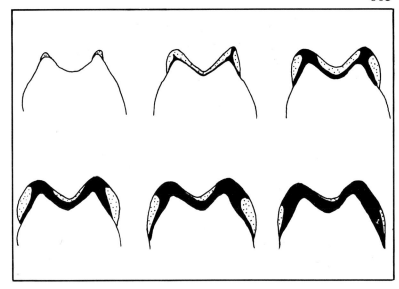

606 Reduced enamel epithelium. Once amelogenesis is complete (for both secretion and maturation), the ameloblasts become flattened. This layer of flattened cells (the reduced enamel epithelium, **A**) still has a role to play in protecting the enamel during eruption and in forming the junctional epithelium (page 281). An amorphous layer approximately 1μm thick forms between the reduced enamel epithelium and the enamel (**B**, enamel space). It may be the last product of the ameloblast or represent enamel matrix that has been extruded during maturation. At the ultrastructural level, the reduced ameloblasts exhibit hemidesmosomes adjacent to the enamel surface from which they are separated by a basal lamina. **C**, connective tissue of dental follicle. (Decalcified section stained with H & E; × 160)

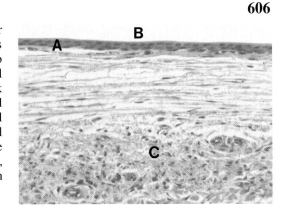

606

The biochemical differences between amelogenins and non-amelogenin proteins is indicated by the differing molecular weights and the amino acid compositions. Note that amelogenins are rich in proline, whereas non-amelogenins have relatively less of this amino acid. Non-amelogenins are rich in glycine and aspartic acid.

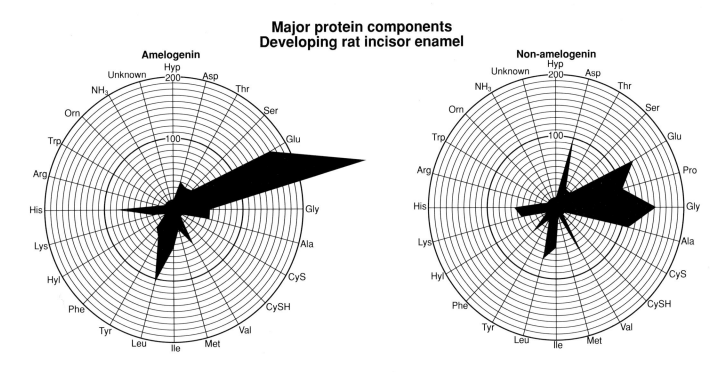

Dentinogenesis

Dentine is the first formed of the dental hard tissues and dentinogenesis begins at the late bell stage of tooth development. Pre-ameloblasts within the enamel organ (see **583**) differentiate before, and have an inductive influence upon, the odontoblasts which secrete dentine. Like the formation of bone or cementum, but unlike that of enamel, dentinogenesis has matrix and mineralisation stages which are both spatially and temporally separated.

607

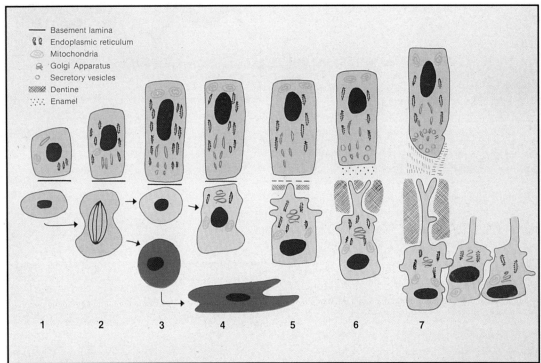

607 Life cycle of the odontoblast (green) and its relationships with the ameloblasts (brown) and the sub-odontoblastic cells (red). The ameloblasts differentiate prior to the odontoblasts. The cell density at the periphery of the dental papilla increases (**1**) and the cells divide (**2**). Some of the daughter cells will migrate to the sub-odontoblastic region (**3**). Others will, after a signal from the ameloblasts, begin their differentiation into odontoblasts. The pre-odontoblasts become columnar, and develop large supranuclear Golgi material and a profuse rough endoplasmic reticulum (**4**). The nucleus moves to the basal third of the cell and a series of processes develop largely but not exclusively at the peripheral end of the cell (**5**). One process becomes more pronounced and it is through this that the matrix is secreted (**5, 6**). The cell body retreats centripetally as more matrix is deposited, leaving behind an elongated process within a dentinal tubule (**7**). After the first layer of dentine is deposited (**5**), the differentiated ameloblast is activated to begin the deposition of enamel (**6–7**).

Dentine formation in the crown

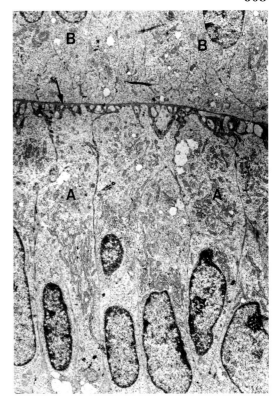

608 The ameloblast-odontoblast interface just prior to dentinogenesis. The odontoblasts (**A**) are columnar and at this stage show all the cytoplasmic characteristics of a synthetic cell, including abundant endoplasmic reticulum and mitochondria, and pronounced Golgi material. Like that of an ameloblast, the nucleus of the odontoblast is basally situated, primarily due to the growth of the distal (secretory) end of the cytoplasm of the undifferentiated mesenchymal cell. At this stage, the odontoblasts form a single layer of cells and are separated from the overlying developing ameloblasts (**B**) by a basal lamina and by a narrow, relatively amorphous layer (*arrowed*). (TEM; × 3,800)

609 Early matrix formation. The odontoblasts begin secretion from the pole of the cell adjacent to the ameloblasts. At this secretory pole, a single, major process (**A**) forms, through which all later secretion will occur. The odontoblast has many minor processes arising from its cell body, but these seem to be primarily concerned with linking odontoblasts to each other and to cells in the sub-odontoblastic region. Many of these smaller processes are linked by gap junctions which are permeable to low molecular weight substances. These junctions may provide the basis for the coordination of odontoblastic activity within the layer. The first dentine formed, the mantle layer (see **292**), differs from subsequently formed tissue primarily in the orientation of the deposited collagen. The Type I fibres (*arrowed*) fan out from the basal lamina (**B**) between the odontoblastic processes, and are approximately parallel to the long axes of the cells. The fibres are embedded in a ground substance rich in glycosaminoglycans. In this first formed layer, there may be some contribution to the tissue from the sub-odontoblastic cells. This does not continue for long, as the odontoblasts develop between themselves a complex of junctions which separate the secretory process from the synthesising cell body. It has also been suggested that, because of the presence of fibronectin in the mantle dentine, the epithelial cells of the enamel organ may also contribute to the formation of mantle dentine. All later secretion occurs through the odontoblastic process and the mechanical properties of the layer may also control the entry of calcium ions during mineralisation. Morphologically, the odontoblast is still differentiating during the early stages of dentine formation. Initially, the large secretory process has a terminal arborisation with a number of small branches. These are lost as the process retreats away from the dentine–enamel junction. This gives the mantle layer a characteristic it retains in the fully formed tissue, many small, branching tubules.

Shortly after dentine formation begins, the ameloblasts phagocytose the basal lamina (see **596**). The junctional region between the forming dentine and enamel will consist of intermixed products of the two tissues. (TEM; × 9,500)

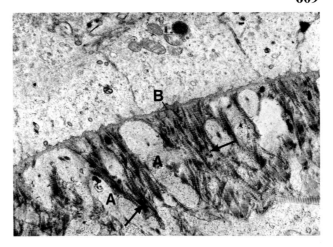

610 Silver stained corkscrew fibres (of von Korff). In formalin-fixed, acid decalcified dentine, coarse black-stained fibres are seen in the mantle region (corkscrew fibres of von Korff). While ultrastructural techniques confirm the existence of collagen fibres parallel to the cells in first-formed dentine (see **609**), they also show the fibres to be much straighter and finer than the silver-stained structures. It is probable that the 'harsh' silver makes the fibres appear much thicker than they really are. (Silver impregnation; × 200)

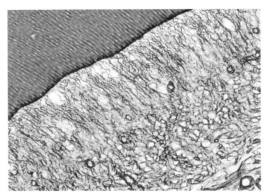

265

Dentine formation progresses by the central migration of the odontoblast layer and by continued secretion from the odontoblast process. The odontoblast is functionally differentiated into a synthetic body and its secretory process. The process is devoid of rough endoplasmic reticulum and other synthetic organelles, but contains numerous microtubules and microfilaments responsible for the transportation of secretory granules. Exocytosis occurs at various points along the process, not just at its end.

The odontoblast provides a classic model for the study of protein synthesis and secretion. Labelled amino acids can be followed as they enter the cell body and are assembled into the collagen precursors in the rough endoplasmic reticulum, then migrate to the Golgi material for glycolisation, triple helical coiling and enclosure in secretory granules. The granules then travel to (and along) the odontoblast process for secretion. Following injection of labelled (tritiated) glycine or proline, collagen can be identified within the extracellular compartment within about 90 minutes. The matrix deposited prior to calcification is termed predentine. Shortly after mantle dentine secretion has begun, and when the predentine is approximately 5μm thick, mineralisation begins.

During the mineralisation of dentine, the matrix undergoes some modifications. Protein is removed and glycoprotein and phosphoprotein added. This accounts for the clear difference in staining properties between calcified dentine and predentine even in sections in which all the mineral has been removed; (see **295**, **613**). In common with bone and cementum, but in contrast to enamel, dentine is almost immediately mineralised to nearly its final level.

611

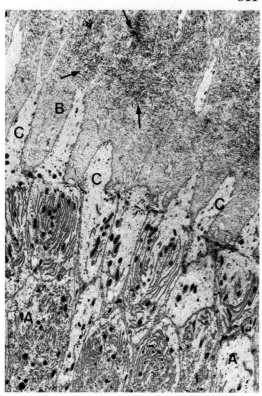

612

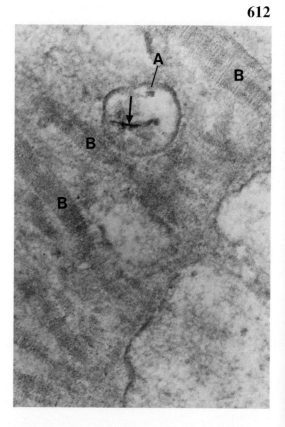

611 Early mineralisation of dentine. Synthetic organelles are abundant in the cytoplasm (**A**). Junctional complexes unite adjacent odontoblasts. The odontoblast process (**C**) projects into the matrix (**B**) with some branching. An outer darker zone in which crystals are being deposited (*arrowed*) can be distinguished from the inner, paler predentine. At this stage, only small groups of crystals have formed. (TEM; × 6,500)

612 A matrix vesicle (A) within mineralising dentine. The precise mechanism of dentine mineralisation remains controversial. Matrix vesicles bud off from the odontoblast processes within the dentine. Collagen fibrils (**B**) can be seen within the predentine. The first crystallites (*arrowed*) are formed within the matrix vesicles. The vesicle walls are then lost and more crystals develop around the original ones. While matrix vesicles are present at the onset of mineralisation, none are seen in the later stages of on-going calcification. Seeding and crystal growth from the original vesicle-derived crystals may explain continued apposition. Non-collagenous proteins such as osteocalcin, dentin phosphoprotein and phosphoporyn have been isolated from dentine and may be implicated in the initiation and continuation of mineralisation. Apposition from a site of initiation occurs in three dimensions forming a spherical mass, a calcospherite. Fusion of adjacent calcospherites results in continuous calcification. As well as this globular pattern, a linear pattern of mineral-isation exists, as reflected in the incremental lines seen in both demineralised and non-demineralised sections. The calcospherite pattern is best seen in the circumpulpal dentine, i.e. just below the mantle layer. The globules decrease in size as the mineralisation proceeds and the linear process predominates. (TEM; × 70,000)

There is evidence of two morphologically distinct but biochemically different layers in the predentine. The basis of the differences is not entirely clear but indicates that changes occur in the matrix prior to mineralisation. The odontoblast appears to add further components (such as lipids, phosphoproteins and carboxyglutamate proteins) to the matrix. The conversion of predentine to the mineralisable form begins about four hours after its initial deposition in the early developmental stages. As well as the addition of new components, the loss of some tyrosine-containing proteins has been reported.

Mantle dentine varies in thickness from less than one to tens of micrometres and it differs in many respects from the later-formed circumpulpal dentine (see page 140). In particular, the collagen fibres in circumpulpal dentine are now orientated in a network mainly parallel to the pulp surface (and thus perpendicular to the odontoblast processes). They are also derived entirely from the odontoblasts and, unlike mantle dentine, with no contribution from the sub-odontoblastic cells or the enamel organ. In addition, the circumpulpal dentine shows less tubule branching, and mineralisation is more regular with a clearer calcospheritic pattern.

613

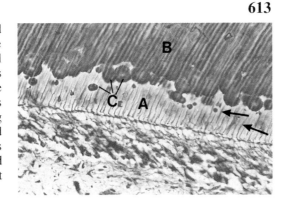

613 Developing circumpulpal dentine. Circumpulpal dentine is formed by the deposition, and subsequent mineralisation, of dentine matrix (the predentine, **A**) as the odontoblasts migrate centripetally into the dental papilla. The size of the papilla (and hence the developing pulp chamber) is thereby reduced and the odontoblasts become crowded together, giving the appearance of a pseudostratified layer several cells deep. Matrix is deposited around the odontoblast processes (*arrowed*) of the retreating odontoblasts, forming the dentinal tubules. The matrix is only mineralised (**B**) after the predentine attains a thickness of several micrometres. This accounts for the difference seen in the staining of the dentine and predentine. The mineralising front shows evidence of both a linear front and calcospherites (**C**). (Sudan black; × 230)

614

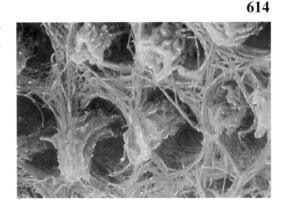

614 Surface of the predentine in circumpulpal dentine. In this colour enhanced micrograph, the collagen fibrils (**brown**) can be seen forming a network arranged perpendicular to the odontoblast processes (**blue**). (SEM; × 4,000)

The crowding of the odontoblasts as they move centripetally on a front of decreasing surface area induces changes in the direction of migration. This is seen in the S-shaped primary curvatures of the tubules which are produced in the circumpulpal dentine (see **268**). Smaller diurnal changes in direction result in the formation of secondary curvatures (see **269**).

615

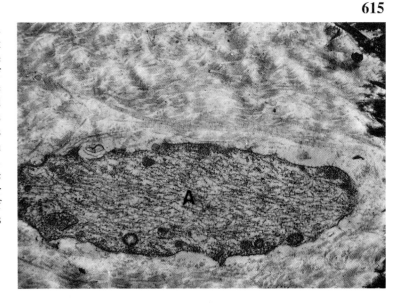

615 Collagen fibrils of predentine adjacent to an odontoblast process. Several vesicles can be seen approaching the surface of the odontoblast process (**A**) prior to exocytosis. Some of these vesicles will contain the precursors of collagen. Other vesicles could contain the elements of glycosaminoglycans which will comprise the ground substance of the dentine matrix. Indentations in the plasmalemma record the site of recently emptied vesicles. The network of collagen fibrils assembled around the process is clearly seen. The orientation of the collagen fibrils is not homogeneous throughout the tissue. It has been suggested that approximately every 20μm there is a somewhat exaggerated and coincident change in their direction. This would correspond to a 5-day cycle of unknown origin. This periodic change might explain the incremental lines originally described by von Ebner (see **298**). An alternative explanation is based upon the supposition of rhythmical changes in the concentration of material in the non-collagenous matrix or in the mineral component. (TEM; × 22,500)

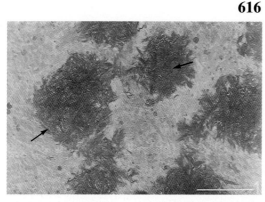

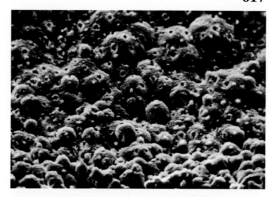

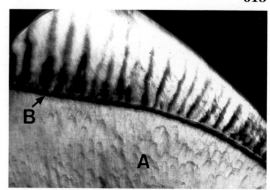

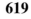

616 Calcospherites (*arrowed*) in calcifying predentine. Many of the crystals in dentine are aligned parallel with the matrix fibres. However, this does not apply to calcospherites. The arrows indicate two neighbouring calcospherites about to fuse. The crystals within each calcospherite are arranged radially and growth is by apposition to the outer surface of the mass. Where fusion does not occur, hypomineralised interglobular dentine will result (see **301**). (TEM; × 1,450)

617 The mineralising front, showing calcospherites. In this anorganic preparation, the predentine layer has been removed and the surface of the calcifying dentine revealed. The surface is irregular due to the presence of numerous calcospherites. Tubules are seen running through the calcospherites. Calcospherites can form around, as well as between, the odontoblast processes. (SEM; × 500)

618 The calcospherite pattern of mineralisation. The use of polarised microscopy through a fully formed tooth can reveal evidence of the pattern of calcospherites in circumpulpal dentine (**A**). Note the spherical junctional regions which outline the original positions of the calcospherites produced during the tissue's development. Variations in both crystal and collagen fibre orientation produce this appearance. At this rotation, the mantle layer (**B**) completely blocks the transmission of the polarised light and appears black. (Ground, longitudinal section of dentine viewed in polarised light; × 25)

619 Pattern and distribution of calcospherites. Most calcospherites are spherical. However, many have an arcade shape such that the round apex of the arcade is directed towards the outer surface of the dentine, and the opening is directed towards the pulp. The size varies considerably; the arcade variety tends to be larger than the spherical variety. The size and shape of the calcospherites seem to be governed by the rate of dentine formation and by the rate at which new calcospherites are initiated. There is a fairly consistent pattern of distribution within the tooth. In the mantle dentine of the crown, in the hyaline layer of the root and in the superficial circumpulpal dentine, the calcospherites are small, spherical and closely packed. In the middle region of the circumpulpal dentine, they are larger, more widely spaced and arcade-like in form (although this region tends to be free of calcospherites towards the root apex). The inner half to two-thirds of the circumpulpal dentine contains spherical calcospherites.

The mechanism underlying the formation of calcospherites has not been investigated, but the presence of these structures is a feature distinguishing dentine from bone and cementum, in which the crystals are uniformly orientated parallel with the collagen fibres.

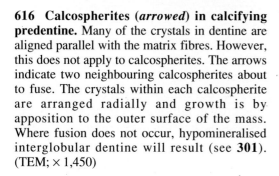

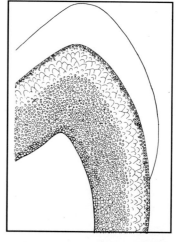

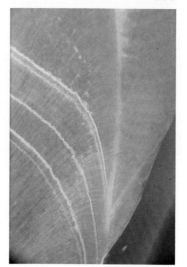

620 Tetracycline lines in dentine. Certain substances (eg the antibiotic tetracycline) are incorporated into the mineralising front of dentine and leave a distinct line. If this line is examined at high power, the calcospheritic and linear nature of the mineralising front may be seen. The micrograph illustrated shows the tooth of an individual who received five separate injections of tetracycline. Although the lines may appear yellow in ground sections viewed in transmitted light, they are more readily identified in fluorescent light. (Ground, longitudinal section; fluorescent light; × 5)

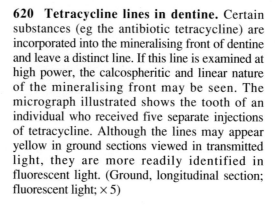

Dentine formation in the root

The basic process of root dentinogenesis does not differ fundamentally from coronal dentinogenesis. However, differences are seen in the early stages. Initial collagen deposition does not begin immediately against the basal lamina of the epithelial cells of the root sheath (see pages 272–273). The space between the initial collagen and the epithelial cells becomes filled with an amorphous ground substance and a fine, fibrillar, non-collagenous material that appears to be formed from the root sheath (and may thus be a form of enamel). These elements form a hyaline layer (page 140) which is approximately 10μm thick. The initial collagen fibres deposited in the root lie approximately parallel to the cement–dentine junction. This contrasts with the mantle dentine in the crown, where the collagen fibres are deposited perpendicular to the enamel– dentine junction. Radicular odontoblasts differ slightly from those in the crown, developing several fine branches which loop in umbrella fashion (**621**). This gives rise to a granular layer (of Tomes), although a large part of this is also thought to be due to the presence of many small, uncalcified interglobular areas. The different character of peripheral radicular dentine presumably relates to the difference between the cells of the internal enamel epithelium (which will differentiate and continue as ameloblasts) and the cells of the root sheath (which lose their continuity soon after dentinogenesis has begun). The loss of continuity of the epithelial cells results in larger numbers of interglobular areas and possibly also in the incorporation of some epithelial remnants in the peripheral dentine. Radicular dentine forms at a slightly slower rate than coronal dentine. Its pattern of mineralisation is similar, although its initial calcospherites are smaller and its interglobular areas are more numerous. In general, root mineralisation proceeds as a continuation of that in the crown, although in multirooted teeth, separate isolated areas of mineralisation may occur.

621

621 Looping and branching in the granular layer of the root. In this preparation, the dentinal tubules have become filled with a silver stain and the tissue has been examined in a thicker than normal section. While this obscures much fine detail by superimposition, it does allow some insight into the three-dimensional arrangement. The peripheral terminations of several tubules may be seen, and a profuse branching in three dimensions can be distinguished. Above the tubules in focus are others below the plane of focus. Here, it may be seen how this arrangement could contribute to the appearance of the granular layer (see page 140). (Silver stain; × 490)

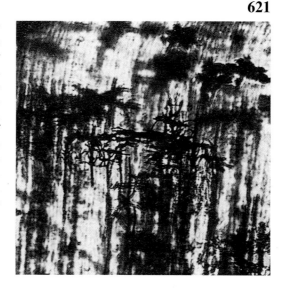

Development of the pulp

The dental papilla is the undifferentiated predecessor of the dental pulp. It is thought that the ectomesenchymal (neural crest) cells provide the initiative for differentiation, at least in part. Although some changes, such as the entry of the first blood vessels, are discernible at the cap stage, cytodifferentiation of the papilla into the pulp begins at the bell stage, when the homogeneous mass of cells starts to change into the organ that will lay down dentine.

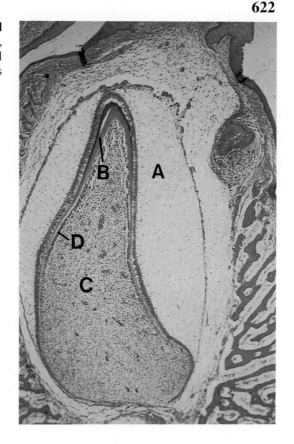

622 The developing tooth at the late bell stage of development (appositional phase). A, enamel organ; **B**, developing dentine; **C**, dental papilla; **D**, odontoblast layer. (Masson's trichrome; × 55)

The small, undifferentiated, ectomesenchymal cells of the papilla are packed closely together with little intercellular material. They are stellate in shape with a relatively large nucleus and little cytoplasm. During growth of the tooth germ, although undifferentiated, the expansion of this cell mass at the cap stage exerts a morphogenetic effect on the enamel organ (see page 255). As the pulp develops, the cytoplasmic component of these central dental papilla cells expands and synthetic organelles appear. The material the organelles produce is released into the extracellular space and consists of fine collagen fibres in an amorphous ground substance. Coarse fibre bundles appear only at about the time that the tooth reaches maturity. In the early stages of pulpal development, the ground substance has a high glycosaminoglycan content relative to that in the mature tooth. The level of glycosaminoglycans increases until the time of eruption and then decreases. The chondroitin sulphates are the main glycosaminoglycans present during pulp development, with only a minor quantity of hyaluronate. This balance is reversed in the mature pulp. The differentiated secretory cells are pulpal fibroblasts. Not all cells undergo differentiation, a proportion remaining as mesenchymal cells retaining the potential to differentiate in later life. Under the influence of the internal enamel epithelium, the peripheral cells of the papilla differentiate into odontoblasts (see page 264). A cell-rich zone develops beneath the odontoblast layer at the time of eruption. It arises by the migration of more central cells rather than by local cell division.

Vascularisation of the developing pulp starts during the bell stage, with small branches from the principal vascular trunks of the jaws entering the base of the papilla. Of these small pioneer vessels, a few become the principal pulpal vessels. These enlarge and run through the pulp towards the cuspal regions. Here they give off numerous small branches, which form a bed of venules, arterioles and capillaries in the sub-odontoblast and odontoblast layers. The vascularity of the odontoblast layer increases as dentine is progressively laid down, probably as the result of the odontoblasts retreating inwards through the vascular bed. Eventually, some capillaries are found immediately next to the predentine surface.

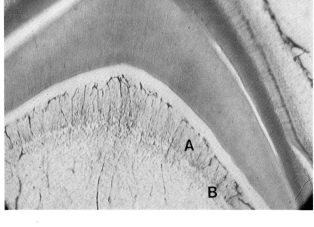

624

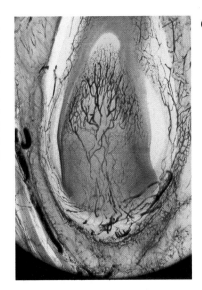

623

623 The vascular pattern within the dental papilla at the late bell stage of development. To highlight the vasculature, Indian ink has been introduced into the vascular system. Note that, as the developing central pulp vessels reach the future cusp regions, they divide into numerous small branches which give off a plexus of venules, arterioles and capillaries. (H & E; × 40)

624 The vascular plexuses in the region of the developing cusp. Beneath the odontoblast layer (**A**) lies the sub-odontoblastic plexus (**B**), from which vessels pass between the odontoblast cells to form an odontoblastic vascular plexus. The vascularity around the odontoblast layer increases as dentine is progressively laid down, probably as the result of the odontoblasts retreating inwards through the vascular bed. Eventually, some capillaries are found immediately next to the predentine surface. (H & E; × 100)

As the dentine thickens and grows inwards, the capillaries next to the predentine are closed off. Occasionally, however, a capillary loop becomes trapped in the dentine.

625

625 Capillary loop (*arrowed*) **in dentine.** (Masson's trichrome; × 20)

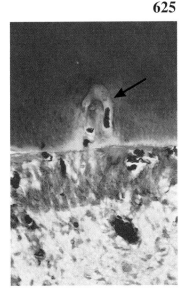

Although nerves are present close to the tooth germ from the very earliest stages of its development, they do not enter the dental papilla until much later, after they have entered the dental follicle. The first fibres to enter the developing pulp are sensory and, although located close to the blood vessels, are not functionally associated with them. The sympathetic fibres follow later. A large number of nerves enter the pulp prior to root formation, but the final pattern, including the formation of the sub-odontoblastic plexus (of Raschkow), is not established until root formation is complete. In the crown, particularly at the cusps, some sensory fibres insinuate themselves between the odontoblast and enter the dentinal tubules. This is an active process and not a mere trapping of these axons during progressing dentine deposition. The time and pattern of appearance of lymphatics in the pulp has not yet been established. The mature pulp contains macrophages, pericytes and lymphoid cells in addition to fibroblasts. These probably enter the pulp with the invading blood vessels.

Development of the root and periodontal ligament

Root development proceeds some time after the crown has formed and involves interactions between the dental follicle, a structure derived from the cervical loop region of the enamel organ (see **579**) called the epithelial root sheath (of Hertwig), and the dental papilla. The onset of root development coincides with the axial phase of tooth eruption.

626 The formation of a single-rooted tooth (A), a two-rooted tooth (B) and a three-rooted tooth (C). At the late bell stage of tooth development, when amelogenesis and dentinogenesis are well advanced, the external and internal enamel epithelia at the cervical loop of the enamel organ form a double-layered epithelial root sheath (see **628**) which proliferates apically to map out the shape of the future root. The primary apical foramen at the growing end of the epithelial root sheath may subdivide into a number of secondary apical foramina by the ingrowth of epithelial shelves from the margins of the root sheath (*arrowed*), which subsequently fuse near the centre of the root. The number and location of these epithelial shelves correspond to the number and location of the definitive roots of the tooth, and may be under the inductive control of the dental papilla. It has been suggested that the ingrowth of the epithelial shelves takes place along paths of low vascularity.

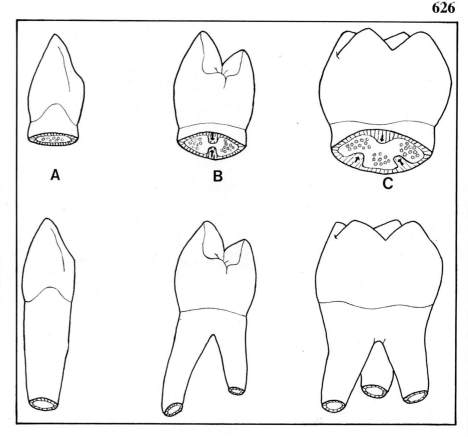

627 Apices of developing roots.
627a—two-rooted tooth.
627b—three-rooted tooth.
When a permanent tooth first erupts, only about two-thirds of the length of the root is complete. A wide, 'open' root apex is present in these situations, surrounded by a thin, regular knife-edge of dentine. It takes about a further 3 years for root completion to occur, when only a very narrow pulp opening exists. Evidence of the addition of root increments may result in the appearance of fine lines running transversely around the root.

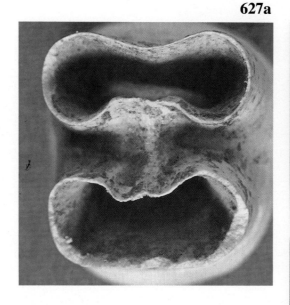 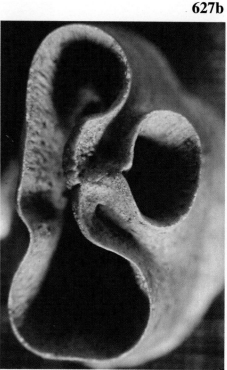

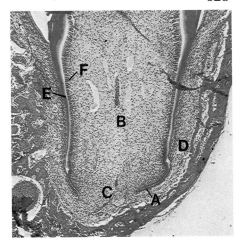

628 The developing root. Growth of the epithelial root sheath (**A**) occurs to enclose the dental papilla (**B**), except for an opening at the base, the primary apical foramen (**C**). Beneath the dental papilla, the epithelial sheath usually appears angled to form the root diaphragm. Note that between the two epithelial layers there is no stellate reticulum or stratum intermedium. The occasional presence of stellate reticulum and stratum intermedium is said to account for the presence of localised areas of enamel (enamel pearls) on the root surface, usually in interradicular regions. The dental follicle (**D**) lies external to the root sheath and forms cementum, periodontal ligament and alveolar bone. E, developing root dentine; F, odontoblast layer. (H & E; × 32)

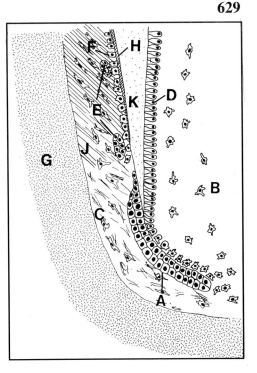

629 Schematic drawing of the developing root. In the region of the root diaphragm, the epithelial root sheath (**A**) is seen as a continuous sheet of tissue sandwiched between the undifferentiated mesenchyme of the dental papilla (**B**) and dental follicle (**C**). Above the root diaphragm, towards the developing crown, the cells of the internal layer of the epithelial sheath induce the peripheral cells of the dental papilla to differentiate into odontoblasts (**D**). Following the onset of dentinogenesis in the root, the epithelial cells of the root sheath lose their continuity, becoming separated from the surface of the developing root dentine to form epithelial rests (**E**) in the periodontal ligament (see **402**). The mesenchymal cells of the dental follicle adjacent to the root dentine now differentiate into cementoblasts (**F**), and cementogenesis commences. **G**, developing alveolar bone; **H**, developing cementum; **J**, developing periodontal ligament; **K**, root dentine.

630 The apical region of the developing root, periodontal ligament and alveolus. A, epithelial root sheath; B, dental papilla; C, odontoblasts; D, dentine of root; E, predentine layer; F, cementoblasts; G, developing cementum; H, developing alveolar bone. The tissues of the dental follicle at the developing root apex have been described as comprising three layers (**577**). Adjacent to the epithelial root sheath is the inner investing layer (**I**) of the dental follicle, which is said to be derived from ectomesenchyme (neural crest). Adjacent to the developing alveolar bone is the outer layer (**J**) of the dental follicle, which is separated from the inner layer by an intermediate layer (**K**). Unlike the tissues of the inner layer, the outer and intermediate layers are thought to be mesodermal in origin; their cells contain few cytoplasmic organelles and the extracellular compartment appears relatively structureless. Cells of the inner layer of the dental follicle differentiate into the cementoblasts, which form a layer of cuboidal cells on the surface of the root dentine. In primary acellular cementum, where the collagen is of the extrinisic fibre type (see page 159), the cementoblasts may contribute material towards the ground substance. Later, with the formation of intrinsic fibre cementum, the cementoblasts will also secrete collagen. Once cementogenesis has begun, cells of the remaining dental follicle become obliquely orientated along the root surface (*arrowed*) and show an increased content of intracellular organelles, becoming the fibroblasts of the periodontal ligament. These fibroblasts secrete collagen into the extracellular compartment, which becomes embedded in the developing cementum at the tooth surface and in the bone at the alveolar surface. (H & E; × 150)

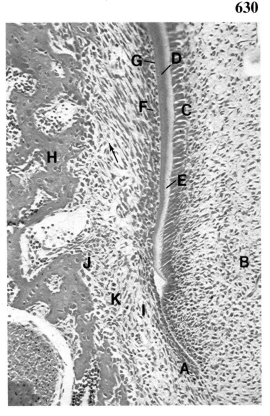

631 The pulp-limiting membrane. There has been controversy concerning the connective tissue immediately beneath the developing root apex. Initially called the cushion hammock ligament, this connective tissue was described as a fibrous network with fluid-filled interstices, with attachments on either side to the alveolar wall. It was thought to provide a resistant base so that forces produced by the growing root were prevented from causing bone resorption and resolved into an eruptive force. This view is no longer held — the thin fibrous membrane seen in this site (*arrowed*) is not attached to alveolar bone, but merges at the sides with the fibres of the developing periodontal ligament. Perhaps, therefore, the structure is more correctly termed the pulp-limiting membrane. It does not appear to be directly involved in tooth eruption as its surgical removal (together with the developing root apex) does not affect eruption. (Mallory's trichrome; × 30)

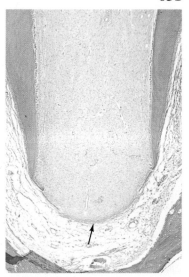

It has been suggested that changes in vascular permeability in the connective tissues around the apex of the developing root can be related to eruptive behaviour. Dense accumulations of tissue fluid (effusions) have been described beneath the growing roots of erupting teeth. Furthermore, when radioactive fibrinogen was used experimentally as a marker, the radioactive label became incorporated rapidly into the effusions, supporting the view that they are vascular in origin. Because effusions were seen to appear when the growing root was situated close to the base (fundus) of the bony tooth socket/crypt, it has been suggested that the effusions might force the root and bone apart and thereby contribute to eruption and enable further root growth. The vascular hypothesis of eruption is considered further on page 287.

Formation of collagen fibres within the periodontal ligament

632 The development of the principal periodontal ligament collagen fibres. Significant differences in this development have been described between teeth of the primary dentition (and also the permanent molars which lack successors) and successional or succedaneous teeth (i.e. permanent premolars).

Stage 1. Prior to eruption, the dento-gingival and oblique periodontal fibres are well developed in the permanent molar. In the permanent premolar only the dento-gingival fibres are organised, the developing periodontal ligament being composed of loosely structured collagenous elements.

Stage 2. As the tooth emerges into the oral cavity, the periodontal ligament of the permanent molar is well differentiated, the oblique fibres being the most conspicuous. However, at this stage in the permanent premolar only the fibres in the region of the alveolar crest are becoming organised. In the periodontal ligament itself, though collagen fibres are developing, they do not yet span the periodontal space.

Stage 3. On reaching occlusion, the fibre groupings in the cervical region of the permanent molar now become organised. In the permanent premolar, while the fibre groups cervically appear prominent, those in the apical part of the root appear relatively undeveloped.

Stage 4. After a period in function, the fibres of both the permanent molar and premolar show the classical organisation of the principal fibres.

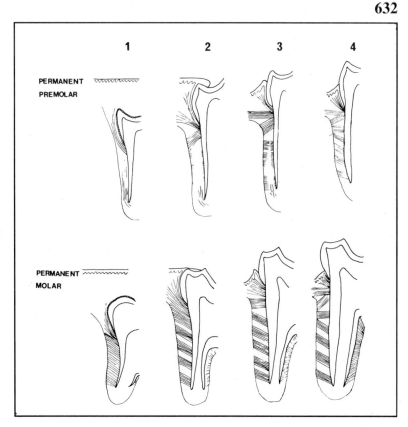

Thus, permananent premolar teeth erupt into their functional position without a well organised arrangement of collagen fibres in the periodontal ligament, unlike deciduous teeth (and permanent molars). This difference in ontogeny has been related to the chronological variation in the sequence of deposition of alveolar bone.

633 Erupting permanent molar (of a marmoset, *Callithrix jacchus*) just emerging into the oral cavity. The coronal half of the periodontal ligament is composed of well-formed, obliquely orientated, principal collagen fibre bundles (Mallory's; × 15)

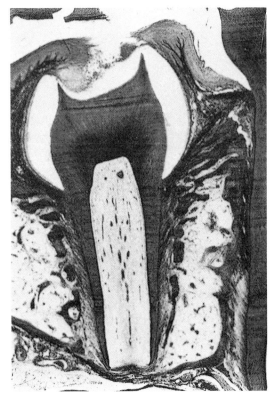

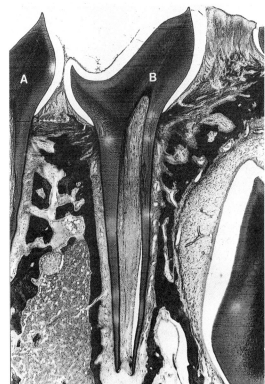

634 Erupting permanent premolar (of a squirrel monkey, *Saimiri sciureus*) just emerging into the oral cavity. Compared with the preceding micrograph, the bulk of the periodontal ligament lacks significant numbers of organised principal collagen fibre bundles passing from the tooth to alveolar bone. (Mallary's; × 35)

It appears therefore that collagen fibres may not be well organised during tooth eruption and this could be significant if it is assumed that collagen has an important role in the generation of tractional forces during eruption (see pages 284–285). However, recent evidence indicates that there are species differences in the ontogeny of principal collagen fibres. Indeed, for some species, the fibres associated with succedaneous teeth may be seen to pass between tooth and bone as the tooth erupts into the oral cavity.

635 Principal collagen fibres associated with an erupting permanent canine (of the ferret *Mustela putorius*) as it emerges into the oral cavity. Compared with the previous micrograph, principal fibres are seen passing from tooth to bone. However, the fibres are not as well organised (in terms of thickness and orientation) as those for the fully erupted tooth illustrated in **636**. (van Giesen; ×150)

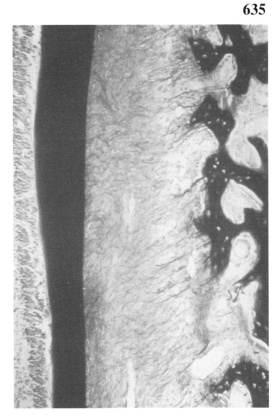

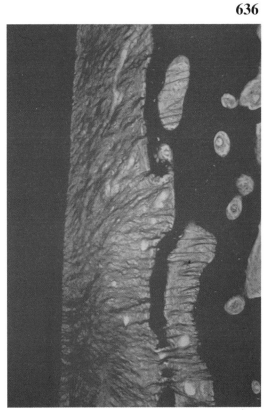

636 Well differentiated collagen fibres for the fully erupted permanent canine of the ferret. (van Giesen; × 130)

There is evidence of a change in the obliquity of the principal collagen fibres and in their dimensions as the tooth reaches its functional position. The inclination of the oblique fibres has been reported to decrease, while the principal fibres are said to thicken with function. However, there may again be species differences.

There appear to be few structural differences between fibroblasts in the developing periodontal ligaments of erupting and fully erupted teeth. However, changes during eruption have been reported for the ground substance and the vascularity of the periodontal ligament (385).

As the tooth erupts, resorption is the predominant pattern of bone activity at the base of the socket (i.e. beneath the developing root). Thus, bone deposition at this site is precluded as a cause of tooth eruption. There are species differences, however, bone deposition being found beneath the erupting permanent premolars of dogs. The different patterns of bone activity in different species may relate to the distance a tooth has to erupt. If the distance is greater than the length of the root then bone deposition is clearly necessary to maintain the normal dimensions of the periodontal ligament at the root apex of the tooth. Remodelling of alveolar bone other than at the socket's base may also be seen during eruption and this relates to the relocation of the teeth during jaw growth and to the establishment of occlusion.

Cementogenesis

Cementogenesis will be considered in terms of the formation of a primary (acellular) cementum and then of a secondary (cellular) cementum (see pages 156–158). Both tissues develop from the activity of the mesenchyme cells of the dental follicle after fragmentation of the epithelial root sheath. As for the development of the crown of the tooth, the hard tissues that comprise the root (cementum and dentine) are formed under the control of various epithelial–mesenchymal interactions (see page 279). Note however, that unlike the crown, the epithelial component of the root is not usually considered to give rise to a calcified tissue.

Primary (acellular) cementum

637

637 The epithelial root sheath. Once the crown has fully formed, the internal and external enamel epithelia proliferate downwards as a double-layered sheet of epithelial cells (the epithelial root sheath) to map out the shape of the root. The root sheath is separated by basal laminae on both of its surfaces from the adjacent connective tissues of the dental follicle and dental papilla. The epithelial root sheath (**A**) induces the adjacent cells of the dental papilla to differentiate into odontoblasts (**B**), which then secrete predentine (**C**) which subsequently mineralises. The cells of the epithelial root sheath, in contrast to those of the enamel organ, do not enlarge during this inductive stage. (TEM; × 5,000)

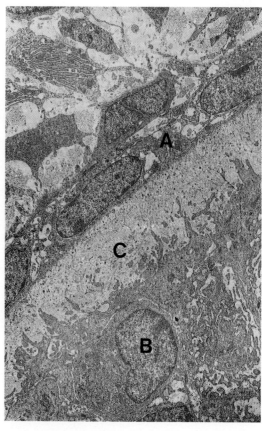

The traditional view of primary cementum formation is that, following the loss of continuity of the epithelial root sheath, the adjacent cells of the investing layer of the dental follicle come to lie on the surface of the root dentine and are induced to differentiate into cementoblasts (see page 273). Much of the collagen in primary cementum is derived from Sharpey's fibres of the periodontal ligament (extrinsic fibre cementum, see page 159) and the cementoblasts secrete little collagen. However, cementoblasts are assumed to secrete components of the ground substance and this is supported by the presence within the cementoblasts of the intracytoplasmic organelles necessary for protein synthesis and secretion.

638

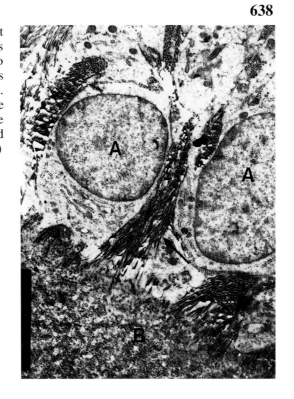

638 Cementoblast and primary cementum. It is not possible at present to distinguish morphologically or biochemically between cementoblasts and fibroblasts, and it is possible that both cell types, when apposed to cementum, contribute to the secretion of cemental matrix. Cementoblasts (**A**) associated with primary cementum are cuboidal and lack cell processes. They contribute little collagen and thus do not have large amounts of the intracellular organelles associated with protein synthesis. Note the periodontal ligament fibres (*arrowed*) passing between the cementoblasts and inserting as extrinsic fibres into the acellular cementum (**B**). (TEM; × 5,000)

Mineralisation of the layer of cementum matrix (precementum or cementoid) does not appear to be controlled by the cells. Indeed, matrix vesicles have not been observed and it is likely that, as with enamel, the presence of hydroxyapatite crystals in the neighbouring dentine initiates mineralisation in cementum. Mineralisation proceeds in a linear fashion and calcospherites are not observed in cementum. There is usually always a thin, unmineralised layer of precementum present on the developing surface of the cementum.

The role of the epithelial root sheath cells in cementogenesis is unclear. However, there is evidence suggesting that, rather than being derived from the mesenchymal cells of the dental follicle, some early cementoblasts may be transformed epithelial root sheath cells. Some epithelial cells may thus contribute material to primary cementum. They may also contribute to the hya-line zone in peripheral root dentine (see page 140).

The traditional view of primary cementum formation has recently been challenged. It has been suggested that the first formed primary cementum is in fact the initial layer of root predentine whose mineralisation is delayed and into which the extrinsic Sharpey's fibres of the periodontal ligament become inserted. Subsequently, this outermost layer (of dentine) would mineralise centrifugally (as opposed to centripetally, for the rest of the dentine). Evidence for this delayed mineralisation comes from studies employing tetracycline, an antibiotic which becomes incorporated into mineralising tissues and which, following microradiographic analysis, shows the state of mineralisation. Clearly, the development of the outer dentine/inner cementum region is not yet well understood.

Secondary (cellular) cementum

Following the formation of primary cementum in the cervical portion of the root, secondary cementum appears in the apical region of the root (at about the time of eruption, when approximately two-thirds of the root has formed). Associated with the increased rate of formation (as evidenced by the thicker precementum layer), cementoblasts at the surface become incorporated into the forming matrix and are converted into cementocytes. Cellular cementum is usually of the mixed-fibre type, containing both extrinsic fibres from the periodontal ligament (arranged more or less perpendicular to the root surface) and intrinsic fibres (arranged more or less parallel to the root surface) which are secreted by the cementoblasts themselves.

639

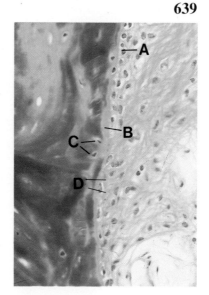

639 Developing cellular cementum. A, cementoblasts; **B**, precementum (unmineralised matrix); **C**, cementocytes within the mineralised cellular cementum. Note that in addition to the collagen fibres secreted by cementoblasts, cementum also contains collagen fibres derived from the periodontal ligament (the Sharpey's fibres, **D**). Because cementum is being continuously deposited, newly synthesised collagen fibres of the periodontal ligament can be attached to the tooth under changing functional situations. Cementoblasts must be continually produced at the cementum surface to compensate for the incorporation of cementocytes into the secondary cementum. (Masson's trichrome; × 230)

640

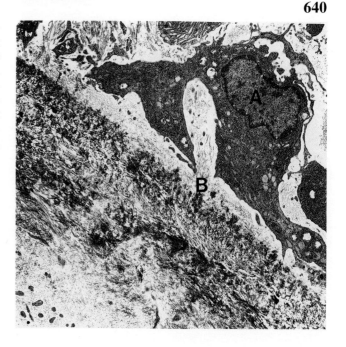

640 Cementoblast (A) associated with the formation of cellular cementum. Cementoblasts are less elongated than periodontal fibroblasts, being squat, cuboidal cells with large nuclei. Like fibroblasts, they contain all the intracytoplasmic organelles necessary for protein synthesis and secretion. The nucleus of a cementoblast is distinctly vesicular with one or more nucleoli. The appearance of a cementoblast will depend upon its degree of activity. Cells actively depositing acellular cementum do not have prominent cytoplasmic processes. However, cells depositing cellular cementum (as illustrated here) exhibit abundant cytoplasm and cytoplasmic processes, and their nuclei tend to be folded and irregularly shaped. **B**, precementum. (TEM; × 4,000).

Acellular cementum may be deposited on top of cellular cementum (**346**). If it is believed that the first formed primary cementum is of dentinal origin, this does not preclude further acellular cementum of true cementoblast origin being deposited superficially after the tooth has erupted.

Intermediate cementum

In the apical half of the roots of most teeth (except incisors) the interface between dentine and cellular cementum is difficult to define and contains cellular debris (possibly epithelial root sheath cells). This zone has been termed intermediate cementum (**357**). It is not clear how it is formed, although there is some evidence that it may be dentinal in origin.

Afibrillar cementum

These localised regions of mineralised ground substance are seen covering cervical enamel (see page 160). It is believed that areas of enamel lose their protective covering of reduced enamel epithelial cells prior to erupting into the mouth, and adjacent cells of the dental follicle secrete afibrillar cementum onto the exposed enamel surface.

Incremental lines in cementum

Cementogenesis occurs rhythmically, periods of activity alternating with periods of quiescence. The periods of decreased activity are associated with incremental lines (**348**) which are believed to have a higher content of ground substance and mineral, and a lower content of collagen, than adjacent cementum.

Epithelial–mesenchymal interactions during cementogenesis

The epithelial root sheath is important in the differentiation of root odontoblasts, as demonstrated by experimental recombinations between isolated epithelial root sheath cells and dental papilla cells (root dentine will only form in the presence of the epithelial root sheath).

The question arises as to whether the presence of root dentine is sufficient to induce dental follicle cells to become cementoblasts. This has been tested by experimental recombinations of slices of root dentine and dental follicle cells. Although occasional formation of bony deposits on the root dentine were observed, cementoblast differentiation and cementum formation were not seen. This demonstrates that the root surface alone does not appear to provide a sufficient stimulus for cementoblast differentiation within dental follicle cells. Indeed, cementum only developed in combinations which included dental follicle cells, root dentine and epithelial root sheath cells. Thus the possibility exists that epithelial–mesenchymal interactions may also occur between the dental follicle and the epithelial root sheath during root development.

Experiments have shown that, when a tooth germ at the early bell stage is dissected from the jaw, it is surrounded by the inner investing layer of the dental follicle. When it is transplanted in this condition, the investing layer has the capacity to give rise to all the investing tissues (i.e. cementum, periodontal ligament and bone). This, however, does not preclude a contribution to the periodontium *in vivo* from the outer part of the dental follicle (**577**). When the dental follicle cells are excluded and the enamel organ and dental papilla alone are transplanted to an ectopic site, there is regeneration of the investing layer of the follicle and a root-related periodontal ligament, but no formation of alveolar bone. Thus, the papillary mesenchymal cells in the region of the root apex may be the source of cells that can migrate to either side of the epithelial root sheath. Depending on the inductive influence of the adjacent tissue, they would then differentiate into odontoblasts on the inner aspect and cementoblasts on the outer aspect of the root sheath.

Development of the dentitions

Description of the development of the dentitions requires consideration of the processes of tooth eruption and of the development of occlusion post-eruptively. Indeed, three distinct phases of tooth development can be recognised which ultimately lead to the establishment of the full dentition. First, there is a phase termed the pre-eruptive phase, which starts with the initiation of tooth development and ends with the completion of the crown (see pages 248–256). Second, there is the phase of tooth eruption (prefunctional phase) which begins once the roots begin to form. Third, after the teeth have emerged into the oral cavity, there is a protracted phase concerned with the development and maintenance of occlusion (the functional phase).

Tooth eruption

Eruption is essentially the process whereby a tooth moves from its developmental position in the jaw into its functional position in the mouth. However, there is no evidence to suggest that eruption entirely ceases once a tooth meets its antagonist in the mouth, and outward axial movements occurring during the functional phase may also be eruptive movements (viz. overeruption following removal of the antagonist tooth in the opposite jaw).

641

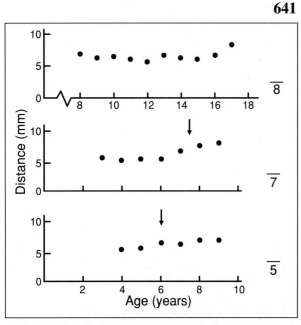

641 Graph illustrating that, throughout the pre-eruptive phase of tooth development, there is concentric growth of the tooth within its follicle without any active bodily movement in a direction indicating eruption towards the oral cavity. The graph plots the mean distance from the mandibular canal (regarded as a fixed point) to the centre point of the developing crown of the tooth for a child who has radiographs taken at various ages. The upper graph is for the permanent mandibular third molar, the middle graph for the permanent mandibular second molar, the lower graph for the mandibular second premolar. Arrows indicate age at crown completion.

642

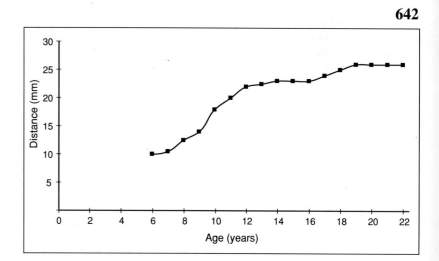

642 Graph showing the mean distance from the mandibular canal to the occlusal surface for a permanent mandibular second molar during its eruption. Note that there are two stages of active eruption of this tooth. The first stage occurs between 6 and 12 years when it is emerging into the mouth. A later second stage occurs at about 16 years in association with the adolescent growth spurt.

While the main direction of the eruptive force is axial (i.e. related to the long axis of the tooth), movement also occurs in other planes, accounting for tilting and drifting. Eruption rates of teeth are greatest at the time of crown emergence. Rates also differ according to tooth type. Permanent maxillary central incisors are reported to erupt at about 1mm/month; the rates for mandibular second premolars have been determined to be as great as 4.5mm in 14 weeks. For permanent third molars, where space is available, eruption rates of 1mm in 3 months have been recorded. In crowded dentitions, however, the rates are less than 1mm in 6 months.

As a tooth approaches the oral cavity, the overlying bone is resorbed and there are marked changes in the overlying soft tissues. The enamel surface is covered by the reduced enamel epithelium, which is a vestige of the enamel organ.

643

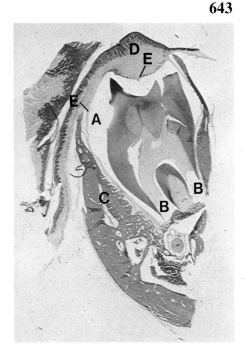

643 An erupting deciduous molar prior to its emergence into the oral cavity. A, enamel space; **B**, developing roots; **C**, developing alveolar crypt; **D**, oral mucosa and overlying connective tissue; **E**, reduced enamel epithelium. (Decalcified, transverse section through jaw; H & E; × 4)

644

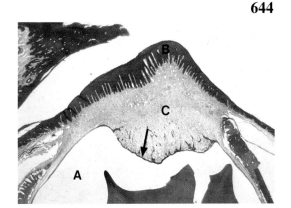

644 The soft tissues overlying the enamel space (A) of an erupting tooth. As the tooth erupts, the outer cells of the reduced enamel epithelium (*arrowed*) proliferate into the connective tissue (**C**) between the cusp tip and the oral epithelium (**B**). It has been suggested that these proliferating epithelial cells secrete enzymes which degrade collagen. Reduced enamel epithelial cells may also be concerned with the removal of breakdown products resulting from resorption of connective tissue. Depolymerisation of ground substance has been detected in the connective tissue overlying erupting teeth. Although a relationship between the degeneration of the connective tissue and the pressure exerted by the underlying erupting tooth has not been established, ischaemia is thought to be a contributory factor. That pressure alone is not entirely responsible is indicated by the finding that there is always evidence of some new collagen formation in this region. (H & E; × 10)

645

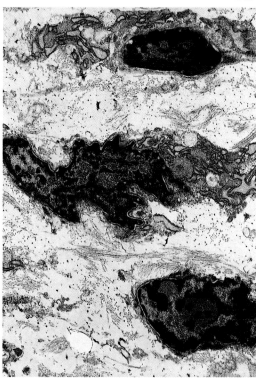

645 Fibroblasts in the connective tissue overlying an erupting tooth. Many of the fibroblasts in this region cease fibrillogenesis. They actively take up extracellular material (as evidenced by intracellular collagen profiles — see **392**) and synthesise acid hydrolases. Eventually, the nuclei become pyknotic and the cells degenerate (as illustrated here). (TEM; × 10,000)

646

646 The development of the dento-gingival junction during the eruption of a tooth. The red outline delineates the oral epithelium, and the green outline indicates the reduced enamel epithelium. As the tooth approaches the oral epithelium, the cells of the outer layer of the reduced enamel epithelium and the basal layer of the oral epithelium actively proliferate and eventually unite. The epithelium covering the tip of the tooth then degenerates at its centre, enabling the crown to emerge through an epithelial-lined pathway into the oral cavity. Further emergence of the tooth results from active eruptive movements and passive separation of the oral epithelium from the crown surface. When the tooth first erupts into the mouth, the reduced enamel epithelium is attached to the unerupted part of the crown, thus forming an epithelial seal — the junctional epithelium. It is generally believed that the reduced epithelial component of the junctional epithelium is eventually replaced by oral epithelium. With continued eruption, as more of the crown is exposed, a gingival crevice is formed. **R.E.E.**, reduced enamel epithelium.

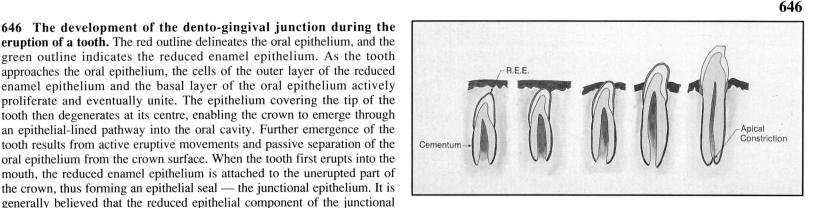

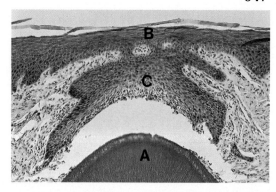

647 An erupting tooth (A) about to emerge into the oral cavity through an epithelial-lined pathway as a result of fusion of the oral epithelium (B) and the reduced enamel epithelium (C). (H & E; × 12)

For the eruption of a permanent tooth, where there is a deciduous predecessor (i.e. excluding the permanent molars), the roots of the deciduous tooth must be resorbed to allow for

shedding. Another specialised feature associated with the erupting permanent tooth is the presence of a gubernacular canal.

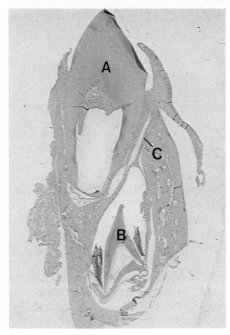

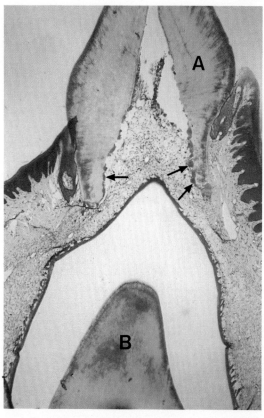

648 Buccolingual section through an erupted deciduous canine (A) and its erupting successor (B). Initially, each deciduous tooth and its developing permanent successor share a common alveolar crypt, the permanent tooth germ being situated lingually to the developing deciduous tooth (see 582). With continued growth this relationship changes and the permanent tooth comes to lie near the root apex of the deciduous tooth within its own bony crypt. Note that the alveolar crypt of the permanent tooth is not complete, there being the opening of a canal in its roof, through which the dental follicle of the tooth germ communicates with, and is attached to, the overlying oral mucosa. This canal has been termed the gubernacular canal (C). (Decalcified section; H & E; × 4)

649 Buccolingual section through a resorbing deciduous tooth (A) and its erupting successor (B). During the early eruptive stages of the permanent tooth, the bone separating it from its deciduous predecessor is resorbed. Following this, resorption of the hard tissues of the deciduous tooth takes place by the activity of multinucleated osteoclast-like cells termed odontoclasts (*arrowed*). The vascular, resorbing tissue has been termed the resorbing organ of Tomes. (Decalcified section; Masson's trichrome; × 70)

For a deciduous incisor or canine, root resorption initially occurs on the lingual surface adjacent to the developing permanent tooth. With subsequent movement and relocation of the teeth in the growing jaws, the developing permanent tooth comes to lie directly beneath the deciduous tooth and further resorption occurs from the apex. For a deciduous molar, root resorption

often commences on the inner surfaces where the permanent premolars initially develop. The premolars later come to lie beneath the roots of the deciduous molar and further resorption occurs from the root apices. The shift in position of the deciduous tooth relative to the permanent successor may account for the intermittent nature of root resorption.

The initiation of root resorption may be an inherent developmental process or it may be related to pressure from the permanent successor against the overlying bone or tooth. To assess which of these explanations is correct, permanent tooth germs have been surgically removed, when it was seen that

resorption of the deciduous predecessors still occurred, though this was delayed. These findings are also consistent with the clinical observation that shedding of a deciduous tooth still occurs but is retarded where the successor is congenitally absent or occupies an abnormal position within the jaw.

It has been suggested that increased masticatory loads affect the pattern and rate of deciduous tooth resorption. Indeed, it has been shown that, if deciduous teeth are splinted following the removal of the developing permanent teeth, there is less root resorption compared with removal of the permanent teeth alone.

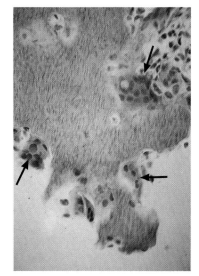

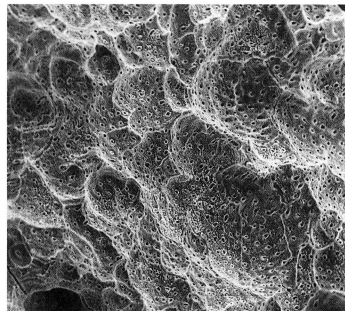

650 Resorbing dentine. Multinucleated osteoclast-like cells (*arrowed*) lie within resorption lacunae (Howship's lacunae). These cells have been termed odontoclasts. Odontoclasts, like osteoclasts, differentiate from circulating monocyte-type cells. They are vacuolated and have long cytoplasmic processes. In an electron micrograph, the cytoplasmic projections form a brush border with the tooth surface. The odontoclasts have an abundance of ribosomes and a large number of mitochondria. (H & E; × 215)

651 Resorbing surface of a deciduous tooth showing Howship's lacunae. Dentinal tubules are seen as small circular openings. Compared with lacunae in bone (**443a**), those in resorbing teeth tend to be larger and more spherical (Anorganic specimen; SEM; × 400)

Resorption of deciduous teeth is not a continuous process. During rest periods, reparative tissue may be formed leading to a reattachment of the periodontal ligament. The tissue of repair is cementum-like and the cells responsible for its formation are similar in appearance to cementoblasts (**358**). If the repair process prevails over the resorption, the tooth may become ankylosed to the surrounding bone, with loss of the periodontal ligament.

652 Fusion between dentine (A) and bone (B). This is a section through an ankylosed root. Ankylosis may also be caused by trauma and/or infection of a tooth. Where a deciduous tooth becomes ankylosed and cannot move, its position within the jaw remains constant so that, with increasing height of the alveolar bone, it appears to sink gradually below the level of the adjacent teeth. Such ankylosed teeth are referred to as 'submerged' teeth. The submergence may continue to such an extent that the teeth become completely buried within bone. (Decalcified section viewed in blue light; × 150)

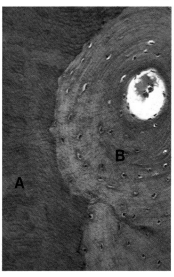

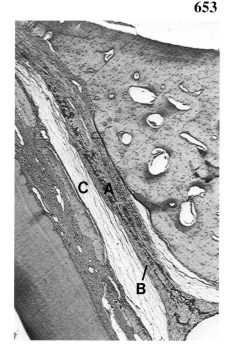

653 A gubernacular canal and its contents. The gubernacular canal (**648**) contains the gubernacular cord. The cord is comprised of a central strand of epithelium (derived from the dental lamina, **A**) surrounded by connective tissue. The connective tissue is organised into inner (**B**) and outer (**C**) layers. Collagen fibres of the inner layer show greater organisation and run mainly parallel to the long axis of the epithelium. In the outer layer, the collagen fibers are fewer and less organised. Differences between the layers can also be discerned with respect to the vasculature, the vessels in the outer layer being larger. During eruption, the gubernacular cords decrease in length but increase in thickness. In addition, they become less dense. Surgical removal of the cord does not prevent eruption of the permanent tooth. (H & E; × 25)

Mechanisms of tooth eruption

Tooth eruption is traditionally considered to be a developmental process whereby the tooth moves in an axial direction from its position within the alveolar crypt of the jaw into a functional position within the oral cavity. However, eruption can be regarded as a lifelong process since a tooth will often move axially in response to changing functional situations (e.g. overeruption resulting from the removal of an antagonist, and compensatory eruption related to attrition).

The rate of eruption represents a balance between forces tending to move the tooth into the mouth (eruptive force) and forces tending to prevent this movement (resistive force). Resistance may be produced by overlying soft tissues and alveolar bone, the viscosity of the surrounding periodontal ligament and occlusal forces. Thus, changes in the rate of tooth movement may be brought about by changes in either the eruptive forces and/or the resistive forces. At present, little is known about the nature, source and magnitude of either the eruptive or resistive forces. Furthermore, it is not known whether the forces are of the same nature and value at various stages of the eruptive cycle. By and large, this situation results from difficulties encountered in producing experimental systems which isolate for study single possible agents associated with the eruptive process.

All tissues within the vicinity of the tooth thought capable of generating a force have, at one time or another, been implicated in the eruptive process. The theories advanced to explain the mechanism of tooth eruption can be divided into two main groups. One view suggests that the tooth is pushed out as a result of forces generated beneath and around it, either by alveolar bone growth, root growth, blood-pressure/tissue fluid pressure, or cell proliferation. Alternatively, the tooth may be pulled out as a result of tension within the connective tissue of the periodontal ligament. Although no one theory is yet supported by sufficient experimental evidence, this brief review will show that the eruptive mechanism (a) is a property of the periodontal ligament (or its precursor, the dental follicle); (b) does not require a tractional force pulling the tooth towards the mouth; (c) is probably multifactorial in that more than one agent has important contributions to the overall eruptive force; and (d) could involve a combination of fibroblast activity (although the evidence to date remains poor) and vascular and/or tissue hydrostatic pressures.

Role of the periodontal ligament in eruption

654 Experiments involving root resection or root transection of the continuously growing incisors of rodents or lagomorphs indicate that the periodontal ligament is the probable source for the generation of the forces responsible for eruption. Root resection involves the surgical removal of the proliferative odontogenic tissues at the base of the continuously growing incisor; root transection involves cutting the incisor into proximal and distal portions. Both surgical procedures result in a situation where the tooth (or the distal segment following transection) remains merely as a fragment attached to the jaw by a periodontal ligament, but without the possibility of root growth and with degeneration of the pulp. Furthermore, there can be no contribution to eruption from bone growth as none occurs at the base (fundus) of the socket. The resected and transected incisors continue to erupt to the point where they are exfoliated from the socket. The radiograph illustrated here is of the transected incisor of a rabbit. Note that the distal segment (**A**) has continued to erupt to the alveolar crest from the site of transection (*arrowed*) without any contribution from the proximal segment (**B**) which has been pinned. That the movement is eruption-like and not an artifactual exfoliation is indicated by experiments which show that the resected incisor changes its rate of movement in response to factors which similarly affect the normal tooth.

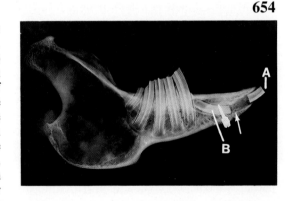

654

655 Although the periodontal ligament is implicated in the generation of the eruptive force, recent experiments show that, for teeth of limited growth, this property can be undertaken by its developmental precursor, the dental follicle. When a developing unerupted tooth is surgically removed and replaced by a silicone replica (**655a**), the replica (**655b**) will erupt provided that the dental follicle is retained. This experiment confirms that rootless teeth (both experimentally-produced and clinically-observed) can erupt, and that the eruptive mechanism is present in a connective tissue (periodontal ligament or dental follicle) which need not gain attachment to the tooth.

655a

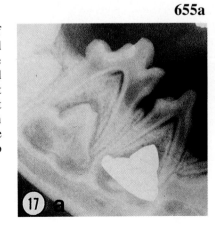

655b

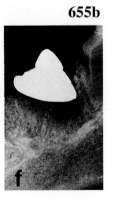

656 Investigation into the eruptive behaviour of the continuously growing, lathyritic incisor confirms that the eruptive force is unlikely to involve a tractional element that pulls the tooth towards the oral cavity. Lathyrogens are drugs that specifically inhibit the formation of collagen crosslinks, thereby disrupting the fibre network in the periodontal ligament. The graph shows that the eruption rates of the lathyritic incisor are unaffected, provided that occlusal forces (which could traumatise the already weakened ligament) are reduced by regular trimming of the tooth to the gingival level. Thus, the lathyrogen experiments support the experiments on rootless teeth which are teeth of non-continuous growth. Further evidence against a tractional eruptive force comes from study of the development of the periodontal ligament (see pages 274–275), which indicates that some teeth can erupt in the absence of well developed periodontal fibres. These studies also disprove the once strongly held belief that contraction of periodontal collagen fibres is responsible for generating the eruptive force.

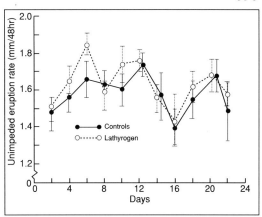

657 Although the opinion is held that the force effecting eruption is derived from a single source (i.e. a prime mover), it is conceivable that more than one agent contributes to the overall force. That eruption is multifactorial is evident when considering the variety of processes that must be involved to produce and sustain eruption. Indeed, four processes seem to be necessary. First, there must be the mechanism itself that generates the eruptive forces. Second, there are processes whereby eruptive forces are translated into eruption by movements through the surrounding tissues (e.g. overcoming the resistance of the tissues to eruption). Third, eruption must be sustained by processes that enable the tooth to be supported in its new position. Fourth, eruption occurs alongside a process of remodelling of the periodontal tissues to maintain the functional integrity of the system.

Experiments support the view that eruption is multifactorial; based upon study of the interactions of various drugs/hormones known to influence eruption, they suggest that there are at least two factors involved — a cortisone-sensitive factor and a cortisone-insensitive factor. The graph shows that when a drug (cyclophosphamide) is given which severely retards eruption, the remaining component of eruption is no longer affected by cortisone administration which would normally produce a marked increase in eruption. Although it is possible to interpret these data in other ways, subsequent experiments show that the recovery of eruption following root resection also has cortisone-sensitive and cortisone-insensitive phases.

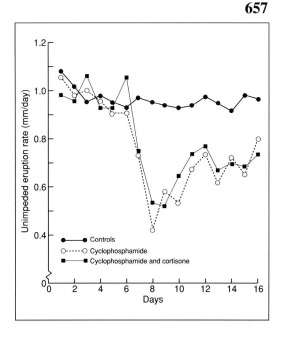

Having established that the connective tissues around the developing tooth are most likely to be the source of the eruptive mechanism, two major systems have been implicated in the generation of the eruptive force. One view holds that the force is produced by the activity of periodontal fibroblasts through their contractility and/or motility. Another view suggests that vascular and/or tissue hydrostatic pressures in and around the tooth are responsible for eruption.

Whatever the system implicated in the eruptive mechanism, the evidence should be judged according to the following five criteria:

1. The proposed system must be capable of producing a force under physiological conditions, which is sufficient to move a tooth in a direction favouring eruption.
2. Experimentally induced changes to the system should cause predictable changes in eruption.
3. The system requires characteristics which enable it to sustain eruptive movements over long periods of time.
4. The biochemical characteristics of the system should be consistent with the production of an eruptive force.
5. The morphological features associated with the system should be consistent with the production of an eruptive force.

The periodontal fibroblast motility/contractility hypotheses

A role for the periodontal ligament fibroblasts in eruption is based upon the notion that these cells can exert a tractional force onto the tooth through the collagen network or through cell-to-cell contacts. This is in some ways analogous to the events occurring during wound contraction, which are thought to be the result of activities of specialised cells termed myofibroblasts. However, the periodontal ligament differs markedly from granulation tissue, and there is considerable evidence against the requirement for a tractional eruptive force acting through the periodontal collagen network (pages 284–285). Reviewing the evidence in terms of our prescribed criteria, there is at present no evidence indicating that the fibroblasts can exert a force under physiological conditions sufficient to move a tooth in a direction favouring eruption. Neither has it been possible to devise procedures to affect selectively periodontal fibroblast activity *in vivo* to assess whether the experimental procedures have predictable effects on eruption. It has been shown that the drug colchicine, by its known disturbance of intracellular microtubules, reduces cell motility and this might explain the drug's significant retardatory effect on eruption. However, colchicine influences more than just cell migration (e.g. it also affects connective tissue turnover). To date, the evidence relating to the fibroblast activity hypotheses relies almost entirely upon consideration of the morphology of the fibroblasts (criterion 5 above) and upon the possible characteristics of the system which would sustain the eruptive forces over long periods of time (criterion 3 above).

658a **658b** **658c**

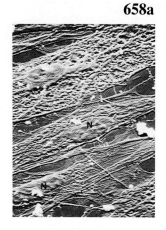 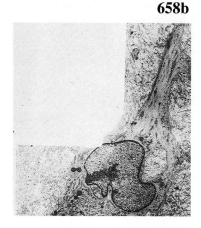 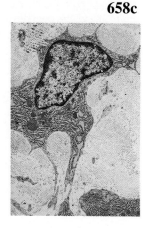

658 The ultrastructural appearance of periodontal fibroblasts. 658a, cells cultured on plastic; 658b, cells cultured in a collagen gel; 658c, cells *in vivo*. When periodontal fibroblasts are cultured on plastic, they assume the appearance and behaviour of migratory cells. They have a highly elongated, shape with numerous, highly polarised arrays of microtubules and microfilaments. Their motility *in vitro* ceases with colchicine. When periodontal fibroblasts are cultured in a collagen gel, they generate tension by their contractility and assume the appearance of myofibroblast-like cells (i.e. fibroblasts with some of the properties of smooth muscle cells, a feature of fibroblasts in granulation tissue). During their contractile phase, these cells possess thick cell coats, considerable amounts of microfilamentous material dispersed throughout the cytoplasm, numerous cell contacts resembling gap junctions, occasional crenulated (folded) nuclei, but little rough endoplasmic reticulum. Their contraction *in vitro* is inhibited when drugs interfering with microfilaments (e.g. cytochalasin) are added to the culture medium. *In vivo*, however, periodontal fibroblasts show features neither of migratory cells nor of myofibroblasts. Instead, they tend to be rounded or flattened in outline without polarity of shape, they have relatively little microfilamentous material (and then primarily as stress fibres beneath the cell membrane, a feature of cells generally exhibited 'after' migration/ contraction), they have only infrequent gap junctions (but more cell contacts in the form of simplified desmosomes) and considerable amounts of rough endoplasmic reticulum. Thus, the periodontal fibroblast *in vivo* shows all the characteristics of a cell actively synthesising and secreting protein rather than of a motile/ contractile cell. Care must therefore be taken in extrapolating from the *in vitro* to the *in vivo* situation. (SEM; **658a**, × 800; **658b**, × 2,500; **658c**, × 2,000)

In terms of criterion 3 (above), there is evidence of sustained migration of periodontal fibroblasts *in vivo*. Studies where the nuclei of cells have been labelled (with tritium-labelled thymidine) indicate that periodontal fibroblasts move occlusally at a rate equal to that of eruption; if the eruption rate is increased there is a concomitant increase in the rate of migration. Although providing some evidence of a shift in the position of periodontal fibroblasts, such work does not in itself indicate whether the cells are moving actively to generate the force of eruption, or whether they are merely being transported passively within the ligament, the eruptive force being generated by another mechanism.

Other morphological features of the periodontal fibroblasts argue against their involvement in the generation of the eruptive force. The large numbers of cell contacts (not a usual feature of fibroblasts in a mature connective tissue) might indicate that a force could be generated through cell-to-cell contacts. However, the contacts are simplified desmosomes and not the fibronexus usually seen for myofibroblasts in contracting wounds. Furthermore, many of the simplified desmosomes for periodontal fibroblasts are located at right angles to the long axes of the cells, and they lack any recognisable microfilament bundles — arrangements which do not seem suited to transmit a tractional force directly through the cells themselves.

One way of assessing the contribution of the periodontal fibroblasts to eruption involves analysing quantitatively the structure of these cells in different periodontal ligaments and in teeth exhibiting different eruptive behaviours. The findings of studies using this approach also provide evidence against the periodontal fibroblast motility/contractility hypotheses. For example, there are no differences in the cells and their various organelles when periodontal fibroblasts in rapidly erupting and fully erupted teeth are compared.

286

The periodontal vascular/tissue hydrostatic pressure hypotheses

An eruptive force might be generated via the periodontal vasculature either directly through blood pressures or indirectly by influencing periodontal tissue (hydrostatic) pressures. Whether acting directly or indirectly, the periodontal vascular hypotheses clearly do not require a tractional mode of activity within the periodontal tissues (see pages 284–285).

That vascular pressures can alter the position of a tooth in its socket is shown by the fact that a tooth moves in synchrony with the arterial pulse. Furthermore, spontaneous changes in blood pressure have been shown to influence eruptive behaviour, and at death, when the arterial blood pressure is zero, eruption ceases. Therefore, there is some evidence that, without experimental intervention, vascular/tissue pressures can produce a force sufficient to move a tooth in a direction favouring eruption (criterion 1 above). Experimental alterations to the periodontal vasculature following the administration of vasoactive drugs or interference with the sympathetic vasomotor nerve supply also result in predictable changes in eruption-like behaviour (criterion 2 above).

659

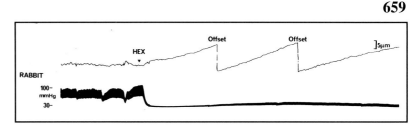

659 Effects of a hypotensive agent on an erupting tooth. Using a sensitive displacement transducer, it is possible to continuously monitor eruptive behaviour (note the minute markers on the time scale). Following the administration of a hypotensive drug (e.g. hexamethonium-hex), as a probable result of increased capillary and periodontal tissue hydrostatic pressures, there is a marked increase in the rates of extrusive, eruption-like movements.

660

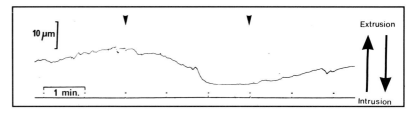

660 Effects of stimulation of the cervical sympathetics on an erupting tooth. During the period of stimulation (*arrowed*), as a probable result of vasoconstriction and decreased capillary and periodontal tissue pressures, note that eruption ceases and the tooth shows a significant intrusion into its socket. Once the stimulus is removed, eruption recommences.

To sustain eruptive movements according to the vascular hypotheses, it is necessary to postulate that periodontal tissue pressures are high, that there are pressure differentials along the periodontal ligament, and that changes in such pressures change eruptive behaviour (criterion 3 above). Indeed, there is evidence to support all three postulates. However, there remains debate as to whether periodontal tissue hydrostatic pressures are supra-atmospheric or subatmospheric.

To assess whether the biochemical composition of the periodontal ligament is consistent with the production of an eruptive force by 'vascular' means (criterion 4 above), analysis of the periodontal ground substance at different stages of tooth development has shown that a proteoglycan, with possibly significant osmotic influences on the tissue, increases in quantity during the active phase of eruption (**385**).

Quantitative electron microscopy of the periodontal vasculature (criterion 5 above) has shown that, for both the degree of vasculature and the numbers of fenestrations on the capillaries, marked changes occur with different phases of eruption. For the non-continuously growing molar of the rodent, the number of fenestrations is three times greater during eruption than after eruption. In addition, for the continuously growing incisor of the rodent, the fenestrations are relatively low in number near the alveolar crest (approximately $1 \times 10^6/mm^3$ of tissue) but are high near the root base of the erupting tooth (approximately $4 \times 10^6/mm^3$), perhaps providing evidence for differential vascular activity along the periodontal ligament. Thus, whilst no single piece of evidence briefly reported here for a role in eruption of the vascular elements of the periodontal ligament is incontrovertible, the sum of the evidence does suggest that it could provide one factor in the multifactorial mechanism of eruption.

Some observations have been made on the rate of emergence of human teeth into the oral cavity. Initially, there is a period of slow eruption when the crown is carried towards the oral mucosa. For permanent teeth, this period may take between 2 and 4 years. A tooth erupts most rapidly as it enters the oral cavity, at which time the length of its root is about two-thirds complete. Eruption then slows as the tooth approaches the occlusal plane. Once the tooth has emerged into the oral cavity, it may take 1–2 years to reach the occlusal plane. The emergence of the crown is partly due to axial movement of the tooth (active eruption) and partly due to retraction of the adjacent soft tissues (passive eruption). For human maxillary incisors, the maximum eruption rate at the time of crown emergence is about 1mm per month. For maxillary third molars, the maximum rates are seen in spaced dentitions and are less than half that recorded for incisors. In crowded dentitions, the rates are even lower (less than 1mm in 6 months).

Table 19: Chronology of tooth development and the order of eruption.

Chronology of the deciduous dentition

Tooth	First evidence of calcification (months in utero)	Crown completed (months)	Eruption (months)	Root completed (years)
Maxillary				
A	3–4	4	7	$1\frac{1}{2}$–2
B	$4\frac{1}{2}$	5	8	$1\frac{1}{2}$–2
C	5	9	16–20	$2\frac{1}{2}$–3
D	5	6	12–16	2–$2\frac{1}{2}$
E	6–7	10–12	21–30	3
Mandibular				
A	$4\frac{1}{2}$	4	$6\frac{1}{2}$	$1\frac{1}{2}$–2
B	$4\frac{1}{2}$	$4\frac{1}{2}$	7	$1\frac{1}{2}$–2
C	5	9	16–20	$2\frac{1}{2}$–3
D	5	6	12–16	2–$2\frac{1}{2}$
E	6	10–12	21–30	3

Unless otherwise indicated all dates are *postpartum*. The teeth are identified according to the Zsigmondy System.

Chronology of the permanent dentition

Tooth	First evidence of calcification	Crown completed (years)	Eruption (years)	Root completed (years)
Maxillary				
1	3–4 months	4–5	7–8	10
2	10–12 months	4–5	8–9	11
3	4–5 months	6–7	11–12	13–15
4	$1\frac{1}{2}$–$1\frac{3}{4}$ years	5–6	10–11	12–13
5	2–$2\frac{1}{2}$ years	6–7	10–12	12–14
6	Birth	$2\frac{1}{2}$–3	6–7	9–10
7	$2\frac{1}{2}$–3 years	7–8	12–13	14–16
8	7–9 years	12–16	17–21	18–25
Mandibular				
1	3–4 months	4–5	6–7	9
2	3–4 months	4–5	7–8	10
3	4–5 months	6–7	9–10	12–14
4	$1\frac{3}{4}$–2 years	5–6	10–12	12–13
5	$2\frac{1}{4}$–$2\frac{1}{2}$ years	6–7	11–12	13–14
6	Birth	$2\frac{1}{2}$–3	6–7	9–10
7	$2\frac{1}{2}$–3 years	7–8	12–13	14–15
8	8–10 years	12–16	17–21	18–25

All dates are *postpartum*. Teeth are identified according to the Zsigmondy System.

Because no individuals are exactly alike in their development, the times given in Table 19 are approximate. Variations of 6 months either way are not unusual, but the tendency is for teeth to erupt late rather than early. By and large, the development of the permanent dentition is more advanced in girls; there does not appear to be any sex difference in the development of the deciduous dentition.

Since the sequence of development and eruption of teeth is under genetic control, and since chronological age is an unreliable guide to the progress of development of an individual child, dental age is a useful index of maturity, especially when used in conjunction with skeletal age. Dental age may be estimated clinically by a visual assessment of the stage of eruption of the dentition or, more satisfactorily, by a radiographic assessment of both the stages of development of the crowns and roots and the stages of eruption.

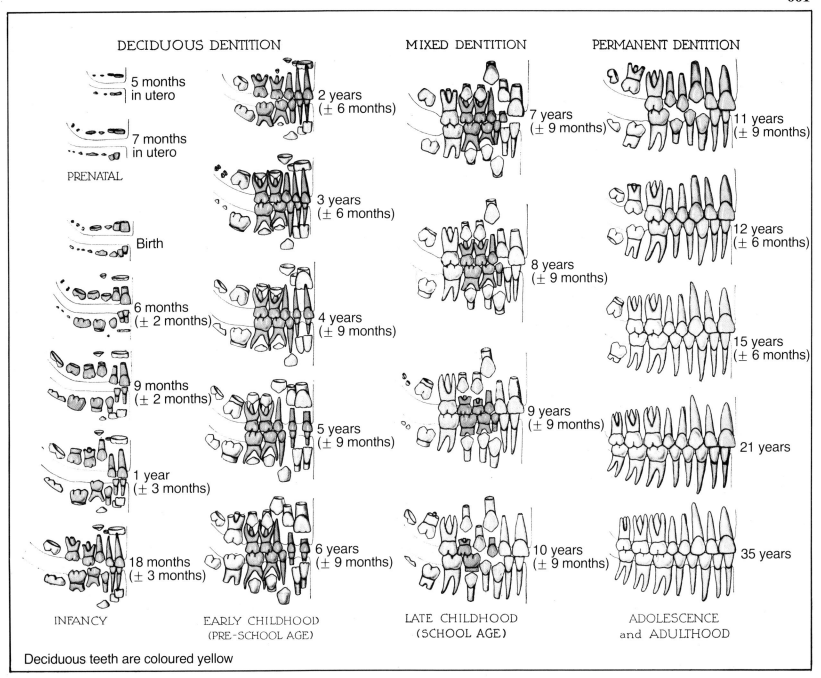

DECIDUOUS DENTITION   MIXED DENTITION   PERMANENT DENTITION

5 months in utero

7 months in utero

PRENATAL

Birth

6 months (± 2 months)

9 months (± 2 months)

1 year (± 3 months)

18 months (± 3 months)

INFANCY

2 years (± 6 months)

3 years (± 6 months)

4 years (± 9 months)

5 years (± 9 months)

6 years (± 9 months)

EARLY CHILDHOOD (PRE-SCHOOL AGE)

7 years (± 9 months)

8 years (± 9 months)

9 years (± 9 months)

10 years (± 9 months)

LATE CHILDHOOD (SCHOOL AGE)

11 years (± 9 months)

12 years (± 6 months)

15 years (± 6 months)

21 years

35 years

ADOLESCENCE and ADULTHOOD

Deciduous teeth are coloured yellow

661 Development of the human dentition.

Radiographic appearances of the dentitions at varying ages

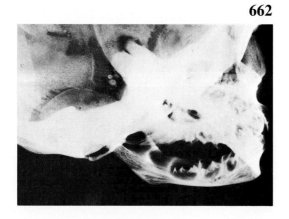

662 The dentition at birth — a lateral oblique view of the skull.

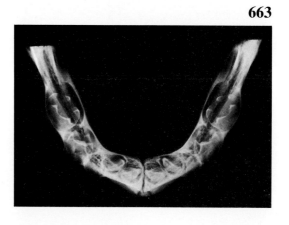

663 The dentition at birth — an occlusal view of the mandible.

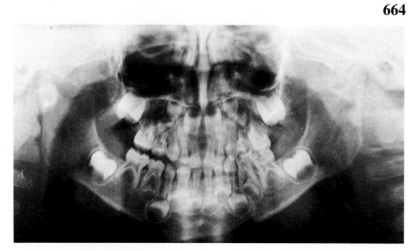

664 Dental age $2\frac{1}{2}$ years.

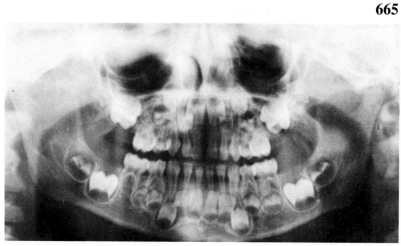

665 Dental age 4 years.

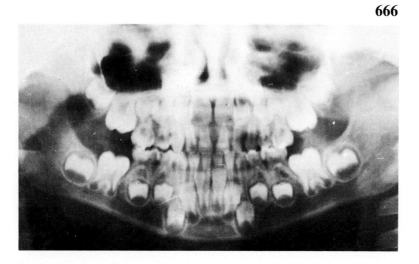

666 Dental age $5\frac{1}{2}$ years.

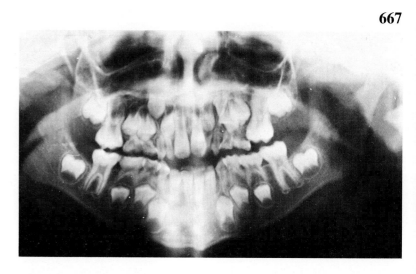

667 Dental age 7 years.

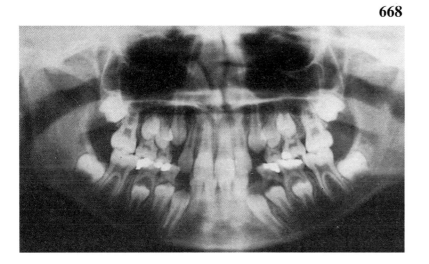

668 Dental age 9 years.

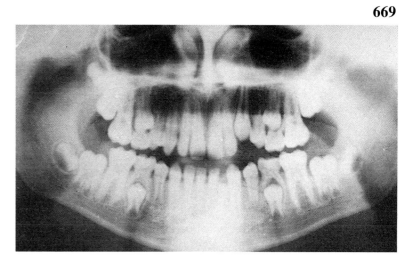

669 Dental age 11 years.

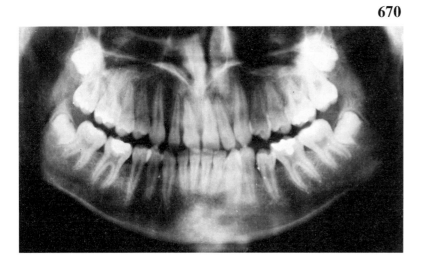

670 Dental age 14 years.

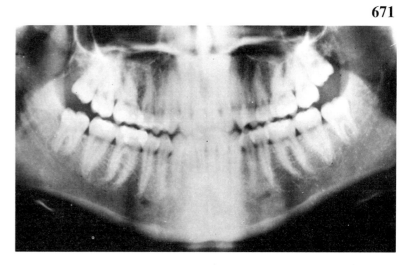

671 Dental age 19 years.

Development of occlusion

At birth, the oral mucosa over the developing alveoli is greatly thickened to form the maxillary and mandibular gum pads. They show a series of elevations, each of which corresponds to an underlying deciduous tooth. The elevations associated with the second deciduous molars do not, however, become prominent until the age of about 6 months.

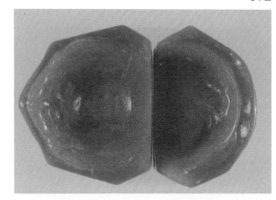

672 The gum pads. The maxillary and mandibular gum pads rarely come into occlusion, the space left between them being occupied by the tongue. The maxillary gum pad overlaps the mandibular gum pad both buccally and labially, the overjet usually being considerable. Beneath the gum pads there is generally considerable crowding of the developing teeth, especially the incisors. However, during the first year of life the gum pads grow rapidly, especially in lateral directions, thus providing space for the developing teeth.

The maxillary and mandibular alveolar processes are not well developed at birth. Occasionally a 'natal tooth' is present. This tooth is usually a supernumerary tooth, formed by an aberration in the development of the dental lamina, but occasionally it is merely a very early, but otherwise normal, central incisor.

The deciduous teeth start to erupt at the age of 6 months and the deciduous dentition is complete by the age of 3 years. At this time, the occlusion of the deciduous dentition differs from that of the permanent dentition in the following respects:

1. The incisors are more vertically positioned within the alveolus and are often spaced.
2. The overbite is usually greater.
3. There may be significant spacings distal to the mandibular canines and mesial to the maxillary canines (the anthropoid or primitive spaces).
4. Although the anteroposterior relationships of the deciduous arches have not been adequately assessed, it appears that the distal edges of the maxillary and mandibular deciduous molars are flush and the mesiobuccal cusps of the maxillary first and second deciduous molars occlude in the buccal grooves of the mandibular first and second deciduous molars respectively.

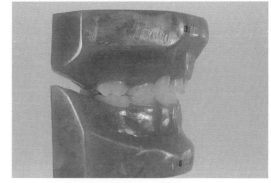

673 Models showing the occlusion of the deciduous dentition at 3 years. Note that the incisors are vertically positioned and that the distal edges of the maxillary and mandibular deciduous molars are flush.

Several changes occur in the deciduous occlusion before the appearance of the permanent teeth. These result from changes in the dental bases. As the dental arches become wider and longer, so the deciduous teeth become more spaced. Since there is a greater forward growth of the mandible compared to the maxilla, the lower arch moves forwards relative to the upper, so that an edge-to-edge incisor relationship is obtained. As a further consequence, the distal surfaces of the deciduous second molars may now show a slight mesial step from maxilla to mandible, the mesiobuccal cusp of the maxillary second deciduous molar lying distal to the buccal groove of the mandibular second deciduous molar. As the deciduous teeth approach the end of their functional lives, they may show signs of considerable wear (the enamel of deciduous teeth being softer and thinner than the enamel of permanent teeth).

674 Occlusal relationships of the deciduous and permanent molars. The flush terminal plane relationship is the usual relationship in the deciduous dentition. When the first permanent molars start to erupt, their relationship is determined by that of the primary molars. The molar relationship tends to shift at the time the second deciduous molars are shed and the adolescent growth spurt occurs. As shown in the illustration, the change in molar relationship depends upon whether there is leeway space for tooth movement and upon mandibular growth. (Modified after Moyers R.E., *Handbook of Orthodontics* (3rd edn), Year Book Medical Publishers.)

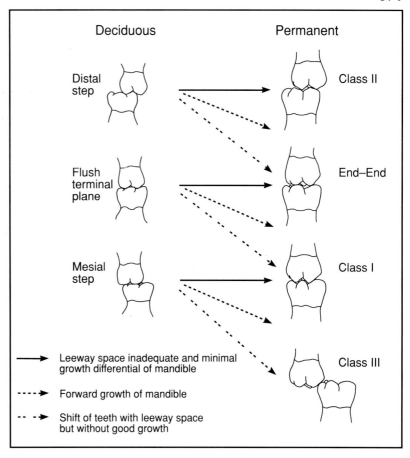

After the age of 6 years, the dentition is said to be mixed, comprising both deciduous and permanent teeth.

The first molars are the first permanent teeth to erupt. Initially, they have a cusp-to-cusp relationship (the flush terminal plane, see **674**) which is governed by the position of the deciduous second molars. The first molars take up their normal adult relationship once the deciduous second molars are shed. The permanent incisors erupt between the ages of 6 and 9 years. Since the permanent incisors are much larger than their deciduous predecessors, they are accommodated into the dental arches not just by the utilisation of the space left by the deciduous predecessors, but also by lateral growth of the alveolar arches and the greater proclination of the permanent incisors. In their developmental positions, the lateral incisors are overlapped by the central incisors, being positioned more palatally. As a rule, space is made for the lateral incisors as the central incisors erupt. However, should there be insufficient growth of the alveolus, the lateral incisors may continue to lie in their developmental, palatal positions (**675**). Frequently,

when the permanent incisors erupt, they fan out (incline distally) so that there may be a significant space or diastema between the central incisors. This appearance has been termed the 'ugly duckling' stage and is said to result from pressure on the roots of the permanent incisors from the developing permanent canines. The diastema usually closes following eruption of the permanent canines. The canines and premolars, which usually erupt between the ages of 9 and 12 years, are readily accommodated into the dental arches, since the combined mesiodistal diameters of the deciduous canines and molars is generally greater than that of their permanent successors. Any leeway space that remains is usually taken up by forward movement of the first permanent molars. By the age of 12 years, all the deciduous teeth have been shed to be replaced by permanent teeth, and henceforth the occlusion appears similar to that in the adult (see pages 44–52). Space is provided for the permanent molar teeth by continued growth of the mandible and maxilla.

675 The developmental positions of the crowns of the permanent teeth (red) relative to the functional positions of the crowns of the deciduous teeth (black). Note the lingual positioning of the permanent teeth (particularly for the maxillary lateral incisors). Arrows point to spaces between the deciduous canines and the first molars for the lower jaw and between the deciduous lateral incisors and canines for the upper jaw which are termed 'primate spaces', so named because they are most marked in the dentitions of primates. The primate spaces are usually seen from the time the teeth erupt. Developmental spaces between the incisors are often present at eruption, but become larger as the child grows and the alveolar processes expand. Generalised spacing of the primary teeth is a requirement for proper alignment of the permanent incisors.

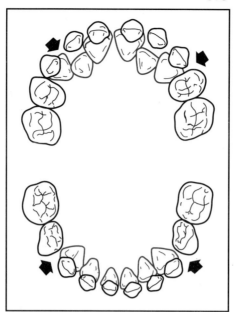

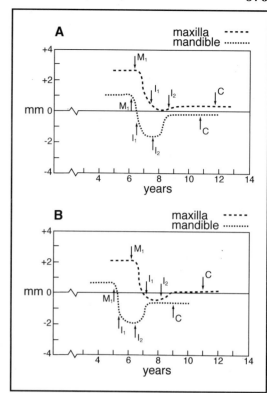

676 Graphic display of the average amount of space available within the dental arches for boys (A) and for girls (B). The arrows indicate the timing of eruption of the first molar (M_1), central and lateral incisors (I_1 and I_2), and canines (C). Note that for both sexes the amount of space for the mandibular incisors is negative for about 2 years after their eruption. Thus, a small degree of crowding in the mandibular arch at this time is not unusual. (Modified after Moorress C.F.A. and Chadha J.M., Angle Orthod.)

Although there is a tendency for the mandible to grow slightly further forward than the maxilla after the age of 12 years, usually there is no appreciable occlusal change. During the later stages of facial growth, there may be an accompanying uprighting of the incisors, with the result that they become more crowded. It has been suggested that mesial drift may take up any remaining space in the arches or even be responsible for some late crowding.

Once a tooth reaches its functional position, it is believed to occupy a position of equilibrium between the soft tissues of the cheeks and lips externally and the tongue internally (**80**).

The movement that has attracted the most attention during a tooth's functional phase is mesial drift. Mesial drift may involve considerable bodily movement of the tooth. It has been reported that, between the ages of 6 and 18 years the first permanent molar drifts approximately 4mm in a mesial direction. Four hypotheses have been postulated to account for this movement, although the precise mechanism is still unknown:

1. The mesial inclination of teeth produces a resultant force during biting that favours mesial drift.
2. The action of certain jaw muscles, particularly the buccinator, 'propel' the teeth forwards.
3. Bone deposited preferentially on the distal surface of the sockets pushes the teeth mesially.
4. Contraction of the transseptal fibre system pulls the teeth mesially.

Comparative
dental anatomy

Dentitions of mammals

Compared with non-mammalian vertebrates, the dentitions of mammals are generally characterised by being heterodont (having teeth of different shapes) and diphyodont (possessing two sets). The mammalian dentition is composed of four different morphological types — incisors, canines, premolars and molars — the premolars and molars having a more complicated form associated with the ability to masticate food. The teeth are restricted to two rows, one in the mandible, the other in the maxilla. In adult placental mammals there is usually a maximum of 11 teeth in each jaw quadrant:

$$I\tfrac{3}{3} \ C\tfrac{1}{1} \ P\tfrac{4}{4} \ M\tfrac{3}{3}$$

In non-mammalian vertebrates the teeth are used mainly for prehension, the prey being seized head first and swallowed whole. Jaw activity is associated with relatively simple up and down movements with little lateral displacement. In mammals the shape of the molar teeth becomes broadened so that, with forceful jaw closure, food can be squashed between opposing occlusal surfaces and partially divided by the penetration of cusps. The ability to masticate food produces a significant gain in digestive efficiency, which is considered necessary for the high rate of metabolism associated with homeothermy.

Other features associated with mastication which are peculiar to mammals include: temporomandibular jaw articulation; salivary glands; prismatic enamel; diphyodonty; a secondary palate; significant muscle development associated with lips, cheeks, tongue and muscles of mastication; and a gomphosis type of tooth attachment (see pages 188–189). The development of the muscles of mastication and a temporo-mandibular articulation allow the force of the bite and the range of movements for chewing to be increased. Saliva moistens and lubricates the food during mastication; its enzyme content allows digestion to commence at an early stage in the mouth. The prismatic arrangement of enamel and its greater thickness in mammals is said to be more efficient in resisting masticatory loads and attrition than non-prismatic enamel. The development of a secondary palate is thought to be related to the necessity of maintaining ventilation during prolonged masticatory periods. The development of muscles within the lips, cheeks and tongue is associated with manipulation of the bolus within the mouth. The change from polyphyodonty (many sets of teeth) to diphyodonty has been related to a 'grinding-in' period necessary to produce an efficient cutting or grinding tooth surface, it seeming inefficient to replace such teeth too frequently. The gomphosis type of attachment may be associated with the increased stresses and strains brought to bear on the tooth during mastication.

Dentitions of animals commonly used in dental research

Rodents

Rodents are a heterogeneous group whose dentitions are reduced in tooth number (compared with the archetypal mammalian dentition) and whose most conspicuous feature is the possession of continuously growing incisors. Many rodents are monophyodont, having only a single set of teeth.

677a **677b**

677 Laboratory rat (*Rattus norvegicus*).

$$I\tfrac{1}{1} \ C\tfrac{0}{0} \ P\tfrac{0}{0} \ M\tfrac{3}{3}$$

The dentition of the rat is monophyodont. The conspicuous, continuously growing (and erupting) incisors are constantly worn to a chisel-shaped edge. The upper incisors are more curved than the lower. The surface enamel contains an iron pigment which imparts a yellow-orange colouration. The upper incisors overhang the lowers, which necessitates the mandible being brought forward in gnawing. This movement is reflected in the elongation of the condyles in the anteroposterior plane. The incisors are separated from the cheek teeth by a diastema. Intrusion of the cheeks into the diastema separates the dentition into an anterior gnawing compartment and a posterior grinding compartment. The molars are teeth of limited growth. Enamel is not formed on the tips of the molar cusps. The molar cusps are joined by transverse ridges. When these ridges become worn, gradually widening areas of dentine are exposed, surrounded by rings of enamel. This arrangement of tissues is said to increase masticatory efficiency. The chronology of development of the mandibular molars is shown in Table 20 on page 299.

678 The continuously growing maxillary rat incisor, showing the distribution of tissues. In essence, this tooth presents root tissue (i.e. dentine and cementum, **A**) on its lingual side and crown tissue (i.e. dentine and enamel, **B**) on its labial side. **C**, dental pulp. **D**, enamel space. On the lingual side of the tooth, a true periodontal ligament (**E**) passes from the cementum to the alveolar bone, while connective tissue intervenes labially between (though it is not attached to) the enamel surface and the alveolar bone. In the region of the proliferative 'root' apex, structures homologous with an epithelial root sheath (**F**) and an enamel organ (**G**) continually produce new dental tissues to compensate for attritional loss. In the laboratory rat, incisor teeth in occlusion erupt at a rate of about 400µm/day (impeded eruption rate). If the teeth are cut out of occlusion, their eruption rate attains levels of about 1mm/day (unimpeded eruption rate). To prevent pulp exposure during continuous incisor eruption, secondary dentine (**H**) is continually deposited beneath the incisal edge. (H & E; × 8)

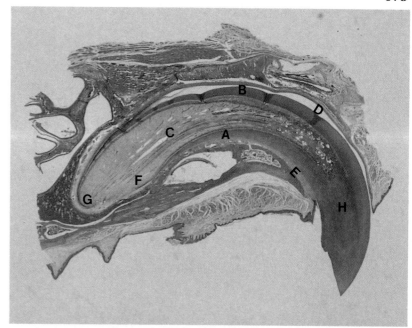

679 Cross-section of the mandibular incisor of a rat. The developing enamel matrix (**A**) is limited to the labial surface of the tooth. The remainder of the dentine (**B**) is covered by a very thin layer of cementum (**C**). A true periodontal ligament (**D**) is only present in association with the cementum-covered component of the tooth. A loose connective tissue (**E**) separates the enamel from the surrounding socket wall. **F**, ameloblast layer; **G**, odontoblast layer. (Masson's trichrome; × 40)

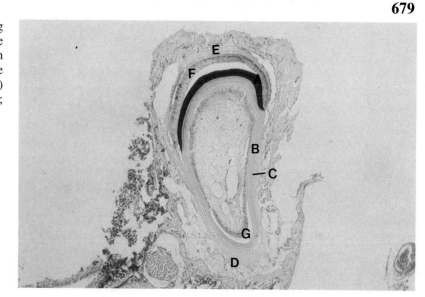

The dentition of the mouse (*Mus musculus*) is similar to, but obviously smaller than, that of the rat. The mouse also has deciduous incisors. The guinea pig (*Cavia*) possesses an additional functional anterior cheek tooth (premolar) in each quadrant. The incisors of the guinea pig are unpigmented. Both the incisors and the molars of the guinea pig are of continuous growth. The guinea pig is born at a relatively advanced state of development with all teeth erupted. Indeed, some of the teeth may even be worn. The anterior cheek tooth has a deciduous predecessor, which is shed *in utero*. This deciduous tooth exhibits wear facets, showing that attrition can occur *in utero*.

Table 20: Chronology of development of the mandibular molars of the rat (the maxillary molars pass through the various stages approximately 1 day later).

Developmental stage	First molar	Second molar	Third molar
Initial appearance of tooth germ	13	14–15	20
Onset of mineralisation	20–21	1–2	13–14
Completion of crown	11	13	21
Emergence into oral cavity	19	22	35
Functional occlusion	25	28	40

Figures above the dotted line are days *in utero*; those below are days *post-partum*.

Lagomorphs (pikas, hares and rabbits)

Despite the apparent resemblance of their dentitions to those of rodents, rabbits are placed in a separate Order (*Lagomorpha*), as other features show that they are but remotely related.

680

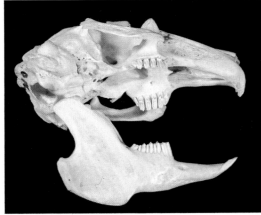

680 Rabbit (*Oryctolagus cuniculus*).

$$I\frac{2}{1} \; C\frac{0}{0} \; P\frac{3}{2} \; M\frac{3}{3}$$

Unlike rodents, rabbits possess a small pair of additional incisors lying behind the large, continuously growing upper incisors. The incisors are unpigmented. All the cheek teeth are of continuous growth.

The deciduous dentition of a rabbit has the formula:

$$DI\frac{2}{2} \; DC\frac{0}{0} \; DM\frac{3}{3}$$

681

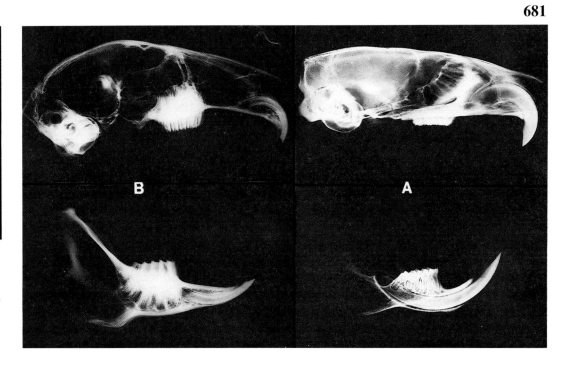

681 Radiograph of the jaws of a rat (A) and rabbit (B). Note that only the incisors of the rat are of continuous growth, whereas all the teeth of the rabbit are of continuous growth.

Carnivores

Carnivores, as the name suggests, are predominantly meat eaters. They show several dental specialisations, particularly enlarged canines and the presence of carnassial teeth.

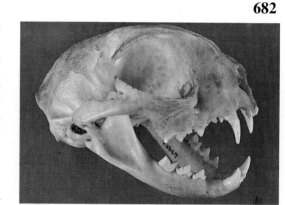

682 Domestic cat (*Felis catus*).

$$\text{I}\tfrac{3}{3}\ \text{C}\tfrac{1}{1}\ \text{P}\tfrac{3}{2}\ \text{M}\tfrac{1}{1}$$

The incisors are small and arranged more or less in a straight line. The canines, often used as offensive weapons, are large, pointed teeth, the mandibular tooth fitting into a diastema in front of the maxillary canine. Both the canines and incisors are used for tearing flesh. The cheek teeth are reduced in number. The last maxillary premolar and the mandibular first molar are specialised to form elongated, blade-like carnassial teeth. These teeth are used for cutting up prey by a scissor-like function. The teeth immediately anterior to the carnassials, though smaller, have a carnassial-like function. The maxillary molar tooth is a small, rotated, instanding tooth which, by contacting the posterior element of the mandibular carnassial, appears to act as a stop. Jaw movement is primarily of the hinge type, though a small degree of lateral movement can occur. To stabilise the temporomandibular joint, the mandibular condyles are transversely elongated and fit into a deep, close-fitting mandibular fossa with flanges both in front and behind.

The deciduous dentition has the formula:

$$\text{DI}\tfrac{3}{3}\ \text{DC}\tfrac{1}{1}\ \text{M}\tfrac{3}{2}$$

The upper carnassial tooth is the middle one of the three deciduous molars, and the lower carnassial tooth is the second deciduous molar. Thus, the permanent carnassial teeth erupt one tooth position behind the deciduous carnassial teeth.

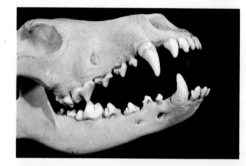

683 Dog (*Canis familiaris*).

$$\text{I}\tfrac{3}{3}\ \text{C}\tfrac{1}{1}\ \text{P}\tfrac{4}{4}\ \text{M}\tfrac{2}{3}$$

The dentition of the dog (family *Canidae*) reflects a more omnivorous diet than that of the cat. Compared with the cat, there is a greater number of teeth. The anterior teeth are similar to those of the cat. Opposing premolars do not occlude. The carnassial teeth are less sectorial than those of the cat. The presence of extra molar teeth, especially the broad maxillary first molar, provides an additional grinding surface.

The formula of the deciduous dentition is:

$$\text{DI}\tfrac{3}{3}\ \text{DC}\tfrac{1}{1}\ \text{DM}\tfrac{3}{3}$$

The first permanent premolar, as in other placentals with four premolars, has no deciduous predecessor.

Table 21: Eruption dates for the dog.

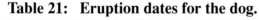

	Deciduous teeth	*Permanent teeth*
First incisor	4–5 weeks	4–5 months
Second incisor	4–5 weeks	4–5 months
Third incisor	4 weeks	4–5 months
Canine	3–4 weeks	4–5 months
First molar	4–5 weeks	4 months
Second molar	3–4 weeks	$4\tfrac{1}{2}$–6 months
Third molar	3–4 weeks	6–7 months
First premolar		4–5 months
Second premolar		5–6 months
Third premolar		5–6 months
Fourth premolar		5–6 months

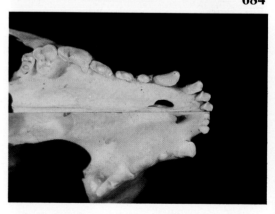

684 Comparison of the upper jaw of a dog (top) and a cat (bottom) viewed occlusally.

The ferret (*Mustela putorius*).

$$I\tfrac{3}{3} \ C\tfrac{1}{1} \ P\tfrac{3}{4} \ M\tfrac{1}{2}$$

This is a small carnivore whose dentition resembles that of the cat.

Ungulates

685 The domestic pig (*Sus scrofa*) is a member of the even-toed ungulates (*Artiodactyla*).

$$I\tfrac{3}{3} \ C\tfrac{1}{1} \ P\tfrac{4}{4} \ M\tfrac{3}{3}$$

The upper central incisors are the largest incisors. Their roots are separated but, because they are inclined mesially, their crowns meet in the midline. The third incisors are the smallest. The lower incisors are deeply implanted and are almost horizontal; they are used for rooting up the ground in search of food. The canine teeth or tusks are of continuous growth; in the male they are well developed and project out of the mouth in an upward and outward direction; in the female they are considerably reduced. The convex surface of the canine is covered with enamel, the concave surface with cementum. Except for the maxillary fourth premolar, which is molariform, the premolars are somewhat narrow, cutting teeth, which increase in size from before backwards. The molar crowns also increase in size from before backwards and have cone-shaped cusps (bunodont). Four main cusps may be distinguished in each molar, although each cusp has numerous accessory cusplets. The formula of the deciduous dentition is:

$$DI\tfrac{3}{3} \ DC\tfrac{1}{1} \ DM\tfrac{3}{3}$$

A selectively bred pig, the miniature pig, is available for research. It has all the dental features of the domestic pig, but is only approximately one-third of its size.

685a

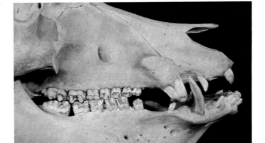

685b

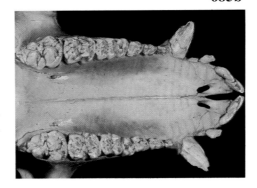

Table 22: Eruption dates for the pig.

	Deciduous teeth	*Permanent teeth*
First incisor	2–4 weeks	12 months
Second incisor	1½–3 months	16–20 months
Third incisor	before birth	8–10 months
Canine	before birth	8–10 months
First molar	5–7 weeks	4–6 months
Second molar		
(maxillary)	4–8 days	8–12 months
(mandibular)	2–4 weeks	
Third molar		
(maxillary)	4–8 days	18–20 months
(mandibular)	2–4 weeks	
First premolar		5 months
Second premolar		12–15 months
Third premolar		12–15 months
Fourth premolar		12–15 months

686 The sheep (*Ovis aries*).

$$I\frac{0}{3} \ C\frac{0}{1} \ P\frac{3}{3} \ M\frac{3}{3}$$

The sheep has proved a useful model for the study of inflammatory periodontal disease, as this occurs naturally — a condition known as 'broken mouth'. There are no anterior teeth in the upper jaw; instead there is a horny pad. The mandibular canines are incisiform and join the procumbent incisor teeth to form a row of eight anterior teeth that help to crop the grass on which the animal feeds. The cheek teeth are described as being hypsodont, having long crowns and short roots. This allows the teeth to erupt slowly over long periods, thus compensating for wear incurred during mastication. The cusps of the cheek teeth are crescent-shaped (selenodont) and, with wear, a darker central area surrounded by ridges of enamel develops, representing secondary dentine. Coronal cementum is present. The deciduous dentition has the formula:

$$DI\frac{0}{3} \ DC\frac{0}{1} \ M\frac{3}{3}$$

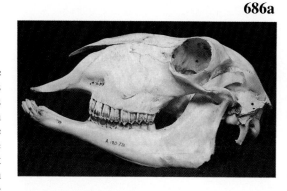
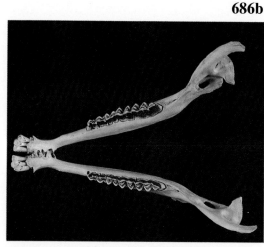

New World monkeys

The New World monkeys are classified into two families, the *Cebidae* (e.g. squirrel monkey) and the *Callithricidae* (e.g. marmosets).

687 Squirrel monkey (*Saimiri sciureus*).

$$I\frac{2}{2} \ C\frac{1}{1} \ P\frac{3}{3} \ M\frac{3}{3}$$

The diet of the squirrel monkey, as for all New World monkeys, consists mainly of fruit and insects. The incisors are spatulate. The canines are large and tusk-like, the maxillary canine being separated from the lateral incisor by a diastema which accommodates the mandibular canine. The premolars are bicuspid, the buccal cusp being the most prominent. The mandibular first premolar, however, is unicuspid. The buccal and lingual cusps of both the second and third mandibular premolars are united by a transverse crest. Typically, the mandibular premolars have two roots, and the maxillary premolars have three roots. The molars decrease in size from before backwards and have four sharp cusps. The reduced upper third molar, however, tends to have three cusps. The mesiopalatal cusp (protocone) of each upper molar is joined to the distobuccal cusp (metacone) by an oblique ridge. The upper molars have three roots, the lowers two. The deciduous dentition has the formula:

$$DI\frac{2}{2} \ DC\frac{1}{1} \ M\frac{3}{3}$$

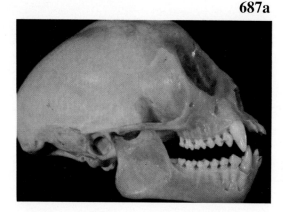
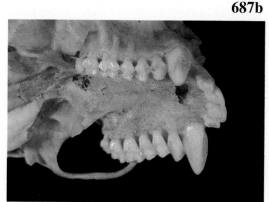

The *Callithricidae* comprise the marmosets and tamarins. The dentitions are similar to the *Cebidae* except for the absence of third molars.

Old World monkeys (*Cercopithecidae*)

The dentitions of Old World monkeys differ from those of New World monkeys in many respects. In Old World monkeys only two premolars are present in each jaw quadrant. The mandibular first premolar of Old World monkeys is a sectorial tooth. Unlike New World monkeys, the cusps of the molars of Old World monkeys are connected by distinct transverse ridges (or lophs) and the third molars are well developed.

688 Stump-tailed macaque (*Macaca arctoides*).

$$I\frac{2}{2} \; C\frac{1}{1} \; P\frac{2}{2} \; M\frac{3}{3}$$

The incisors are spatulate. The canines are long, dagger-like teeth, being especially prominent in the male. The maxillary canine is separated from the incisors by a diastema. The well-marked groove on the anterior surface of the maxillary canine is said to help guide the mandibular canine into occlusion. The maxillary premolars and mandibular second premolar are bicuspid. The mandibular first premolar is a highly specialised sectorial tooth. Its crown slopes sharply backwards to leave a wedge-shaped space between it and the crown of the mandibular canine into which the maxillary canine occludes. It has been suggested that the posterior edge of the maxillary canine may be sharpened against the sloping surface of the mandibular sectorial premolar. Each maxillary molar has four cusps, the anterior and posterior pairs of cusps being linked by transverse ridges. Viewed occlusally, the crowns show distinct buccal and lingual constrictions in the midline, giving the teeth a characteristic bilophodont appearance. The maxillary first molar is the smallest molar, the second and third molars being approximately equal in size. The mandibular molars are also bilophodont and increase in size from before backwards. The mandibular third molar has an additional posterior cusp (hypoconulid). The maxillary molars and premolars have three roots, and the mandibular molars and premolars have two roots. The dental formula for the deciduous dentition is:

$$DI\frac{2}{2} \; DC\frac{1}{1} \; DM\frac{2}{2}$$

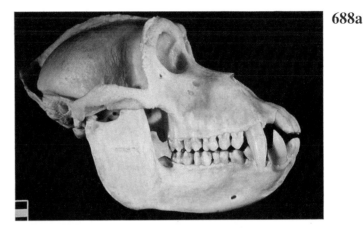

688a

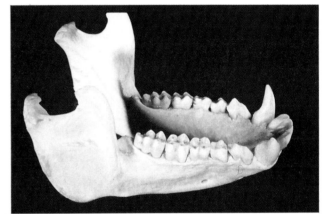

688b

Table 23:   Eruption dates for rhesus monkey (*Macaca mulatta*).

	Deciduous teeth	Permanent teeth
First incisor	1–5 weeks	32 months
Second incisor	2–7 weeks	37 months
Canine	8–17 weeks	47 months
First molar	8–19 weeks	20 months
Second molar	15–32 weeks	42 months
Third molar		79–90 months
First premolar		48 months
Second premolar		48 months

The evolution of man

Modern man (*Homo sapiens*) belongs to the order *Primates*. This order is one of the most ancient of the mammalian orders. For purposes of classification, the living primates are divided into two suborders (Table 24): the *Prosimii* (or lemur-like primates) and the *Anthropoidea* (containing monkeys, apes and man). Further subdivisions lead down to families. The diet of primates consists mainly of fruit and vegetables. In some, however, the diet may be insectivorous or omnivorous.

Table 24: Classification of living primates.

Order	Suborder	Family
Primates	Prosimi	Tupaiidae Lemuridae Daubentonidae Lorisidae Tarsiidae
	Anthropoidea	Cebidae Callitricidae Cercopithecidae Hylobatidae Pongidae Hominidae

Homo sapiens is the only living species in the family *Hominidae*, although fossil remains of other species and genera have been discovered.

When a putative hominid fossil is uncovered (most commonly fragments of the jaws and teeth), anthropologists attempt to age the specimen (using an array of techniques relating to geological information and radiometric dating) and then ascertain those features that are ape-like and those that are man-like. Thus, before describing the fossil crania of hominids, it is necessary to provide some information concerning the skulls and dentitions of the extant great apes and to outline the features which distinguish them from man (see Table 25, page 307).

There are three genera within the family *Pongidae*: the orang-utan (*Pongo*), the gorilla (*Gorilla*), and the chimpanzee (*Pan*). The dental formula for all these apes is:

$$I\tfrac{2}{2}\ C\tfrac{1}{1}\ P\tfrac{2}{2}\ M\tfrac{3}{3}$$

The living Pongidae

689a & b Orang-utan (*Pongo pygmaeus*). This 'oriental' ape is found in the forests of Borneo and Sumatra; it is mainly fruit-eating (frugivorous). The skull shows marked sexual dimorphism in terms of size, and there are pronounced bony crests for muscle attachments (e.g. sagittal crests on calvaria). The foramen magnum is positioned well back and the mastoid processes are poorly developed. The mandible is robust and there is a simian shelf (*arrowed*). This shelf is a ridge of bone lying in the midline on the inferior aspect of the medial surface of the mandible. It is a site for muscle attachments and corresponds in the human to the genial spines. It has been suggested that the shelf strengthens the front of the mandibular arch in order to support the large canines. The face is moderately prognathic (i.e. the jaws project forwards beyond the cranium) and has a distinct dish-like profile.

689a

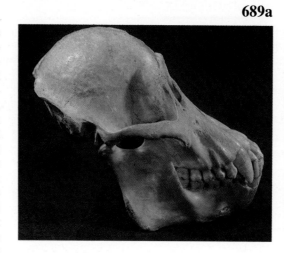

689b

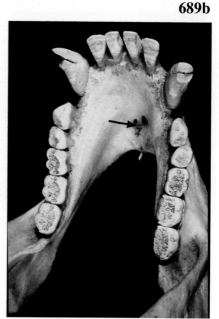

690 Chimpanzee (*Pan troglodytes*). The chimpanzee is the smallest of the great apes. It is widely distributed across equatorial Africa. In addition to *Pan troglodytes* (illustrated here), there is a species of pygmy chimpanzee (*Pan paniscus*) which is restricted to certain regions of central west Africa. The face, like that of the other apes, is prognathic. One feature in helping to distinguish the skull of the chimpanzee from that of the orang-utan relates to the orbit. In the chimpanzee, the width of the orbit is greater than the height; in the orang-utan the reverse is the case, and the orbits appear closer together due to the narrowness of the intervening bones. The mastoid process is absent or small in the chimpanzee, and there are pronounced crests on the cranium.

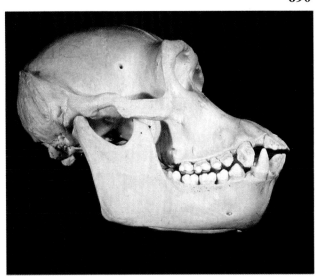

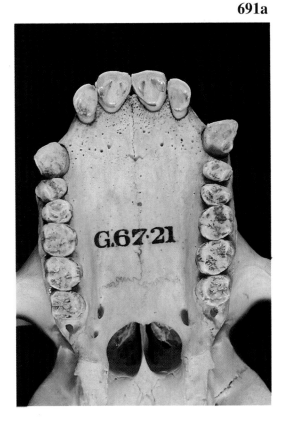

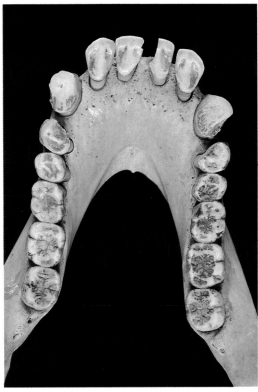

691a & b The permanent dentition of the chimpanzee shows some similarities to that of man. However, the following differences can be noted. The incisors are spatulate, procumbent and meet edge to edge. The maxillary second incisor is only slightly smaller than the first incisor, unlike the situation in the orang-utan where the second incisor is considerably smaller. The canines are powerful, pointed teeth. Sexual dimorphism is evident in adult apes. An aspect of this is the large size of the maxillary canines in the male. Between the maxillary canine and maxillary lateral incisor is a space (diastema) to accommodate the mandibular canine. The mandibular first premolar is essentially unicuspid. The maxillary premolars have three roots, the mandibular premolars two. In both jaws the second molar is the largest tooth. All the mandibular molars bear five cusps. There is considerable wrinkling of the enamel.

692a & b Skull and deciduous dentition of chimpanzee. The juvenile skull of the chimpanzee is more like the human skull than is the adult chimpanzee, there being less development of the facial complex (hence the neurocranium appears comparatively large). Furthermore, the dental arch is less U-shaped and more parabolic. The deciduous dentition of the great apes is:

$$\text{DI}\tfrac{2}{2}\ \text{DC}\tfrac{1}{1}\ \text{DM}\tfrac{2}{2}$$

The deciduous incisors are similar in shape to those of man, although they are disproportionately smaller compared to the permanent incisors. The canines remain proportionately large, but there is no sexual dimorphism. The diastema between the maxillary lateral incisor and canine is still a conspicuous feature in the deciduous dentition. The morphology of the deciduous mandibular first molar differs from that of man in that there is a greater disproportion between the anterior trigonid element, which is high, and the posterior talonid element, which is low and without cusps. Compared with the corresponding human tooth, the maxillary first deciduous molar of apes has a more pointed buccal cusp and a reduced palatal cusp. As in the human, the second deciduous molars closely resemble the first permanent molars. Note the gubernacular canals (*arrowed*) leading down to the underlying permanent teeth.

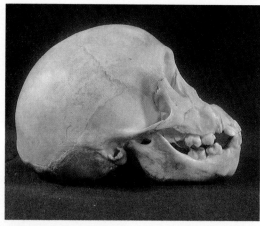

692a

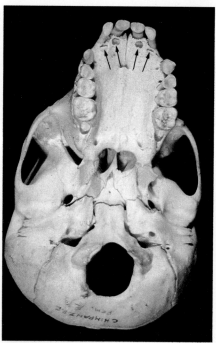

692b

693a & b Lowland gorilla (*Gorilla gorilla*). The gorilla is the largest of the great apes. The lowland gorilla (illustrated here) inhabits the forests of western Africa, and the highland gorilla is found in eastern equatorial Africa. The skull is very large (especially in males) and the face very prognathic. The crests on the skull for muscle attachments show some sexual dimorphism. For example, a sagittal crest is always found in males but less frequently in females. Although a mastoid process is often absent, in some specimens it may even be pronounced. The mandible is much longer than that of the orang-utan. The dentition in general conforms to that of the Pongidae. Unlike the orang-utan, both maxillary and mandibular canines show sexual dimorphism. In addition, the mandibular first premolar is more sectorial. For the molars, the maxillary teeth have pronounced oblique ridges on their occlusal surfaces and the mandibular molars show the standard five-cusp dryopithecine pattern. Note the crenellated folds of enamel at the bases of the cusps of the molars.

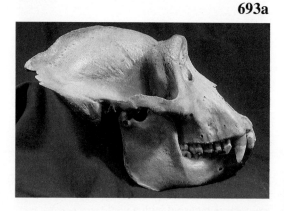

693a

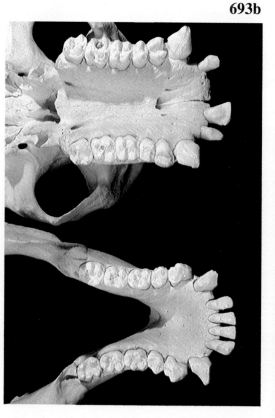

693b

Table 25: The principal differences between the skulls and dentitions of the great apes and man.

Feature	Apes	Modern man
Cranial capacity	Small (400–500cm^3)	Large (1300cm^3)
Facial skeleton	Prognathic	Flat and beneath neurocranium
Orbital regions	Marked supra-orbital ridges	Ridges frequently absent
Crests (ridges) for muscle attachment	Prominent to reflect greater development of masticatory apparatus	Absent
Premaxillary/maxillary suture	Present	Absent
Mandible	Square and massive	Gracile
	Simian shelf	Genial spines
	No chin	Chin present
	Shallow mandibular notch	More pronounced mandibular notch
	Coronoid process taller than condyle	Condyle taller than coronoid process
Dental arches	U-shaped	Parabolic
Incisors	Large and procumbent	Smaller and more vertically inclined
	Maxillary and mandibular incisors meet edge to edge	Maxillary incisors usually overlap the mandibular incisors anteriorly (overbite)
Canines	Large, especially in males (sexual dimorphism)	Smaller, minimal sexual dimorphism
	Erupt late, sometimes after the third molars	Erupt relatively early
	Maxillary canine and lateral incisor separated by a diastema	No diastema
Premolars	Maxillary premolars have three roots; mandibular first premolar has three and second premolar two roots	Usually have one root, except for the maxillary first, which has two
	Mandibular first premolar is predominantly unicuspid; second premolar is bicuspid with a well developed talonid	Mandibular premolars are similar in shape and are bicuspid
Molars	Second molars largest	First molars largest
	Mandibular molars all have five cusps	Second and third mandibular molars usually have four cusps
	Cusps more pointed	Cusps more rounded

The fossil evidence for the evolution of man

Archaeologists and anthropologists have made considerable progress in unravelling the history of man's evolution. And yet so few fossils have been discovered that the story remains incomplete and controversial.

It has been estimated that the Earth is about 4000 million years old and that the Primates only evolved during the last 70 million years. Estimates of the age of modern man vary. However, new fossils suggest that anatomically modern *Homo sapiens* was present at least 100,000 years ago.

The fossil record is thought to begin in Africa, where primate and hominid fossils have been discovered with remarkable frequency. The oldest fossils regarded as ancestral to great apes and man belong to a group known as the *Propliopithecidae*. These creatures are thought to have lived about 30 million years ago. Later, between 20 and 10 million years ago, are found a group of apes which includes *Proconsul*, *Kenyapithecus* and *Sivapithecus*. It is not until about 5 million years ago that the first hominids are found, the australopithecines.

Propliopithecines

Remains of the genera *Propliopithecus* and *Aegyptopithecus* have been found in the Fayum region of Egypt and dated to about 30 million years ago, during the Oligocene period. They share important features with both Old World monkeys and apes, and must lie close to the ancestry of all later, higher primates. They were probably herbivorous and/or frugivorous and were tree-living quadrupeds.

The remains of *Aegyptopithecus* are slightly younger than *Propliopithecus* and are more complete. The facial skeleton exhibited marked prognathism. The dental formula was typically hominoid, there being only two premolars in each quadrant. There were projecting canines, a sectorial mandibular first premolar tooth, and mandibular molars that increased in size from before backwards and that possessed a dryopithecine (five cusp) pattern.

It is not certain when the great apes evolved from the Old World monkeys, although it is likely that this occurred in the Middle Oligocene (about 30 million years ago).

Miocene apes

The classification of the many apes known from the Miocene period, 20 to 10 million years ago, is in a state of flux. Generic names are numerous, but some may be congeneric (i.e. of the same genus).

Proconsul

694a & b *Proconsul* is the name given to a group of apes which lived in Africa between 22 and 14 million years ago and contained at least five species. It represents the earliest known ape. It had a V-shaped dental arch, large canines, a sectorial premolar and five-cuspid mandibular molars. Its teeth were covered with thin enamel. It was arboreal, with a cranial capacity of about 170cm³. *Proconsul* has been the subject of considerable debate. It has been thought that from the group arose the gibbon (*Hylobatines*, the lesser apes) and the great apes and humans.

694a

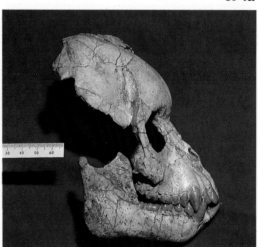

694b

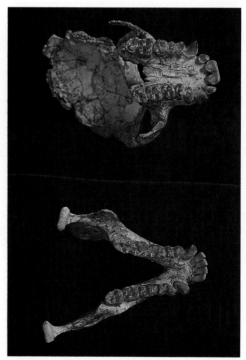

Between 14 and 8 million years ago, in the Miocene period, three important new groups of fossils appear: *Kenyapithecus*, *Sivapithecus* and *Dryopithecus*. The precise relationship between these types of Miocene apes is unclear. During this period, apes were encountered for the first time outside Africa.

Kenyapithecus

Kenyapithecus was an African ape that probably lived within, and at the edge of, forests about 14 million years ago. It is thought to have been an arboreal quadruped and to have eaten seeds and nuts, which were gathered on the ground in the open areas around rivers and lakes. From the fragmentary remains, the jaws of *Kenyapithecus* appear relatively robust. Among the more hominid-like features were the anterior position of the canines and the reduced size of the anterior teeth. However, the canines still projected above the occlusal plane. The cheek teeth had flat, broad, chewing surfaces and thick enamel, suggesting that the diet was coarse. The gradient of tooth wear along the molars was very marked. This pattern of wear indicates that, unlike present-day apes, there was a considerable interval of time between the eruption of successive molars. The dental arch was V-shaped, the tooth rows being straight and slightly divergent. The shape of the jaws suggests that *Kenyapithecus* had diminished prognathism. Among its more ape-like features were the projecting canines and the presence of a diastema. The crown of the mandibular first molar was unicuspid. Although *Kenyapithecus* was once thought to be the most likely candidate to represent the earliest ancestral hominid, this is now regarded as unlikely. A less advanced, older, but closely related group is represented by *Heliopithecus*.

695a

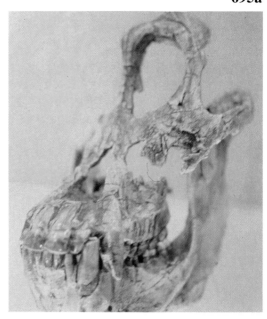

Sivapithecus

Remains of these apes have been found from between about 14 and 7 million years ago. Now included within the group are specimens of a smaller ape, *Ramapithecus*, once thought to be distinct.

695a *Sivapithecus* **(Potwar Plateau specimen).** This is the oldest ape found outside Africa, remains having been discovered in Greece, Turkey and Indo-Pakistan. It was a relatively large ape and there is evidence that there was considerable sexual dimorphism. Illustrated is a recently discovered specimen from Pakistan, which has been dated at 8 million years. Unlike other *Sivapithecus* fossils, this specimen contains part of the face as well as the jaws. The cranial capacity was approximately 300cm³. Dental and cranial features show similarities with the orang-utan (e.g. the similar outline of the orbital and nasal cavities, and the absence of a frontal sinus). The enamel was extremely thick (see page 317). Consequently, it is unlikely that the sivapithecines are hominids. They may be on a line leading to the evolution of the oriental apes (including the orang-utan). This is supported by evidence from the analysis of blood proteins from the extant primates, which suggests that the orang-utan split from the line leading to man approximately 10 million years ago. For this reason, some believe that the orang-utan should not be grouped in the same family as the African apes.

695b

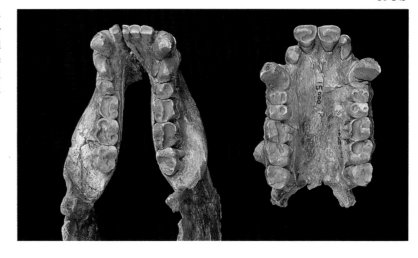

695b The maxillary and mandibular dentitions of a *Sivapithecus* **from the Potivar Plateau, Pakistan.** Note the well marked diastemata, the parallel molar tooth rows and the relatively large molars whose thick enamel shows heavy attrition. The small lateral maxillary incisors are an orang-like feature.

Dryopithecus

Dryopithecus was a European ape that lived between 11 and 9 million years ago. However, it is quite distinct from *Kenyapithecus* and shows some similarities with *Proconsul*, although the more robust cranial features may indicate that its diet was coarser. *Dryopithecus* could be regarded as an emigrant hominid from Africa which did not evolve into any species living today.

The fossil record is poor for the crucial period (12 to 4 million years ago) in the evolutionary history of the hominids. However, studies comparing blood proteins from living primates indicate that the final split between man and his present relatives, the African apes, was much later than was once thought. Palaeoanthropologists now place this divergence as occurring between 5 and 8 million years ago.

Australopithecines

These were the first undisputed hominids. The name means 'southern ape'. They were confined to Africa and lived between about 5 and 1 million years ago. Their environment was probably grassland and open woodland. Available evidence indicates that the australopithecines were bipedal. Indeed, the discovery of fossil footprints dated to about 3.6 million years ago at Laetoli in Tanzania confirms this view. Some anthropologists consider that the use of, and ability to make, tools may have been established by these creatures, the

oldest known stone tools being about 2.5 million years old. There is controversy concerning the relationships between the australopithecines. This is complicated by the existence of considerable sexual dimorphism, particularly in *Australopithecus afarensis*. Furthermore, there is no consensus concerning their precise location along the evolutionary path leading to man. Several australopithecines have been described: *A. afarensis*, *A. aethiopicus*, *A. africanus*, *A. robustus* and *A. boisei*.

Australopithecus afarensis

To date, this appears to represent the oldest and most primitive australopithecine. Remains of this hominid have been found in eastern Africa and date to between about 3–4 million years ago. Despite being small-brained (cranial capacity 375–500cm^3), they were bipedal, as evidenced from the discovery of much of the skeleton of one individual and from the chance preservation of fossil footprints. The dentition, however, still showed primitive ape-like features. The jaws

were comparatively large and prognathous. The dental arch was V-shaped, being narrow anteriorly. The teeth were large. The canines projected beyond the occlusal plane and a diastema was present. The mandibular first premolar was commonly unicuspid. One specimen comprises the most complete skeleton yet discovered. Named 'Lucy', the remains have been dated to about 3 million years ago. She was about 20 years old, weighed roughly 30kg and was 1.1m tall.

696

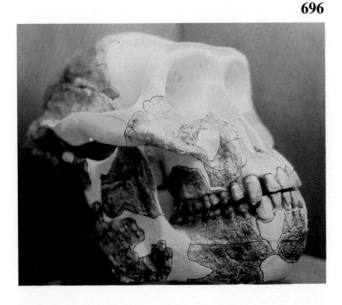

696 Reconstruction of the skull of *A. afarensis*. This reconstruction was possible by combining various fossil remains.

697

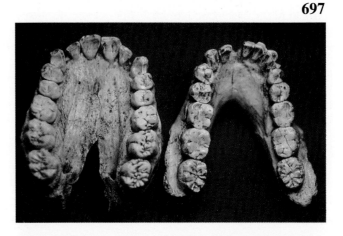

697 Maxillary and mandibular dentitions of *A. afarensis* from Hadar. Compared with the more robust australopithecines (**700**), note the comparatively large anterior teeth and the small posterior teeth. The premolars are relatively small. The maxillary molars have four cusps, and the mandibular molars have five cusps. The second molars are larger than the first.

Australopithecus aethiopicus

A recently discovered skull of a robust australopithecine (WT 17000) from Kenya has been dated to about 2.5 million years of age and assigned by some to the species *A. aethiopicus*. The species may have evolved from *A. afarensis*, and may be ancestral to the later robust australopithecines.

Australopithecus africanus

698a

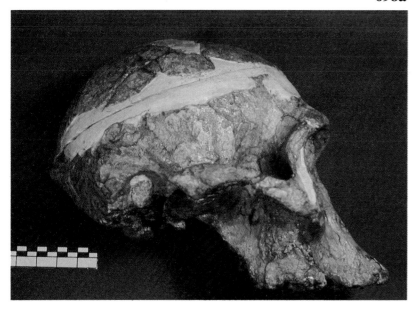

698b

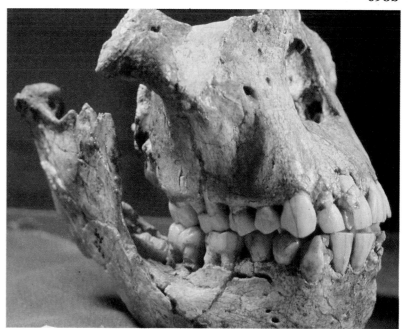

698c

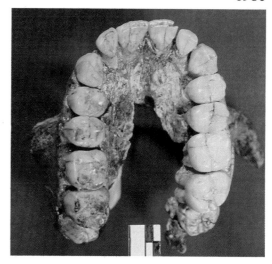

698 Australopithecus africanus. 698a, specimen STS 5; **698b**, STS 52a and b; **698c**, STS 52a maxilla. The remains of this gracile hominid have been limited mainly to southern Africa, and date to between 3.5–2.5 million years ago. Recently, remains have also been claimed to occur in eastern Africa. *A. africanus* was small (1.2–1.4m in height), had a somewhat rounded skull with a short muzzle and a cranial capacity of 400–500cm³. Only moderate brow ridges surmounted the orbits. Compared with *A. afarensis*, the teeth showed more hominid features. The incisors were spatulate and vertically implanted in the jaws. The canines were short and barely projected beyond the adjacent teeth. There was no diastema between the incisors and canines. The dental arch was more curved, like the human arch. The mandibular first premolar was bicuspid. The molars were larger than in later hominids but morphologically were very similar to those of *Homo*.

699

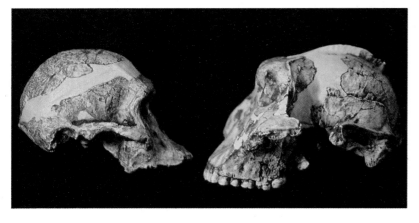

699 Comparison of the sizes of the skulls of *A. africanus* (left) and *A. boisei* (right).

Australopithecus robustus

Australopithecus robustus, as the name implies, was a more robust and larger form than *A. africanus* (see **699**). Found in southern and eastern Africa, its remains have been dated to 2.5–1.5 million years ago. It would appear to be younger than *A. africanus*. Male specimens appear to have been about twice the size of females. It had a flatter and slightly larger skull (cranial capacity 500cm^3), with prominent sagittal and nuchal crests associated with maximising areas for muscle attachment. Although the incisor teeth were similar to those of *A. africanus*, the cheek teeth were much larger, with molariform premolars. The cheek teeth also had a thick covering of enamel and were subjected to considerable wear, indicating a tough vegetarian diet. The heavy buttressing of the face and the large attachments for the masticatory muscles confirm the tough diet.

700a

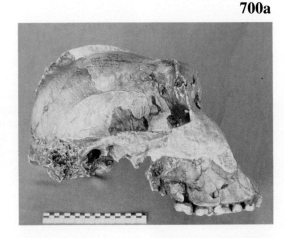

700b

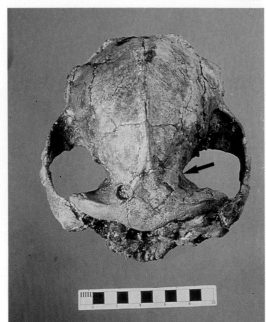

700c

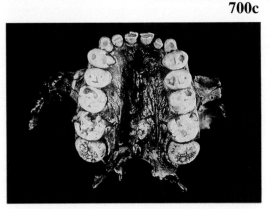

700 *Australopithecus boisei.* **700a**, lateral view of specimen OH5; **700b**, superior view of KNM-ER 406; **700c**, occlusal view of OH5. This fossil represents an even more robust form than *A. robustus*. The specimen referred to as Olduvai Hominid 5 (OH5) is about 1.8 million years old and comprises an almost complete cranium, probably of a young adult male. It was found in Olduvai Gorge, Tanzania. The presence of a sagittal crest indicates well developed temporalis muscles, and the cranial vault is low. Heavy buttressing is seen in the cheek region and the zygomatic arch stands well away from the temporal fossa to allow the large, anterior temporalis muscle to pass between. This feature is associated with a narrow post-orbital constriction (*arrowed* in **700b**). The cranial capacity is approximately 530cm^3, but this increase, compared with the other australopithecine species, may simply reflect the increased body size. The molars and premolars are enormous relative to the incisors and canines, and broad compared with those of other australopithecines. This probably reflects the coarse nature of the vegetarian diet. Note the wrinkling of the third molars. Two additional skulls have recently been found in East Turkana: an almost complete skull of a male, somewhat similar to the original specimen, and one half of the skull of a female. The female skull lacked a sagittal crest and was more gracile.

There is controversy concerning the phylogenetic relationships of the australopithecines. Did *A. africanus* arise from *A. afarensis* or from a separate, and as yet undiscovered, stock? Do *A. robustus* and *A. boisei* represent separate genera? Some anthropologists place both the robust types (*A. robustus* and *A. boisei*) into a separate genus called *Paranthropus*. Some evidence in support of this is derived from estimates of the chronology of dental development. In *Paranthropus*, first incisor and first molar crown completion and eruption times are concordant. In *A. africanus,* the incisor takes considerably longer to form and erupts later. Recent fossil finds in West Turkana suggest a close relationship between *A. afarensis* and *Paranthropus*.

There is general agreement that the robust forms (*A. robustus* and *A. boisei*) are an offshoot and not in the direct line leading to *Homo sapiens*. This is because of their specialised cranial and dental morphology as well as the fact that they co-existed with later and more advanced forms such as *Homo habilis* and *Homo erectus*. There is less agreement as to whether a line from *A. afarensis* to *Homo habilis* passed through *A. africanus*, or whether the latter was, like the robust forms, also an offshoot from the main stream. Recent fossil finds suggest that the genera *Homo* and *Australopithecus* may have diverged about 2 million years ago.

Homo

It is difficult to decide which hominid fossils should be regarded as the earliest members of the genus *Homo*. This is mainly because of the problem of defining the characteristics distinctive of *Homo*. Besides physical features, cultural and behavioural considerations are also involved. There is also the problem of morphological variation in the fossils. However, three species of *Homo* (a cerebral, dextrous, tool-making, habitual biped) are recognised: *Homo habilis*, *Homo erectus* and *Homo sapiens*.

Homo habilis

The remains of a gracile hominid type, which has some features of *Australopithecus* and others of *Homo*, has been found in southern and western Africa. The specimens have been dated to between 2–1.5 million years ago, and most anthropologists have designated them to a species called *Homo habilis*. There is evidence that *H. habilis* may have been a more efficient biped than the australopithecines, and that he was also a tool-maker.

701a

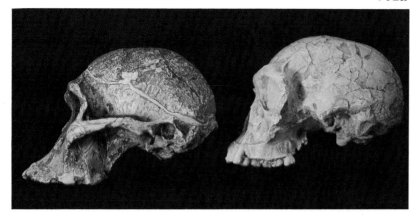

701a Homo habilis (specimen 1813, right) compared with *A. africanus* (left). Among the cranial features which distinguish *H. habilis* from *Australopithecus* are its greater cranial capacity (ranging from about 550–750cm^3), its more rounded head, its less massive jaws and its smaller, less projecting face.

701b

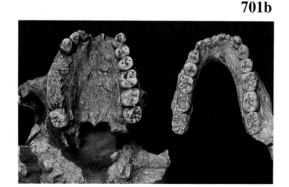

702

701b Occlusal view of dentition of individual assigned to *Homo habilis*. The maxilla on the left (KNM-ER 1813) is from Koobi Fora, Kenya, and dated about 1.9 million years old. The mandible on the right (OH 13) is from Olduvai Gorge, Tanzania, and dated about 1.7 million years old. Note the parabolic dental arches, the small canines, the absence of a diastema, and a particular feature of *H. habilis* specimens — the relatively narrow (bucco-lingually) human-like cheek teeth.

702 KNM-ER 1470. This is a fairly complete skull resembling *H. habilis* (but with a larger cranial capacity of 750cm^3) and named after its catalogue number in the Kenya National Museum. It was found in Kenya and is about 1.8 million years old. The supra-orbital ridges are poorly developed. There are no indications of a nuchal crest or of other sites of very powerful muscle attachments. No teeth were recovered with the specimen, although from the size of the sockets the teeth appear to have been large.

The various specimens that have been attributed to the group *H. habilis* display a wide range of dental characteristics and cranial capacities. Some have small brains but human-like teeth, while others have large brains but less human-like teeth. Recently discovered material from the Koobi Fora and West Turkana areas of Kenya may help to clarify the features specific to this group. Until such clarification is forthcoming, some anthropologists will continue to regard *H. habilis* as an advanced australopithecine. Increasingly, there are those who consider that the two species of early *Homo* exist among the remains presently attributed to *Homo habilis*.

Homo erectus

This hominid was similar in size to modern man. It represents the first widely distributed human species, evidence suggesting that they migrated from Africa (where the oldest specimens occur) into south-east Asia, China, and perhaps even into Europe. Although it is generally believed that they lived from about 1.8–0.3 million years ago, there is some evidence that they may have survived until as recently as 200,000 years ago. Early *H. erectus* was apparently contemporaneous with *H. habilis* and was certainly contemporaneous with late examples of *Australopithecus robustus/Paranthropus*. *H. erectus* has been linked to the first use of fire.

For many reasons, members of the *H. erectus* group are unarguably placed in the genus *Homo*. Compared with *Australopithecus*, *H. erectus* was taller and more completely adapted to bipedal locomotion. The skull had a greater cranial capacity (850–1050cm^3), there was a relatively smaller face and smaller teeth, and the dental arch was parabolic. However, it differed from *Homo sapiens* in that it had brow ridges, a long, low skull, a more projecting face, a thicker zygomatic arch, and an angled occiput with a well developed ridge. The mandible was large, with a thickened body, often multiple mental foramina, and no chin.

703

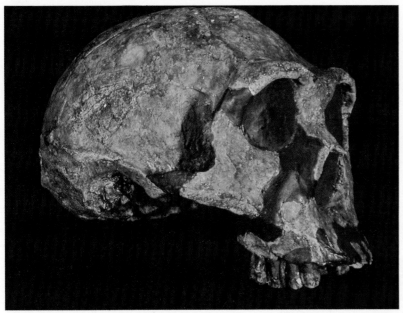

703 *Homo erectus* from Kenya (Specimen KNM-ER 3733).

704

704 *Homo erectus* from China (Zhoukoudian). The specimens from Asia are mainly between 200,000–700,000 years old. The marked flattening of the profile of the cranial vault and the receding forehead are apparent. A ridge or sagittal keel is seen running along the tip of the skull. The bregma is the highest point on the skull. There are very prominent supra-orbital ridges and, when viewed from above, a post-orbital constriction is evident. The occipital region is angled and there is a prominent horizontal ridge (the occipital torus) for the attachment of powerful neck muscles to help support the cranium (which is not as perfectly balanced on the vertebral column as in *Homo sapiens*). The broadest part of the low-vaulted skull is towards the base. The size of the mastoid process is variable. Just above the external auditory meatus, the parietal bone is thickened to form the angular torus.

The dentition of *Homo erectus* is essentially similar to that of modern man, the dental arch being parabolic. However, the teeth differ from modern man in the following respects: (1) they are larger; (2) the maxillary central incisors are more shovel-shaped (see page 41); (3) the canines are more robust; (4) cingula are present around the cheek teeth and there may be some wrinkling of the enamel; (5) the mandibular second and third molars tend to possess five cusps rather than four cusps; (6) there is some degree of taurodontism (i.e. the pulp chamber extends well into the roots).

The crania of late specimens of *H. erectus* appeared rounder and higher, and in some cases had smaller supra-orbital ridges and a greater cranial capacity (up to 1250cm^3).

Controversy exists concerning the relationships between the various geographical groups of *H. erectus* and their positions along the evolutionary pathway leading to *H. sapiens*. This is mainly due to the considerable morphological variation encountered. As the oldest specimens that have been found are limited to Africa, it must be assumed that *H. erectus* evolved there and subsequently migrated out to Asia and Europe. The Asian population (from Indonesia and China) forms the most homogeneous group and shows little variation over a period of about 0.5 million years. Their skulls exhibited features (sagittal keel; marked occipital torus; angular torus; tympanic plate which was thick and robust) not all found in other groups of *H. erectus*. For these reasons, some have suggested that there may be more than one species of *H. erectus*, and further that *H. erectus* in Asia was an offshoot which became extinct, *H. sapiens* evolving from *H. erectus* populations in Africa and Europe.

Homo sapiens

There are obvious gaps in the fossil record relating to the evolutionary changes which took place from *Homo erectus* to *Homo sapiens*. Even if more specimens were available, difficulties might still exist in classification because of the problems associated in defining the precise differences which distinguish *H. erectus* from *H. sapiens*. Among the cranial features distinguishing *H. sapiens* is the increased cranial capacity (about 1300cm^3), the high domed forehead, the small nasal opening, the absence of brow ridges and the occipital torus. The broadest part of the skull is towards the parietal eminences. In addition, the jaws became less robust and the teeth a little smaller. The specimens dating from this period include fossils from Britain (Swanscombe and Pontnewydd), Germany (Heidelberg and Steinheim), France (Arago) and Greece (Petralona) as well as some from Africa. They tend to show features transitional between *H. erectus* and *H. sapiens*. Some authorities have used the term 'archaic *H. sapiens*' when referring to such material, while others have classified it as 'Preneanderthal'.

The final emergence of modern *Homo sapiens* is complicated by the appearance of Neanderthal man.

705

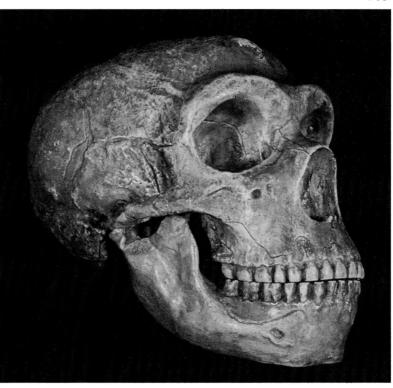

705 *Homo sapiens neanderthalensis*. Neanderthal man is an archaic subspecies of *H. sapiens*. Neanderthals appeared in Europe and the near east about 100,000 years ago. Culturally, they have provided the first intentional burials. They had long, low, robust skulls with prominent occiputs and well developed supra-orbital ridges which were divided centrally and extensively pneumatised by the frontal air sinuses. The cranial capacity was as great as 1600cm^3. The nasal cavities were particularly capacious. The mandible did not exhibit a well defined chin. The anterior teeth were comparatively large. The teeth were positioned more anteriorly than in *H. sapiens*, so that the mental foramen came to lie at the level of the first permanent mandibular molar (rather than the level of the first/second premolar), and there was a distinct retromolar space between the third molar and the anterior border of the ramus. The molars were often taurodont, the pulp chambers extending well into the root area. The great emphasis on the use of the anterior dentition resulted in a substantial midfacial prognathism. The group apparently became extinct about 30,000 years ago. It appears likely that Neanderthal man was not a direct ancestor of modern *H. sapiens* but may have been a cold-adapted subspecies. Alternatively, he could even have been a distinct species. The unearthing of typical Neanderthal remains in France (St.-Cesaire) less than 35,000 years old indicates that Neanderthal man was contemporaneous with modern *H. sapiens*, and therefore did not directly give rise to *H. sapiens*. Furthermore, preliminary studies on recent finds from the Kebara cave in Israel indicate that Neanderthals and modern man may have co-existed for some considerable time.

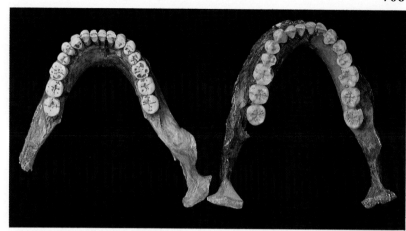

706 Comparison of the mandibles of a Neanderthal (left) and early modern (right) specimens. The Neanderthal mandible is from Regordon, France, and may be about 60,000 years old. The early modern mandible is from Qafzeh, Israel, and is about 100,000 years old. The Neanderthal dentition is positioned anteriorly and there is an associated large retromolar space. Despite the overall modernity of the Qafzeh dentition, the teeth are large.

Two different models have been put forward to account for recent human evolution. These are the 'multiregional model' and the 'single origin model'. For the multiregional model, recent human geographical variations are regarded as having evolved after the radiation of *Homo erectus* from Africa. As a consequence of the radiation, local differentiation led to distinct regional populations. For the single origin model, however, it is proposed that there is a relatively recent, common ancestral population for *H. sapiens* which already displayed most of the anatomical characteristics shared by

modern man. Accordingly, it is proposed that all anatomically modern varieties of *H. sapiens* originated in Africa after 200,000 years ago, with subsequent radiation leading to the geographical establishment of modern racial characteristics outside Africa. Recent genetic, fossil and archaeological studies add weight to the single origin model. They indicate that modern man reached western Asia shortly afterwards, subsequently spreading throughout most of Eurasia and reaching Australia about 40,000 years ago, and probably the Americas by about 30,000 years ago.

707 Early modern *Homo sapiens* from Qafzeh (9), Israel. This skull is an example of a very early modern human from Israel, dated at about 100,000 years old. It has a very modern cranium, combined with a prognathic face and very large teeth. Note the presence of a chin, the high forehead and the small brow ridge. The rest of the skeleton is completely modern in its anatomy.

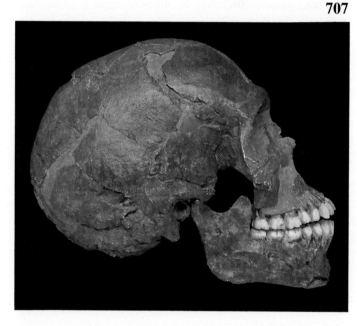

The first appearance of modern *Homo sapiens* in Europe was about 40,000 years ago (Cro-Magnon man). Cro-Magnon man probably arrived in Europe from south-west Africa and rapidly replaced Neanderthal man, who had been continuously present in Europe, evolving over a period of hundreds of thousands of years. Where specimens of Cro-Magnon man are seen to have

more primitive, Neanderthal-like features, this does not necessarily mean that they were derived from definite Neanderthal stock; they could have evolved from more primitive ancestors, or from cold adaptations in parallel with Neanderthals in Europe.

Dental enamel and hominoid relationships

Studies have been undertaken to investigate the significance of the structure of enamel in determining hominoid relationships. The parameters which have at present been assessed are tissue thickness, prism pattern and incremental markings. It has been suggested that the prism patterns within enamel are a reflection of the thickness of the tissue. Pattern 1 and pattern 3 enamel (see **203**) are found in all hominoids. Pattern 3, however, predominates in the deep layers and is associated with Hunter–Schreger bands (see page 120). Pattern 1 is present superficially and as a very thin layer immediately adjacent to the enamel–dentine junction. In these regions there are no Hunter–Schreger bands. Pattern 3 enamel is associated with a cross-striation repeat interval of about 5µm. Pattern 1 enamel has a cross-striation interval of 2.5µm. The cross-striation intervals therefore indicate that, in hominoids, pattern 3 enamel forms between two and three times faster than pattern 1.

Thin enamel is found in gibbons, chimpanzees and gorillas. Enamel of intermediate thickness occurs in the orang-utan. Thick enamel is found in *Homo* which (like the gibbon) has pattern 3 enamel accounting for about 95% of the enamel thickness. Thick enamel also occurs in *Sivapithecus* (including *Ramapithecus*) which, like humans, is comprised almost entirely of pattern 3 enamel with only a very thin covering of pattern 1 enamel. The thickest enamel of all occurs in *Australopithecus boisei* (**708**). These data have been interpreted as indicating that the ancestral condition for dental enamel is the thin, fast-forming pattern 3 enamel found in the gibbon. During evolution this changed to a thick form of pattern 3 enamel for the precursors of the apes and *Homo*. This change has been retained in modern man but enamel thickness has been secondarily reduced in the African apes and, to a lesser extent, in the orang-utan.

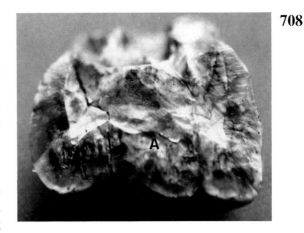

708

708 Fractured surface of a maxillary first premolar crown from Australopithecus boisei (KMN-ER 733D). The enamel (**A**) may be up to 3mm thick.

Assessing the rate of dental development in fossil hominids

It is possible to use incremental markings in enamel (i.e. cross-striations, enamel striae and perikymata — see pages 117–119) to assess the time taken for teeth to form and also to provide information to help age juvenile fossil hominids. For human teeth, some striae do not reach the surface beneath the incisal edge of cusp.

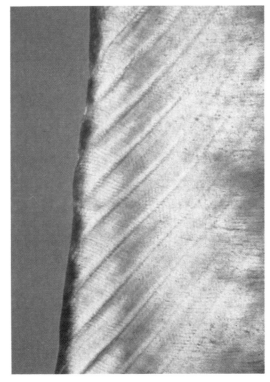

709

709 Section of the crown of a modern tooth showing striae of Retzius at the enamel surface. There are about seven cross-striations between adjacent striae, confirming the view that striae are approximately weekly incremental lines (i.e. circasepta). (Ground longitudinal section; × 80)

710 Crown surface of modern human permanent lower incisor showing perikymata. The circaseptan enamel striae are manifested at the enamel surface as perikymata. Note these are closer together in the cervical region, indicating a slowdown in the rate of enamel formation (i.e. the distance between cross-striations becomes smaller). In the case of unworn incisors, between 25 and 30 striae remain hidden before the remainder reach the surface (see page 118). The hidden striae represent about 6 months' growth. When this is added to the number of visible perikymata on the surface (plus a few months for tooth development prior to the onset of mineralisation), a reasonable estimate of the length of time taken for crowns to form can be made. (Montage SEM; × 10)

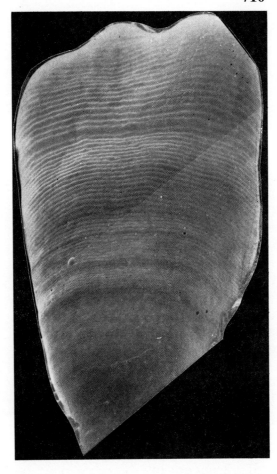

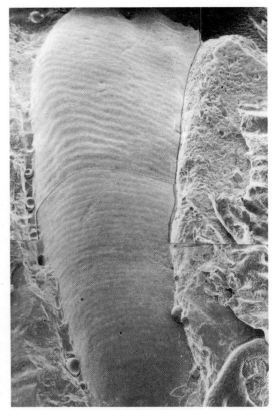

711 Crown surface of mandibular right permanent incisor of *Australopithecus boisei* (SK62). Using non-invasive techniques, replicas of the surfaces of fossil teeth can be obtained which demonstrate the presence of striae. This has allowed the time of emergence of the first permanent molar to be calibrated in fossil hominids. Known periods for incisor crown formation can then be cross-matched with events such as first molar eruption. Apes erupt mandibular first molars at approximately 3½ years of age; for humans this occurs at close to 6 years of age. From such work, there is evidence that the growth periods of the australopithecines were markedly abbreviated relative to those of modern man, and in this respect were more similar to modern great apes. This information has consequences for the estimates of age at death of juvenile fossil hominids, which were previously based on dental eruption, maturation and dental wear criteria used for modern man. Indeed, the use of such criteria has led to overestimates of the age at death.

712 Fractured enamel surface from *Australopithecus boisei*. Although rare fossil teeth have yet to be sectioned in order to examine enamel structure, some information may be gleaned from fractured teeth. Here, cross-striations can be clearly identified and it has been shown that, liked modern human enamel, there are approximately seven cross-striations between each enamel stria, confirming that in fossil teeth, the interval between successive perikymata represents approximately one week. (SEM replica; × 30)

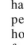

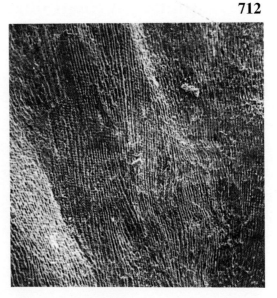

Index

Location references are page numbers.

326